# IF YOU WANT
# GOOD PERSONAL HEALTHCARE
## – *SEE A VET*

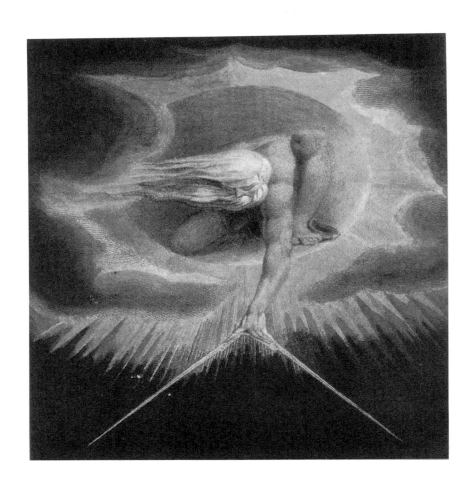

The Beginning. Imagination and Apotheosis:
William Blake, *The Ancient of Days* 1794

# IF YOU WANT GOOD PERSONAL HEALTHCARE

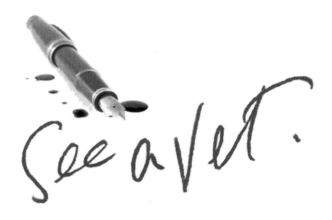

## Industrialised Humanity:
Why and how should we care for one another?

# DAVID ZIGMOND

First published 2015 by New Gnosis Publications,
Whitstable, U.K.
© David Zigmond 2015

ISBN-13: 978-1506173382
ISBN-10: 1506173381

Printed by CreateSpace

# Contents

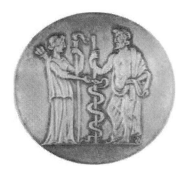

# Introduction

This anthology covers many writings from my first forty-five years in medical practice. It is intended to be the first of a series: other volumes will follow at similar intervals.

The long period covered is reflected in the length of the book. This may be problematic and I have considered several options – for example, a much briefer selection, or a division of volumes by assigning eras or categories. But such easier accessibility incurs losses: not only the Gestalt of the evolution of ideas, but also the interconnectedness of expanding and propagating perspectives: Holism. For the patient reader, therefore, I hope this large whole will bring more than the sum of its many parts.

But other readers have many different preferences and proclivities. I accept that many may wish for shorter works with less elaborate framing. For them I have divided this long anthology into three separate books: *The Psychoecology of Gladys Parlett*, *From Family to Factory* and *Bureaucratyrannohypoxia*.

For those who choose this longer compendium, you may sense that it was carefully written, in clusters of activity, over many years. It is probably best read in a similar manner. Few readers will wish to ingest it in a steady, linear fashion. Instead, I suggest approaching it as a *Meze*: a large, varied platter to be sampled, savoured, contemplated and enjoyed according to the reader's changing inclination and appetite. To guide the reader's choices I have employed devices which I explain later.

From the beginning of my medical work I have always had interests beyond the biomechanical. Fifty years ago I thought this hinterland was often unwisely disregarded: this is even more so now. My long explorations of this hinterland have invoked a medley of heart, soul, relationships, intuition, semiotics, imagination, intellect (philosophical v pragmatic intelligence) and meaning. Many would name this medley 'holism', but I am wary: I do not want to differentiate or offer yet another brand or package. Yet, whatever we call these things, they are substantial – if elusive – essences of our humanity. Throughout my writings I argue that our incorporation of such essences into our many practical tasks constitutes the imperilled art of medicine. I wish to explore with you, too, two important primary principles. Firstly, how these elements – of humanity, art and healing – are not themselves directly measurable or manageable. Secondly, and consequently, we can never successfully proceduralise or industrialise them. Later articles consider how the attempt to do so leads to perverse results.

My *Acknowledgements* are many, and I have separately sectioned them.

The number and variety of articles is now very large. This can seem confusing and overwhelming. To mitigate this I have dated the articles and written a very brief synopsis of each. These are found in the *Contents* section.

To break up the great steppes of text I have introduced pictures to refresh, contrast, amplify, parody, clarify or puzzle.

The sequence of writings is mostly chronological: the exceptions are explained. To further aid navigation and digestibility I have divided the anthology into three sections.

*Section One* is titled *What can go right*. I start by exploring the limits of the biomechanical approach, and then the very different skills and perspectives we may develop to offset these limits.

The earlier writings in this section are from another era and were written for then respectable, now deceased, mainline medical journals. They have a formality and quaint courteous style that I later abandoned. Those with an interest in history, anthropology or archaeology will find here a trove of recorded relics: doctors' white coats, residents' messes, physician superintendents, mental hospitals and babies home-delivered by GPs: the curious reader will find more. Can writing from this very different era now be seriously relevant? Indeed: I think that these earlier articles contain messages and challenges that are now even more urgent. Also remarkable and very pertinent is this: equivalent mainstream journals now would not publish such articles: the writing would be deemed to have inadequate data, evidence basis and academic references. Is such strictness of convention progress? I leave that question with the reader.

I open *Section One* with an *Overture: All is Therapy: All is Diagnosis*. This is a very recent article and I have deliberately placed it to immediately precede the earliest in this anthology. Such juxtaposition of the two ends of a professional lifetime's writing – separated by nearly forty years – highlights not just individual change, but social ones, too. The chosen contemporary article – the herald to its ancestors – is itself a kind of viewing-platform for history: it describes three episodes from my own sixty-year experiences with doctors – as a child in the 1950s, being a doctor now, and going to the doctor now, for my own healthchecks. These autobiographical vignettes thus serve as historical snapshots: they sample, at different places and times, what is happening to human relationships and meaning in healthcare. Section One offers many other engagements with these Leitmotifs.

*Intermezzo* is not primarily about healthcare but a brief encounter with some of our richer human complexity: often such are decisive but unspoken aspects of our fate. Shimmering chimera are often vital subtexts to our health, yet our schematised healthcare has become increasingly illiterate of such subtext. This growing discrepancy is addressed in later writings.

*Section Two* is titled *What has gone wrong*. Round about the millennium I had a belated awakening: I slowly discerned the institutional changes that were gathering throughout our Welfare services, and then the depersonalising consequences. In many ways this depersonalisation can be seen as what happens when we attempt to short-circuit or eschew certain kinds of understanding. What are these? They are for the same kinds of human variety and complexity that are poorly served by biomechanics and quantifiable science – the kinds of understanding I was developing as a younger practitioner: Section One of this anthology.

Section One thus starts by considering healthcare blessings we may confer on one another if we develop our capacities for resonance, imagination and creative tolerance of ambiguity. Section Two then describes the curses we unleash if we neglect or proscribe these capacities.

These later, post-millennium, essays can also be seen as broader profiles: of what can go wrong in technologically advanced societies when we do not know how and when to constrain manipulative and managerial thinking, language and activity.

Even in the one decade these later articles were written, computer use has increased massively. Section Two surveys not only the burgeoning follies that come from attempts to industrialise and commodify healthcare; I also wish to portray how these are fuelled and amplified by insentient computer use. I believe this has accreted to perilous proportions, yet remains little discussed. For this reason I have used a later article – *Where in the World are You?* – to introduce the otherwise time-ordered pieces collaging our many guises of unintended human disconnection.

*Section Three* carries the mission and title of *What we may do*: my missives to newspapers, journals, politicians and colleagues. These sample recent efforts to galvanise and broaden thought and debate. Generally the letters to colleagues are longer and more detailed. Those to newspapers are necessarily brief, pithy and skeletal. The long submission to the Health Secretary – *Five Executive Follies* – serves as both an extended critique and then summary of the problems of the 3Cs in healthcare: Competition, Commissioning and Commodification.

Remarkably replies from politicians were almost all diplomatic feints: self justifying, aphoristic and urbanely dissembling. Senior NHS managers mostly did not respond: I have included the one candidly thoughtful reply.

Sections Two and Three thus have much description and analysis of the difficult relationship between individuals and institutions. I have therefore had to use some technical and institutional terms, though I have tried to reduce these to a minimum. To further aid the reader there is a Glossary of key terms.

\*

The *style of writing and format* require some introductory comment.

My longer articles and letters often include stories or descriptions of events to illustrate, clarify or reify theory. I believe this kind of interpersonal 'biopsy' can be much more effective than its conventional scarcity would suggest. Human experience is primary; theories and systems, however effective they might be, are secondary and artefactual. In our increasingly virtual world we are apt to forget this important principle. My narratives may be a reminder.

Personal identifications are disguised, but the stories, descriptions and dialogues are as accurate as this human can make them.

\*

Lastly some *notes about language*. Firstly a minor point. I tend to use a generic 'he', rather than the now almost conventional 'he/she' as the latter looks/sounds cumbersome/ugly, to me.

Secondly, a more major point, for me: I like rich, polyvalent, carefully expressive language, as this not only communicates complex realities better, it makes it more possible for us to perceive them. Restricted and impoverished language does the reverse. The science of medicine can function with a plain, if arcane, prosaic vocabulary: the art of medicine needs always to expand this. My language therefore aspires to both the poetic and precise.

In an amply humanised healthcare we need wide, connected spans of mental life and language.

# Prelude
# Personal reflections
## Depersonalised Times

My life, conceived just after World War Two, has an almost exact parallel span to our National Health Service. This infant, yet revolutionary, giant first delivered me, then immunised and protected me against previously rampantly lethal diseases, and finally has provided me with the core of my very interesting healthcare work for several decades.

On an infinitely greater scale, the story of the NHS also parallels the 'Developed World's' triumphs, struggles, follies and conundrae – of our increasingly technologised individual and social lives. So, the triumphs and tribulations of our healthcare are often those of our culture. This has become increasingly apparent to me as I have witnessed, then striven to understand, how increasing investment in, then dependence on, technology has often been followed by impoverishment of human understanding and connection.

What has happened? Yes, first we must recognise how biomedical sciences and Information Technology have brought about miraculously life-changing and life-saving procedures. In my lifetime I have seen the introduction of polio vaccines and antibiotics in my childhood, renal dialysis in my youth, then transplantation and coronary artery surgery: all have become commonplace yet massive blessings, available for all who may need them. But these bright blessings of technological manipulation have often come at the price of human connection and understanding. It is not just the horror-headlines of stark neglect or cruelty; more commonly our human losses are concealed by 'Service Development' – for example, our long-trusted Family Doctor becomes a short-term Primary Care

Service Provider; at the time of our emotional breakdown our psychologist gives us an interrogatory standard questionnaire, not a delicate personal encounter. Unless we are very careful, our healthcare becomes expediently defined by a series of impersonal procedures which then largely extinguish more delicate networks of personal relationships and understandings.

Procedures are increasingly the hardy offspring from the recent royal marriage between Evidence Basis and Managed Service Delivery. Via the hegemony of the procedure, personal medicine becomes Public Health: personal language and understanding becomes displaced by the technical and formulaic. You can read about this in *Language is Not Just Data: it is a custodian of our humanity.*

Let us return to the very beginning, to the combining title of this anthology: *If You Want Good Healthcare, see a Vet.* You may initially think this is mere facetious banter or meretricious wit: read on. I hope to show you how the statement, beyond any theatrical effect, has substantial literal truth. This cymbal-clashed greeting thus introduces several decades of mostly quieter exploration of the nature of relationships and the meaning of meaning in healthcare.

To reword and expand the title's aphorism with less stark flourish: Vets are, generally, better at holistic, imaginative, empathic care than contemporary doctors.

Does this notion still strike you as hyperbole?

Well consider this: I have spent many years observing how a wide range of healers work. A suburban Vet recently invited me to spend time in her surgery. What I witness is charming and disarming, and then disturbing. I am immediately engaged by *her* engagement with the variety of domestic animals and their owners: it seems to me that she offers for each a fresh and deft weft of listening, watching, feeling, thinking, 'vibing' and imagining. She weaves these multifarious strands with affection, wit and warmth. Her human and animal charges sense this: they are, generally, soon comforted and stilled. In her many years and roles as a Vet, she has rarely been scratched or bitten and has never yet been eaten. Anchoring this deeply intuitive yet informed holism is her quick and dextrous ability to enter the 'mind-set', the experience, of the animal: there is no explicit communication. If you are interested in a fuller description you will find this in the article with the same title: *If You Want Good Personal Healthcare, see a Vet.*

To range further: our capacity for such accurate empathic, creative leaps – then to subject them to empirical scrutiny – is one aspect of holistic or humanistic practice: we cannot manage these without the risk of using imagination.

To say that imagination is important in understanding experience – one's own and others' – is hardly original, but I realised just how important it was when I was at Medical School in the 1960s. I witnessed many examples of how the inordinate application of scientific method and thinking in matters of human complexity could short-circuit richer, imaginative contact with others.

My ideas crystallised with experience. In the mid-1970s I was working as a fledgling psychiatrist on a Unit that did much work with 'physical' doctors. We very selectively attempted to discern when a patient's illness indirectly expressed or concealed important *personal meaning*, and whether that meaning could be usefully understood and addressed.

In 1975 I cared for a man who, shortly after his retirement became, for the first time, mentally and physically very ill. Through our conversations it became clear to us both that it was the sharing of the meaning of these convergences that largely healed him. This led to my first article: *The Medical Model: its limitations and alternatives* and subsequent articles on Psychosomatics. This earliest article was the progenitor of many far-travelled but related themes. Egregiously, such sophisticated psychomatics has since perished. If you read *Words and Numbers: servants or masters?* you can find out why.

Such imaginative capacities were more valued when I was a young doctor, but they have become progressively lost or discouraged. Much medical practice may be better managed, but it is also more dehumanised. *No Country for Old Men* portrays how this has happened, personally and professionally.

But is this, again, hyperbole? Consider this second example: I currently attend, as a patient, my local health centre (previously GP surgery) for risk-factor monitoring and management. Fortunately, I am not (yet) asking for anything more. On arrival, there is now almost no personal reception: registration and conveyance to consultation are now electronically automated. In the last year I have had two appointments with a nurse, and one with a doctor. They are polite and businesslike in their prepacked interrogation, instruction and advice. I sense that they do not much sense how and when to vary their packages. They discover almost nothing about me. Remarkably they seem not to notice that, at the top of all the screens they bring up, my full name is preceded by 'Doctor'. Their lack of curiosity about me has generated in me a lot of curiosity about them, and about the loss of healthy curiosity that is essential to any common humanity. You can read about these particular encounters in *All is Therapy: All is Diagnosis*.

This anthology offers many thoughts about the origin and cost of such losses. I hope these offerings may help some, in some kind of restitution.

# Acknowledgements

To start, let me short-circuit convention.

I wish to share fairly the various errors and follies in this long anthology. Many years have spawned even more people who have not merely tolerated my preoccupations, but have actively encouraged them.

In the early 1970s I had four mentors who modelled how to combine the divergence of compassionate imagination with the convergence of scientific discipline: Doctors David Trounce, Donald Woods, Gerald Goldberg and Roger Tredgold. Forty years later my memories and deep gratitude remain clear and detailed.

In more recent times I have had many friendly colleagues in healthcare and academia who have catalysed, guided and nourished discussions about complexity. I hope they, too, benefitted from our often sprawling explorations. So I wish to thank Robin Hobbes, Sue Wheeler, Christopher Cordess, Richard Donmall, Janet Wingrove, Noel Hodson, Pauline Hodson, Gaie Houston, Martin Baggaley, André Tylee, Andrew Margo, John Sloboda, George Blair, Nick Kendrick and Susan Joekes. Often our conversations have germinated tendrils of development long after our meetings.

As I am an Internot, my public viability in the 21st Century has been far from assured. Several people have saved me from more severe oblivion and isolation. Mark Alder has made available many of my writings on the Internet: in view of my obstinate resistance and antipathy to electronic communication I deserve rather less than his assiduous and painstaking talents. Likewise Jacki Reason for some years has deciphered and packaged my many notebooks of chiaroscuroed pencil writing: she has been my electroamanuensis. Jacki and Mark have thus enabled an Internot survival in this Internetted 21st Century: my gratitude is deep and awkward.

Philosopher and writer Peter Wilberg as well as Karin Heinitz of *New Gnosis Publications* have provided a very human net of intelligent support, suggestions and evident pleasure in sharing humanistic values. Likewise my colleagues William House and David Peters at the *British Holistic Medical Association*: it is a necessary pleasure for me to have such long-term colleagueial resonance and consonance. Edwina Rowling has provided another very human link with the *Journal of Holistic Healthcare*. For me this is a welcome respite: thirty years ago I had many interesting discussions with editorial staff, often over an elegant table-clothed working lunch. In recent years my articles have instead been silently and electronically phagocytosed before being incorporated into a journalistic greater whole: a faceless, voiceless, personless – and rather joyless – experience. Yet despite my Cyberspaced anomie I am nevertheless grateful to the many other journals for their agreement to republish in this anthology.

Ian Lee, Ruskin Kyle and Joseph Zigmond helped with the book's cover, pictures and graphics.

Professor André Tylee patiently explained to me, and others, that I have Black Sheep Personality Disorder. Any jest on his part is surpassed by consummate wisdom. On the larger scale he enabled the psychiatric categorisers to triumphantly claim yet more territory. On the much smaller personal scale he provided me with an epiphany to explain my past and an epigram to embolden my future. As a fashion-mullah said: 'If you've got it, flaunt it!' Hence this anthology; without the diagnosis, I might still be a fugitive yet Internetted Internot.

To finish, let me rejoin convention – my deep gratitude to family: our universal source, and usually final solace. At this stage of my life and writing I cannot possibly recall who they all are; but they have been far less busy than me, so they will remember. Amidst some inevitable sorrows my family relationships have generated much of my spark, current and the loving homeostasis necessary for my offerings to others. They have also taught me, time and again, that curiosity, receptivity and understanding of otherness must always precede and exceed our design and intent for those others.

David Zigmond
April 2015

# Glossary
# of Institutional Terms

Much of the writing of Sections Two and Three encounters our increasing and severe healthcare conundrae: these are largely consequent to our over-industrialisation of the Medical Model. This has become particularly clear in the cultural and political turmoil besetting Britain's National Health Service.

The interest and importance of these issues extends far beyond this already vast arena, but the organisational events are very complex and often difficult to understand: examples may need explanation. This is even more likely for readers who are not healthcare workers or British residents. As a bridge to clarity and comprehension, I have constructed this critical glossary of key terms. Many of the italicised words are cross-referenced: this helps to give an outline of the current System's skeleton. Some key terms are worth highlighting but are widely known and understood: for economy of space I have italicised but not glossaried these.

**Algorithm.** A templated and flow-charted system of defined and logical steps prescribed to analyse and manage identified problems. Can be readily diagrammed and computerised. Has rapid appeal due to its standardised reproducibility, apparent clarity, precision and logic. Disadvantages: deals poorly with real-life's ambiguity, variation, meaning and complexity. Can displace individually responsive and intelligent judgement and imagination.

**Appraisals** for healthcare staff. A formal procedure whose purpose is to monitor and assure quality and safety of professional performance and development. Much effort has been made to standardise and, when possible, quantify such complex evaluations. Guidance has been sought from the newer professions of business management and consultancy. The aspiration is far less controvertible than the results: for the formalistic segues easily to the formulaic. Subsequent attempts to make procedure 'fair and comprehensive' commonly become burdensome, blind and bureaucratic. Generally professionals have described their experiences of appraisals as elaborate rituals of proffered compliance and verbalised obedience. Far fewer report the kind of intelligent searching dialogue that will helpfully identify or clarify important problems.

**Balint.** Michael Balint (1896-1970) was a psychoanalyst who, in the 1950s and 1960s, explored the 'subtext' of medical consultations. He started with a small group of London GPs, but his influence expanded to galvanise a generation of doctors to think about inexplicit meaning, encoded actions and attachments, and the possibility of both treatment and illness as kinds of preverbal or paraverbal language. Many GPs experienced their work as enriched and enlightened by such informal and qualitative research. This brief, rich flowering was largely extinguished by the rapid rise of systems that demanded quantification, standardised codes, and mass-reproducibility.

*Evidence Based Medicine* has great difficulty accommodating Balint's subtle invitations to explore meaning.

**Care Quality Commission (CQC).** A governmental network of healthcare inspectors. This is similar in mission to the *Appraisal* of professional individuals, but applied to the healthcare organisation that employs them. As with Appraisals, the task is certainly necessary and important but its sensible and accurate execution very difficult. Again, presentations of formulaic compliance can easily mask deeper lack of integrity. The shocking debacle at *Mid Staffs* examples what can be missed by 'competent' yet routinised methods of inspection.

**Clinical Commissioning Group (CCG).** A recently mandated executive network for deciding, defining, procuring and purchasing the healthcare needs of an allocated geographical population. The boards are now dominated by local GPs but contain other healthcare professionals and lay members. The CCG has replaced the *Primary Care Trust (PCT)*, which was administered, ultimately, by non-clinical managers.

The aspiration – for democratic healthcare decisions that are locally responsive and responsible, and professionally decided – seems laudable. The unravelling reality is less so: multitasking, overmanaged and weary GPs already have much diminished time for their traditional role as personal physicians and cannot give adequate, good attention to this new and very complex task. The result is an expedient short-circuiting to a hastily assembled (and thus often not competent) network of oligarchies that are themselves likely to be in thrall to a very flawed *Internal Market*.

**Cognitive Behaviour Therapy (CBT).** An attempt to schematise and standardise therapeutic psychological contact for the mentally or behaviourally troubled. It is largely based on depersonalised diagnostic categories, focused on the symptomatic and explicit, and guided by *algorithms* and *Care*

*Pathways*. It is readily (if speciously) computer-coded and measurable: CBT thus has appeal to planners, economists, managers and the kinds of practitioners who share their mindset. The limitations are similar to all algorithms and Care Pathways: the model has difficulty with complexity, variation, meaning and imagination – and thus can easily impoverish practitioners' personal resources to deal with these.

**Commissioning.** A currently common term for design, negotiation and procurement of services within the marketised NHS. Like other devices to industrialise and monetarise healthcare it is least problematic when applied to healthcare problems that are generally resolved rapidly and reliably by standardised technical procedure (eg hip replacements). *Pastoral Healthcare* (eg psychiatry) starkly exposes its limitations.

**Commodification.** The attempt to treat and process all healthcare activities as if they are manufactured objects or geophysical resources. This can work relatively well in tasks that have clear and stable boundaries. *Pastoral Healthcare*, by contrast, needs vocational and holistic attitudes that cannot be processed in this way. Nevertheless, commodification makes welcome sense to planners and managers in conducting many aspects of the *Internal Market*. Experiences from frontline health workers are far less tidy: for many years there have been mounting, frustrated expressions of clinical and personal meaninglessness and the stymying of good personal care.

**Community Mental Health Team (CMHT).** Thirty years ago CMHTs were vaunted as a progressive face of the future, consummated by the closure of the old *Mental Hospitals*. Instead mentally distressed patients would be speedily streamed to community-based specialisms. The specialists themselves professionally progress via certified trainings rather than personal qualities or vocation. Recent healthcare management thinking – much derived from 1980s Japanese car manufacturing – promised more efficient, accessible and responsive help. As elsewhere in the NHS, this attempt to industrialise pastoral healthcare produces results that often become inefficient and perverse.

**Evidence-based Medicine (EBM).** This has been introduced into healthcare to optimise the reliability and efficiency of therapeutic interventions. The idea is to invest in language and procedures that are officially sanctioned by scientific rigour, and then *Governance*. Healthcare economists and planners favour EBM because it is apparently objective, clear and unambiguous – and can then extirpate the errors and obfuscations of the personal and subjective. In this way *Quantification*, *Standardisation* and *Commodification* are all expedited. EBM thus becomes a key component in the *Internal Market*.

EBM is yet another example from healthcare of how a model's attractive simplicity may be woefully inadequate for complex realities. EBM has mostly operated from evidence restricted to the quantifiable and reproducible. This makes a base that is deemed 'safe', but is also narrow and rigid. It may be necessary, but it often is not sufficient. Problems arise because EBM may be loaded with an authority it cannot bear. Very often the most important aspects of human experience and variation cannot be directly measured or objectified. This is far more than any administrative anomaly: for the unmappable area is the massive – yet vulnerable – human heart of healthcare. EBM, in compatible areas, may be a valuable guiding principle: aggrandised to wider and rigid diktat, it can do real harm.

**Increased Access to Psychological Treatment Services (IAPTS).** A late parallel, and equivalent, to *CMHTs*. The task focus is therapeutic psychology (not psychiatry). Similar processes are used to identify, stream and manage problems: diagnoses, *Care Pathways* and (especially) the use of *CBT* as a procedural intervention. The system is designed to be easily compatible with electronic informatics, the *Internal Market* and *Payment by Results*. Some also argue that it helps equity and fairness of distribution. The flaws are largely common to those of the *CMHT*.

**Internal Market.** In the early 1990s this was a seminal and radical idea: to introduce monetarist values and mechanisms to nationalised healthcare. The enormous federal cooperative network would be broken up into economically and occupationally autarkic *NHS Trusts*. Wide and informal affiliations were replaced by a complex system of *Purchaser-Provider Splits*, which need tending by ceaseless negotiations to facilitate 'trade' between the Trusts. Computerised, quantifiable data, *Care Pathways* and *Payment by Results* are all necessary developments to service this Internal Market. The idea is to positively influence motivation and focus attention. After more than twenty years' evolution the results are mixed and highly contentious. Many longer-term observers (myself included) assess the losses as much greater than the gains. Since the recent Health and Social Care Act there is now more possibility of an external market: this amplifies contention.

**Mid-Staffs.** Refers to the Mid Staffordshire NHS Trust. In recent years perplexed and appalled attention has focused on the clear and massive failures and abuses of care uncovered in this NHS hospital. The widespread institutional human disengagement has been shocking enough. Further grotesquerie is provided by the attractive and respectable public persona of the Trust: it had received very favourable reports from routine official inspections, eg by the *CQC*. Mid Staffs is one of many egregious examples of concealed inhumanities in current NHS healthcare, though the most notorious. Many see Mid Staffs as being a kind of diabolic iconic: a harsh signal of the consequences of abandoning healthcare's primal task of human recognition and connection. Such abandonment, it is argued, is due largely to the rise of the *Internal Market's* 3Cs (Competition, Commissioning and Commodification) and a culture cowed by managed demands for numerous, rigid and narrow *targets* and *PBR*. Subsequent statements from Mid Staffs' employees have described a bullied and intimidated work culture redolent of factory workers a century earlier.

**National Institute for Health and Care Excellence (NICE).** A governmentally appointed network of experts tasked with evaluating and applying *EBM* in specified areas of healthcare. As its operational nucleus is EBM, it has the same assets, limitations and liabilities. Thus NICE makes its most competent contributions to healthcare problems that are clearly physically defined, and which can then be reliably resolved or contained by standardised physical procedures.

So, NICE-prescribed frameworks usually make good and useful (though not infallible) contributions to the care of, say, Diabetes or Hypertension. Yet this kind of *algorithmic* management fares far less well with the vast human variations of pastoral healthcare (eg mood disturbance or alcoholism) where individual practitioners' wisdom, experience and subtle hues of judgement are central and indispensable.

**Pastoral Healthcare**. A term little used, but increasingly needed. It refers to our guiding human matrix of care: all those personal influences that comfort, heal, guide, contain, encourage, vitalise and illuminate. Pastoral healthcare thus extends far beyond any procedure or formula. Although certainly including such activities as personally attuned 'mental healthcare' or 'psychotherapy', it is not confined to these. Good Pastoral Healthcare is synonymous with the heart, soul and broader intellect involved throughout our encounters with others' distress. Like so many holistic activities, its subtler enactments cannot be readily measured, coded or proceduralised: Pastoral Healthcare thus tends to be neglected, displaced or destroyed by a culture dominated by the *Internal Market* and such satellite procedures as *Payment by Results, Evidence Based Medicine, Quality Outcome Frameworks* etc.

**Payment by Results (PBR).** The intention and thinking behind this kind of infusion of commercial motivation is relatively clear. It often galvanises manufacturing industries. Yet the consequences – when applied to complex human welfare – become frequently obscure, tangled and perverse. Results of complex activities are often difficult to define, measure or predict. Motivation in welfare is – and should be – much broader and more complex than that of commerce. Unbridled PBR in healthcare provides specious statistics, bad science and egregiously perverse incentives.

**Primary Care Trust (PCT).** For several years this body preceded the *CCG* in managing the trade and conduct of Community Practitioners (GPs, Dentists, Pharmacists, District Nurses, Health Visitors, Chiropodists etc). It was managed largely by non-clinicians: the transition to CCGs brings doubtful benefits as few GPs can maintain the long-term personal resources necessary for the complexity and size of the task.

**QUOF (Quality Outcomes Framework).** A complex system of remuneration for GPs, constituting a kind of 'performance related pay'. This is based on electronically guided and recorded *Specific Performance Indicators,* themselves based on *algorithms* and *Care Pathways* designed by governmental think-tanks and committees. The resultant computerised systems monitor and signal how each practitioner is managing each encounter with a patient with a chronic disease or risk. QUOF has thus brought the government and the computer into the centre of the consulting room in an unprecedented way. The results are mixed. The gains are most clear in bringing more vigilant and systematic management to high risk conditions where therapeutics are clearly effective (eg Hypertension and

Coronary Heart Disease), and detection of some other areas of significant risk/poor engagement. The losses are from displacement. Computer informatics and governmentally dictated tasks replace subtle, personally nuanced exchanges that are essential for comfort, understanding and healing influences. Such undesignated 'softer' activities are also essential to NHS staff morale. The QUOF-directed GP has become more of a public health commissar than a personal physician: patients are increasingly 'efficiently' treated, but poorly understood.

# Section One

# What can go right?

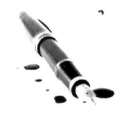

## Author's note

The oldest writings in this first section date from the 1970s. They comprise a selection of articles written for conventional medical journals. This is reflected in the formal style and some of the medical language and terminology. Amidst this I hope that my early development of humanistic themes – of the experiential, the interpersonal and Holism – will be clear and engaging for the non-medical and current reader.

Readers interested in how specific technical developments have changed patterns and problems of practice over this period will find clear examples. For example, in the last thirty years advances in medication have rendered perforated Peptic Ulcers extremely rare and Auto-immune Arthropathies much more treatable; surgical approaches have transformed the relief and prognosis of Angina. So my examples have dated, but original arguments have not. On balance I decided not to make major revisions, and instead confined rewriting to minor tidying and tightening of some of the text, leaving the form, arguments and examples as they were. If the reader is prepared to accommodate this compromise, current cogency may be combined with historical interest.

# Overture

## All is Therapy
## All is Diagnosis

Unmapped and perishing latitudes
of healthcare

.

Advances in medical science have steadily made biomechanical diagnoses and treatments more precise and effective. But this has been achieved, often, by a narrowing of focus so that much human context and meaning becomes unperceived and unconceived. Authentic vignettes from the author's experience – over several decades – illustrate the process and consequences

*'You don't really understand human nature unless you know why a child on a merry-go-round will wave at its parents every time around – and why the parents will always wave back.'*
Bill Tammeus, American Journalist (1945-)

## 1950s. Richness in austerity

The austerity Britain of my childhood sighed wearily: a murky, exhausted wake from the long convulsions of World War II. My surrounding childhood world drew breath amidst a wary stability and peace: many grieved and more were haunted. Less obvious were the wordlessly yet powerfully disturbed: the guilt of the survivors, the partially-sighted resentments of those who sensed infidelities in their absence. My parents – resourceful and uncomplaining people – had their more particular trials and sorrows: my father for a late-war injury which crippled his mobility (and possibly his male self-esteem) for his remaining decades; my mother, much earlier, from her mortally-shattered family who all perished (from 'natural' causes) in her childhood, exposing her as an orphan to the perils of a Depression-ravaged inter-War Britain.

Doctors Paul and Margaret, I think, rapidly sensed and apprised such things even before they knew much of the detail. I remember, as a small boy, feeling protected by their discrete warmth, knowledge and kindness.

Doctors Paul and Margaret were a married couple, our near-neighbours, and together ran a small General Practice from their home. Margaret's consulting room was next to the reception and waiting area. To see Paul we took a few steps outside to a converted garage, where he sat at a handsomely plain and robust oak desk – utility furniture that had served in their thousands throughout the War. The house's domestic hinterland became familiar to me, too: my parents became friendly with Paul and Margaret, I became part of a street-gaggle with their sons.

This interweaving of professional-vocational-locality-domestic-family was, I think, typical of much life – and General Practice – of the time. Amongst better practitioners it led to an unselfconscious integration, an innominate holism, well before common attempts were made to distil, commodify or brand such notions. I think now that Paul and Margaret had a natural understanding – a sense and sensibility – of the unspoken spectres and meanings behind the presented distress or anxiety. Amidst my mists of memory I cannot define clearly the exact times or childhood decisions that led to my later vocations. Yet I think these early experiences, of this couple's benign aura, had a strong inductive influence: even then my innocently receptive eye and mind somehow discerned what I could formulate only much later: that their converged knowledge of the personal and the impersonal could contain, comfort and heal. My early proclivity to such understanding was born of intuition: the vocabulary of scholarship, to describe or explain, would take many more years.

## 2010s. A small Practice: a bridged island

*'The All is alive'*

Thales of Miletus (624-527 BC)


Pam knocks gently, knowing my signs of incipient late afternoon gruff fatigue. Her entrance is welcome: she comes revitalising me with hot tea. Pam has been afternoon receptionist in our small practice for a decade. Her middle age experience and deportment are sparkled by youthful gleams and warmly ironic humour. I greet and test her with a long moan of mock-theatrical self-pity conveying the suffering I so self-effacingly endure for others: I, a broken, groaning dying soldier on the carnaged Crimean battlefield; she, the consoling, saintly Florence Nightingale, The Lady with the Tea. Pam's smile is complex: amusement, commiseration, contrition, teasing tolerance and palliation. I do not need to say much: she understands my need for bantered, boundaried, fleeting tenderness. She heals me a little: it has been a long and difficult day. Her tea and resonance may be almost wordless, but they are powerful: like a life-affirming force-field these help contain and sustain me. Such is well-fared welfare; a benign relay – now I am restored to do the same for others.

Pam waits a few seconds for the first signs of my revival, then refreshed attention. Her expression has solemned and now conveys earnest request.

'What now?!' I ask, part question, part peremptory and pre-emptive retort. 'I thought you'd come just to refuel me … It's been a really difficult day.' I add, now more sharply, to scotch any further demands.

'It's Ruby…' Pam persists: she is kind to me, but resilient too. 'I think you should see her today … I've said you will and asked her to wait: she initially didn't want to, but now she will…'

My exasperation is tinged with hostility; I sigh conspicuously: 'But why today, of all days?!' more a warning than a question.

Pam is unerringly calm: 'Because she looks terrible … she's never been right since Robert (her husband) died so quickly of that cancer, just after Christmas … she's always been quiet and shy, but now she's really gone into herself … She comes regularly, every month, for her usual prescriptions. Before she'd chat a little, but now she hardly looks at us … and today I was quite shocked: she's not just withdrawn – she looks really ill: pale and frail … She's all on her own and hates asking for help … Yes, I think you should see her today, while she's here…'

In this small practice people's faces, voices and stories are seen, remembered and recognised. Receptionists accrue percipient and vernacular understandings of patients and their lives. So when longer and good bonds evolve, so do dialogues rich in personal investment.

While doctors' interchanges often segue rapidly to the technical, the task-focused and the managerial, the receptionist's encounters may linger more freely and naturally.

*

Pam is right.

She ushers Ruby in with patient and tender vigilance. Ruby is weak, pale, sallow and almost extinguished of life-spirit. She crosses the room as if impeded by a dense and invisible gas. Despite this torpor she manages her usual self-abnegation – now it is almost inaudible: 'I did ask Pam not to bother you, doctor … I know you've got a lot to do…' Her voice is enfeebled and leaden, her gaze unfocused, dull and lifeless. She is short of breath.

Soon after I am technically categorising and recording. 'Severe Reactive Depression/Impacted Grief. ?Probably Anaemia ?GI bleeding ?Self-neglect and diet ?Other. Mild Heart Failure.' The medical train is on its tracks. It might not have been if Pam had not looked and thought and cared as she does. Much does not conveniently present as we wish: I must value and protect my receptionists as my social antennae.

I am wondering, too, how could Pam have made this bond of affectionate observation in a now commoner and much larger practice, with its airport-like forms of human processing and (dis)connection? There, I might get home sooner; but what would happen to Ruby?

## 2010s. A larger Practice: impoverishment in plenty

*'Seek knowledge, even if it be in China'*

Muhammad

Soon after the new Millennium I sensed my mortality more sharply. I submitted to conventional sense and decided to register with a GP. I, too, will eventually need more than easy (self) prescription for transient complaints: age begins to perish our seals of denial.

I sought and found a small single-handed Practice with a trail of good repute. Dr F. was a likeable, courteous, thoughtful Frenchman; laconic humour spiced an understated compassion. I did not see him much, but each time I did I sensed a growth of joint interest, memory and understanding. Five years ago I was sorrowed by what he told me: he was leaving his work in the NHS and his life in the UK. He had become increasingly frustrated and demoralised by the progressive loss of personal satisfactions, meaning and connections in his work.

He was emigrating to mainland China, to work as a Family Doctor, to reclaim an ethos, a modus vivendum, he increasingly missed. I think my expression signalled perplexity or incredulity, for he rapidly offered bridging explanations: his wife is Chinese, he had spent years learning the language.

I had not needed him much but had sensed a deep affinity, were I to need him. I felt a gentle pang of sadness; I was grieving for a receding attachment I had never really tested, but which I felt had been quietly there.

We shared a warmly farewelling handshake. I briefly thanked him for his friendly and competent contacts with me; I would be sad not to see him again. His look shared this light, sweet flutter of melancholy and he nodded to signal his confluence: 'Of course, there are many people I shall miss, but I think you understand why I am leaving...'

I did and I do.

*

In more recent times my awareness of my blessings has become both stouter and more tremulous: my gratitude for my particular good health is reluctantly laced with a darkening sorrow: for our universal transience – our eventual and inevitable fragility and extinction. I try to be pragmatic; I can offset this a little. I will submit to the nationally vaunted programmes to monitor and control physical risk-factors: horizoned Black Riders of mortality.

\*

I attend this re-staffed and managed health centre. A young desultorily expressioned receptionist is looking fixedly at a display on a computer screen. I softly cough to signal my presence, but she is a receptionist who is not receptive. Aware of my waiting presence she attempts to rapidly offload me: 'Over there. Check-in is with the computer', she jerks her head to indicate its direction, keeping unbroken contact with her own computer task.

The computer interrogates and briefs me with brief staccato instructions. When satisfied with my identity and appointment it emits a soft chiming sound to tell me that I am temporarily dismissed and where to go while awaiting further instructions.

I sit in a waiting area that has rows of stackable plastic chairs all facing a wall in which there is a large viewing hatch beyond which the (non) reception staff sit. Above the hatch is a horizontally long, thin, electronic screen across which an endless procession of bannered messages loop to inform, mollify, instruct or warn: 'Feeling down? Find out about our Counselling Services … Problems with alcohol consumption? … Are you at risk of HIV? Other sexually transmitted disease? … Has your child had its MMR vaccinations? … Stopping smoking will be the one decision you'll never regret … One consultation is for one patient with one problem …None of our staff will tolerate any form of rudeness, threat or aggression of any kind. Offending patients are immediately removed from our list …'. I am aware of the insidious, silent hegemony of such devices; legal civilian nerve-gases to secure compliance and docility.

\*

There is a louder, sharper chime, to alert attention. Eyes are raised to the screen to be briefed and instructed. My name appears alongside which consulting room I should go to.

I am seeing the Practice Nurse for some routine blood tests. I have never seen her before. She is looking at a computer as I enter the room, I think to brief her about my 'personal' data. 'Good morning', I say, cheerily, I think. She makes a brief, low, rear-throat sound in acknowledgement. This is wordless and her attention remains with her screen. 'I don't have a request form, but I have come for blood tests: Renal-function, Lipid Profile, Uric Acid and HbAIC'. I say this overtly to inform, but I also have my curiosity about her curiosity, or lack of it: will she enquire about my likely knowledge of such things, and the source of it? She does not.

Instead, without looking, she hurls a question across the room. The question is imperative, stark and unredefinable. The voice is loud, rhetorical and with the guttural, gravelly menace that only impatiently direct Ulster citizens can convey to otherwise benign utterances. 'WHICH ARM?' is the sudden and unframed question. My unprepared, then panicked perception back-somersaults to somewhere in the late-1970s' Northern Ireland: I think I am going to be taken out and shot.

I wince briefly, offer my exposed left arm and then regain sufficient composure to have bland but cordial contact with Nurse Q. As my blood flows I become quietly amused by my images: historical memory-shards, relics of harboured hatreds. Now rapidly recovered I ask whether she is from Northern Ireland. Yes, she says, she was brought up and trained in Londonderry, but her secondary home and family have been here, in London, for many years.

She does not ask me about my probable medical knowledge, or anything else about me. She smiles, as if into a mist, when I leave.

*

I phone the surgery to make an appointment to see the new (for me) GP to discuss my blood tests. I am put on hold while waiting to speak to a receptionist. This administrative hiatus is filled by an expedient plug by and for the practice: a softly, even seductively, authoritative female robotic voice begins to inform me of extra clinics and services that may be offered by the practice, which services can be competently dealt with by nursing staff, and what to do about Out of Hours requirements. In these two minutes I have not yet heard threats or ultimata to the deviants or misbehaved: I am relieved. Another voice cuts in: the real voice of a live receptionist. I make my requests clear, succinct and practical and follow these with some questions about the new order: she replies in kind. 'Dr NP (the new Principal) has expanded the practice and is very busy, so it's easier for you to see one of the part-time assistants. I'll book you to see Dr A: she's very nice...'

*

I come to see Dr A. I do not now expect anyone to recognise or greet me in the practice beforehand. The computer and I, now better acquainted, perform our brief chimed procedure and I go to the waiting area to discern my name from the bannered attempts to crop-spray my mind and conduct.

A more commanding chime now beckons my encounter with Dr A. As I enter she turns a brief, warm but tiredly unfocused smile toward me with a simultaneous 'Hello'. She signals to a chair at the corner of her flimsily veneered, already chipped, new desk before turning away again, back to the computer: the anchor-post for her consultation-consciousness. As she is scrolling down my laboratory results, I can see my non-medical details which remain constant at the top of the changing screen contents. My name is preceded by 'Doctor'.

She turns back to me and offers another jading smile. She asks me how I am: I sense this is mostly a courtesy, but also to ensure I do not have another major agenda before she can start on the one she has decided. I do not have one, so now she is free to quickly move us both onto the problem she has identified and dissected.

'Well, I've looked at your recent blood tests ... they're all fine except your sugar, so that's one we have to talk about, because officially you're now a diabetic...'

She goes on to automatically convey structured questions, information and advice about my diet, lifestyle, monitoring regimes and possible future medications. This, I can see, is a generic didactic package she applies to all mild diabetic-risk patients. She has been professionally mannered and clear in her delivery: but it is a delivery and not a dialogue. Fascinatingly (for me) she has learned nothing about me as a person: what kind of life and relationships I have had, what I hope for, what I fear, what brings me joy, what brings me dread – what is likely to sicken me, what to heal me.

Yet within her frame she is a competent didactic teacher, her messages are well rehearsed and well formed. She pauses to see if I understand: I do. I am thoroughly cognisant of what she is telling me: imaginative observation would quickly indicate this. At the end of this auto-piloted freight run she slows a little to tie up this parcel with a faintly simpered, liberal, school-mistress voice: 'Well, I think that's as much as we need to say today – quite a lot, isn't it? – is that ok?' This is a statement and prescription from her, not really a question for me. She tilts her head a little while beaming an unknowing yet coquettish smile: her sweetening and concealment of control is the outer packaging.

She never asks about me being a doctor, and I (partly now for experimental reasons) do not tell her. She shows no curiosity about my personal or occupational life. Dr A acts a role of the agreeably impersonal: I think that she does not know that she does not know me – and can then proceed with her job as if this is of no consequence to either of us.

At present this is, arguably, enough: I do not yet have the kind of dis-ease, disease, dependence or infirmity which requires the kind of personal understandings that can contain, comfort and heal. If I live long enough, I will.

Yes, Dr A's advice is sound, and her prescribed medications far more precise and powerful than anything that was available to my 1950s doctors. Yes, *treatment* is usually much better, but what about *care*? Here there is no such commensurate progress, often the reverse. I know that when my health and life begin to ineluctably unravel, like Ruby, I will want *personal* and personal-*continuity* of care from practitioners with that ethos and vocation: people like Doctors Paul and Margaret.

But in a healthcare world increasingly designed, commissioned, commodified, commercialised and managed by others very different from them, and remote from me, how is this possible? What, instead, will happen?

The portents are already visible, if only we will look.

\*

Healthcare is a humanity guided by science.

# Ω

*'The danger of the past was that men became slaves. The danger of the future is that men become robots.'*

Erich Fromm, *The Sane Society*, 1955

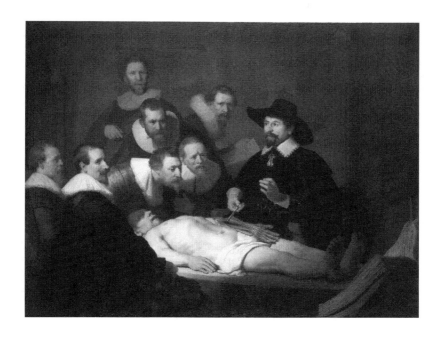

Rembrandt *The Anatomy Lesson of Dr. Nicolaes Tulp* 1632

# The Medical Model
# – its Limitations and Alternatives

## How humanism may synergise biomechanism

## What is the Medical Model?

Although most doctors' working time is spent using the Medical Model, we might find the term difficult to define. This itself reflects particular restrictions of thinking: those conditioned by years of training and modelling ourselves on other doctors. We then find it difficult to stand outside our methodological framework and see other realities.

Here is a preliminary definition: the Medical Model assumes a simple mechanical view of illness and the body it occurs in. Any illness is thus seen simply as a fault in the machine. Although lip-service may be paid to interfering concepts of the mind, the family and the environment, these are uncomfortable bedfellows of the Medical Model and the machine-body continues to be regarded as something that functions autonomously: a hermetic system. Diagnoses therefore tend to be formulated in terms of structural or functional failures of the machine alone. It follows that because treatment methods derive from diagnostic concepts, then medical treatment is likely to be equally mechanistic and exclusive of non-material or psychological factors. The Medical Model sometimes does well with these restrictions: for example, in orthopaedic trauma surgery where the problems are most clearly circumscribed and structural.

## The Reasons We Use the Medical Model

The Medical Model has enticing clarity: it is generally succinct, tangible and understandable: it has easy confluence with a scientific method which relies primarily on objective and measurable observation. This has the advantage of offering terminology, formulations and explanations which can (seemingly) be unambiguously understood and then handled in an identical fashion by all similarly trained people. We therefore have the potential of knowing precisely what others are talking about and what they are doing in defined situations. This makes possible the kinds of standardisation of terminology and concepts that are essential for scientific communication and research. These activities can then give us useful information about general patterns of illness and the effectiveness of therapies.

Less defensible reasons for our inflexible and often inept use of the Medical Model lie in habit and conditioning. Most of us were never encouraged or taught to use anything else. Therefore we have developed skills only within a narrow framework: this we continue to use alone, even when a problem requires alternative or additional methods.

## Some Snares We Fall into Unconsciously

At its best the Medical Model functions extremely well, providing guidelines for processing circumscribed problems and predicting what the outcome will be, with or without intervention. Such important considerations are invoked in the concept of diagnosis. Diagnosis provides powerful navigational aid when we have substantial knowledge about what we are labelling: *Substantial diagnosis*. If, on the other hand, a diagnosis does not offer us accurate information about prognosis and intervention, then we can call this a *Nominal diagnosis* because it gives only an arcane name to something we know very little about. Let us take an example of each.

1. Acute follicular beta-haemolytic streptococcal tonsillitis is a Substantial diagnosis. It tells us with relative certainty what the symptoms and signs are, what treatment is going to be effective and what the hazards are of leaving the complaint untreated. The Medical Model works well here. Our concepts and tools are effective. We know what to do and are rarely surprised by subsequent events if we do the right thing. The patient senses this, and he and the doctor will probably get along well in this situation.

2. Non-articular or seronegative rheumatoid arthritis*[1] is a Nominal diagnosis. It really does not tell us much at all. It does not tell us how the patient's health will be affected in the future. In five years' time he may be perfectly well despite not having any treatment. On the other hand he may be crippled with arthritis, blind with iritis and have an ileostomy because of fulminating ulcerative colitis. Furthermore, he may have developed all this despite the best treatment available. The Medical Model is now working extremely badly. The doctor feels unsure and ineffective and is likely to be on the defensive. The patient senses this and reciprocally lacks confidence. The relationship between patient and doctor is now likely to be more strained. The patient may become 'difficult and demanding'. The doctor attempts to maintain a confident persona by whatever new kinds of investigation and therapy he can think of, because he does not know what else to offer.

### Substantial and Nominal Diagnosis

The two diagnoses here are really quite different in their implication. The 'Substantial diagnosis' offers us extremely helpful information as to what we might do and what we should expect, while the 'Nominal diagnosis' does neither satisfactorily. At best it is a descriptive tag which we attach to some apparently similar phenomena which we do not understand. However, such is the power of words that we equate them with understanding. Just as a religious incantation is intended to dispel evil spirits or attract good ones, so the

---

[1] *Post-scripted note December 2014. In the thirty-eight years since this was written, scientific knowledge has advanced, so that these conditions are now more contained with Substantial (rather than Nominal) diagnoses. Thus the knowledge has grown – the examples are now somewhat obsolete – but the guiding principles remain.

Rather than rewrite the examples, they are retained for historical interest. It is hoped that the underlying argument is unobscured. It remains seminal to this book.

medical incantation of naming the diagnosis is meant to dispel uncertainty and indecision. However, as we can see from the above example it often fails to do this – nevertheless we continue to repeat the ritual and hope the rest will follow.

Many ailments fall somewhere between the Substantial and Nominal end of the diagnostic spectrum. Often a particular illness will shift its position at different times. For example, a man who has the dyspepsia appropriate to a barium-meal proven duodenal ulcer* may well present the doctor with a Nominal diagnosis, as the course of his illness and the efficacy of therapy remain largely unknown. If this same man perforates his ulcer then the situation is one where a Substantial diagnosis becomes very important; treatment is incontrovertible and clear-cut and the prognosis with and without this intervention equally so.

In formulating diagnoses we need to be aware of their position on this spectrum. Are we really making meaningful statements, or are we merely tagging labels onto phenomena we are ignorant about? If it is the latter, who is benefited by the Nominal diagnosis – the doctor, the patient or the institution? Complex terminology is often used as a defence against substantial ignorance. If the doctor is lost, bemused and largely ineffective, then at least he can fall back on some technical words and 'scientific' concepts which he hopes will maintain his position in his own and the patient's eyes as the potent and unassailable authority. Such unconscious defences and collusions are not always a bad thing, but they can often block the doctor's opportunities to explore more fruitful avenues of rapport and investigation.

## What the Medical Model Misses Out

Because it has its roots in the scientific method, the Medical Model functions best when incorporating phenomena that are measurable and quantifiable. That is, it copes well with the physical or organic components of illness, but has much less assurance with other factors, the most important of which are personal and psychological. Most of us are instinctively aware of the importance of external stresses and inner emotional conflicts in the precipitation, course and eventual outcome of many illnesses. Yet the problem of being unable to directly measure stress or emotional conflict is always problematic.

There have certainly been attempts to rate and scale such reactions as fear (anxiety) and dispiritedness (depression), but on scrutiny these endeavours only measure phenomena which are assumed to have a direct relationship with the inner experience, which itself remains elusive and unmeasurable to our tools of scientific enquiry. True, we can measure and classify certain of the simpler aspects of behaviour – that is, reported speech and habits, alcohol consumption, compulsive rituals etc – but never the inner life that motivates them. Rating scores of described experiences are beset with ambiguities and potential distortions. If the usual Medical Model is incapable of dealing imaginatively with these aspects of illness then we have two alternatives. We can ignore the non-organic, non-measurable aspects of medicine and remain always within the respectable territory of scientific convention, or we can use alternative modes and models – we can add to the more traditional medical diagnoses.

Such a whole-person or even whole-family approach to illness has received increasing attention in recent years. Perhaps the most influential work in this area pertinent to the general practitioner was investigated by Michael Balint. Much of his work indicates that the traditional medical diagnosis used alone is often severely limited in the amount of help it gives to the doctor in understanding the patient's illness, what he can do about it, and what he might expect in the future. Balint found that these limitations can be countered by the doctor entering into new, speculative territory where skills of empathetic imagination might attempt to formulate the position of illness within its matrix of family relationships and internal emotional tensions. Such formulations cannot give us the same sort of uniform agreement of the more traditional diagnoses, but this venture offers much else in terms of understanding and influence. The following case illustrates a typical medical formulation, then expanded by humanistic speculation.

## A Case from General Practice

*Mr CT is 65 years of age. One month before his date of retirement he developed ankle oedema and ascites. His general practitioner first saw him late one night when he developed acute and severe dyspnoea. Examination indicated mild hypertension, biventricular cardiac failure and slight cardiac enlargement. Routine investigations yielded only the one additional useful finding that his cardiac failure was probably caused by ischaemic heart disease (ECG evidence). Unfortunately, fairly large doses of Digoxin and diuretics had no effect on his ascites and oedema, although his blood pressure was well controlled with Methyldopa. He had no further attacks of pulmonary oedema.*

*One month later, therefore, he was hospitalised with a view to controlling his right-sided heart failure. Even with complete bed rest and massive doses of Frusemide and Spironolactone this problem was extremely difficult to manage. At this time he became increasingly anxious, irritable and demanding. It became difficult to keep him in bed or to get him to take his medication, which he seemed to view with suspicion. Eventually this ended in a mixed manic-paranoid reaction. He claimed to be in perfect health and said that he was in hospital to help his wife's illness (she was in good health).*

*While embarking on numerous impractical projects simultaneously, he would make grandiose and untrue proclamations about how wealthy and important he was. His distractibility made it difficult for him to sleep or eat, and his motor restlessness made him a difficult nursing problem. At times he showed fluctuating paranoid delusions about the nursing staff, saying that they had poisoned him and stolen his money. On the other hand he became unprecedentedly sexually suggestive and familiar with the same nurses. Although showing undoubted manic signs when interviewed, the depression was just below the surface. He became extremely distressed and tearful when certain important and personal and life topics were discussed. Although Chlorpromazine was needed to contain the immediate situation, the bulk of his improvement came from helping him come to terms with his underlying emotional problems.*

Before we move into this alternative and personal diagnostic area, we might formulate the medical diagnoses thus: mild controlled hypertension with ischaemic heart disease causing decompensated right ventricular failure. Superadded mixed manic-paranoid psychosis.

## Method or Madness?

Let us now look into the story of this man's life and see how his illness fits in. The hallmarks of Mr CT's life were caution, safety, orderliness and continence. He only took the minimum and essential risks in life, and then only with the maximum preparation. He had married 40 years ago and had lived in the same house ever since. Throughout these four decades, he had worked in the same clerical job, though with minor promotions. In his work he was diligent to the point of obsession and found any criticism or disorder highly disturbing. His marriage was contained in a similar framework of orderliness and safety. His wife never worked outside the home because he found the idea threatening. Their life together was safely but drably concordant, and structured by well-worn routine. Their sexual life sounded courteously suppressed and obscured: latterly he had been rendered impotent, probably because of his Methyldopa.

His leisure time similarly drifted: passive and unexplorative. He watched television indiscriminately and fell asleep after supper while reading the *Daily Express*. Occasionally he would potter in the garden, but took little else in the way of physical activity. His lack of pursued hobbies or interests and led to boredom and irritability at weekends: time and freedom became enemies. Anger was never overt; he would similarly avoid or appease any conflict, which he evidently found threatening. In his social relationships he had cordial but ritualised contacts, hence no committed or intimate friends. Because of his passivity and temerity, he felt exploited at work: a cruel consequence of his diligence and compliance. He was resentful that after 40 years of service to his employers, he left with little promotion, perfunctory compliments and a gold watch. Secretly he had hoped for grand applause and a big send-off.

Last, but not least, this man had never been seriously ill.

## Understanding and Management

How does this backcloth help us in our understanding and engagement with this frightened and frustrated man? One of the most striking features about him is his inability to assert himself as an individual, or act in any way that would lead to dissonance with others. His early background can help us understand. He experienced his father as authoritarian, overpowering, distant yet violent when drunk or frustrated. His mother and siblings learned that the only way to be safe was to be silent, obedient and unnoticed. He had carried this legacy of submissive, stoic resentment throughout the rest of his life.

Until the onset of his illness.

In his fantasy life he had vaguely hoped that retirement would bring some of the fulfilment and satisfaction that had always eluded him. The reality turned out to be very different. Even without his illness, his fixation to many years' routine, his inflexibility and lack of creative interests made retirement an extremely demanding testing-ground for this overadapted and underdeveloped man. It is even possible that he recognised this unconsciously, and that his heart-failure represented a lost battleground: the disconsolate 'loss of heart' – that this was all there was to his life.

What is evidently true is that his serious illness then brought to consciousness the possible imminence of his death. This insinuated the futility of his life: all the things he wished he had achieved, yet had avoided. Such a demeaned view of his life was intolerable: a defence was essential. Hence his manic reaction; thence his grandiosity, his multiple and unrealistic plans, his display of hypersexuality and the demanding urges he had kept so well contained for so many years. Equally difficult for him was the way in which physical illness had underlined his shamed self-perception of passivity and weakness; hence the denial that he himself was ill, and that any illness within him was displaced from his wife, or the result of others poisoning him.

Other destabilising facets emerged: the established structure of his marriage had been radically changed. Although a sedentary man, he had claimed the conventionally undisputed dominant marital role: his submissive wife offered him some sense of domestic power. His illness, however, had reversed their roles. Now he was the partner who had to stay at home and be provided for – her role until he fell ill.

He struggled painfully and tearfully with coming to terms with these realities. With a growing sorrowful calm he perceived how his mania and paranoia were defences against his deep-rooted frustrations and sense of loss. It was bravado in the face of grief. He was both grieving and raging for the life he had feared to live, and whose possibilities were now passing.

The human core of this formulation lies outside conventional scientific and medical methods. It can neither be proved nor disproved, because his feelings and his entire inner world cannot be objectively observed or measured. With unprovable plausibility they can be logically inferred; with imagination, intuitively felt. Yet without this meeting in the regions of uncertainty he must endure his grief, fear and primitive anger alone. Enabling him to share these brought compassionate palliation and relief. His manic and paranoid defences became no longer necessary.

Understanding his rage enabled him to metabolise it. He has then been freer to cope with his diminished and disabled life. Although sorrowful he is not now 'ill' in the strict psychiatric sense. Interestingly his heart failure became much better controlled. Has his cardiac function improved because his heart is no longer subject to the autonomic-nervous and hormonal storms that beset it in his previous state of emotional turbulence? Happily he no longer needs major tranquillisers to assure his sanity and stability: his inner healing has now anchored this.

## Conclusion

This case illustrates how the Medical Model can be integrated within a wider framework of alternatives. From a strict scientific view these other concepts do not avail themselves so readily to more direct kinds of empirical testing. Yet the price of ignoring these alternatives is high. Mr CT would probably have continued his mania, paranoia and depression and had a much more turbulent end of life. It is likely, too, that his cardiac failure would have remained intractable: his improvement was definite and otherwise unaccountable.

Such pursuits are subtle: they require more flexibility in approach than we are generally trained for. In return our understanding of, and rapport with, the whole patient becomes richer. The benefits extend beyond prevention or curtailment of significant illness in others – we ourselves derive greater human interest and satisfaction from our work.

Ω

Published in *Hospital Update* 424-427, Aug.1976

# Illness as Strategy
# and Communication

In spite of the vast bulk of literature deriving from psychoanalysis and applicable to medicine, the predominant orientation in the training and practice of doctors remains entrenched in concepts of illness which are mechanistic and unconnected with the patient's emotional and relationship matrix. Perhaps the increasing precision and sophistication of our technology has made other dimensions of illness seem less important in assessment and management.

Modern techniques of diagnosis and therapy are now complex, powerful and, at times, dangerous. Because of these developments, it is hardly surprising that the contemporary doctor may see himself as some kind of biological engineer or technician, whose job it is to rectify faults in the human machine. However, there are emotional factors which are also operative in maintaining this kind of technocracy and alienation between patient and doctor. We can think of these as 'defences' whose function is to protect both parties against distressing and threatening feelings, and also conserve the doctor's position of executive power. I have explored some of these factors in an earlier paper (Zigmond 1977) but here I want to elaborate further the role of illness in meeting the emotional needs of patients. Without this approach, I believe, diagnosis and therapy are often liable to be less effective. Four cases are described later to illustrate this.

## Illness as Strategy

Illness is usually conceived and experienced as a malevolent intrusion by an alien force, which has no connection with the self and its relationship with others. Whatever our knowledge of the mechanics, the illness is felt and thought of as something apart, that strikes us 'out of the blue'. Because of this split we feel that we are at the mercy of the disease process, which seems to have an autonomous, even magical, existence. In the face of illness, therefore, we are all liable to feel helpless and dependent, either on the disease process or on any person who may alleviate it. In psychoanalytic jargon, disease may be said to be 'ego-dystonic', i.e. separate from the familiar complex of volition and experience that we conceive of as 'the self'. Such infirmity, therefore, may compromise our usual traits of independence and individual effectiveness. When ill, we often find ourselves incapable of making decisions or performing the necessary tasks to realize them. A state of regression is engendered, where autonomy is necessarily abdicated. If a man in his 40s, for example, is admitted to a coronary care unit, it is likely that he will be necessarily regressed to the early infant stage. He will be put to bed, washed, and evacuate himself into a bottle or bedpan. Such dramatic and coerced regression may be difficult, but any resistance on his part is likely to have him branded as 'uncooperative'.

Alternatively, however, illness may have its uses. There is a childlike and dependent part in us all, whatever our age or maturity. From the infants we all were, there remains our archaic and relentless drive for recognition, attention and care from those around us. Equally, we may at times feel immense rage and destructiveness towards those who are closest, just as the infant does rather more overtly. Because of societal taboos, such intense dependence or rage is clearly discouraged. Illness, however, is a state where the individual is not thought to be responsible for himself, and thus offers a less stigmatizing and more conventionally acceptable means of regressing into this child-system. Under the cloak of illness we may become helpless, ask others to look after us, act out and abdicate our usual identity-structure. Behaviour which in other circumstances would be criticized or even punished, can be connived at, and often colluded with.

## Illness as Communication

It has already been indicated in which way illness may serve as a conventionally acceptable route to regression that might otherwise be considered dys-social or antisocial. This does not mean, however, that illness communicates only archaic and primitive messages. Very commonly an individual has developed his own specific taboos with particular kinds of feelings. Frequently this is because his parents indicated to him that these feelings would be ignored, belittled or even punished. Such moulding of emotional responses occurs via parental influence in a child's formative years. Explicit pressures such as punishment or mockery are clear, but covert pressures such as a hostile tone of voice or parental indifference are commoner, though sometimes equally damaging. The feelings that are forbidden may range from fear to assertion, from sadness to anger, depending on the parents' area of difficulty. Later on in life this person will be unable to express this particular feeling with direct words and gestures. Instead he will resort to oblique expressions via somatic language which, in his developmental frame of reference, provides immunity from the hurt he received when he was young. In this way psychosomatic illness may be viewed as having its roots in a habitual and compulsive form of body language.

## Case No. 1: A Little Boy Escapes Bellyaching

Stephen, aged seven, is generally a healthy boy who has a good communication with his humorous and intelligent mother. His parents separated when he was an infant. Mother has recently remarried. Stephen is tentatively fond of her new husband but feels insecure with him. In addition, Stephen's real father has fallen into debt and depression and has been unable to pay the usual maintenance, creating an atmosphere of tension and split loyalties for Stephen, who is fond of his father, and has regular contact with him. Because of father's difficulties, he had to defer his weekend visit. The following dialogue then ensued.

Stephen: (plaintively) 'Mum, I feel sick and I've got a tummy ache.'

Mother: (intuitively, noting his empty dinner plate) 'I am sorry Stephen, it's horrible isn't it? . . . I think you're sad and disappointed that daddy's not happy and he can't come today. But it doesn't mean he doesn't love you... I think your tummy ache is saying that you're a bit angry and sad.' Stephen then goes to his mother, sits on her lap, has a cuddle and forgets his abdominal discomfort.

Mother here did not discount Stephen's tummy ache, but more importantly she recognized, validated and accepted his sadness, anger and confusion. Contrast this with a possible and likely alternative:

Stephen: 'Mum, I feel sick and I've got a tummy ache.'

Mother: 'Oh dear, I do hope it's nothing bad . . . you must go to bed, and I'll call the doctor straight away.'

Here the long-term and short-term outcomes are likely to be quite different. Mother only takes Stephen's stomach ache seriously because she herself cannot cope with unhappy and distressed feelings. Her implicit message to Stephen is, 'I don't mind you having stomach ache, but don't show me your unhappiness, because I don't know how to deal with it'. Stephen now learns that overt communication of distress, anger and sadness cannot be displayed; he must settle for tummy ache instead, if he is to evoke mother's protection and concern. As an adult he may well be getting antacids from his general practitioner every time his dyspepsia indicates sadness and frustration that he feels inwardly compelled to bear alone. In this latter situation, the alert and empathetic general practitioner will be able to verbalize and accept the patient's distress and frustrations, thereby rendering them more tolerable to the patient himself. The doctor who is able to recognize, validate and hold a patient's unhappiness, performs much the same function as a parent with a child who is afraid of being overwhelmed by the intensity of his feelings. Once confirmed and shared, some resolution or subsidence of emotional problems may be possible. This is a cornerstone of psychotherapy at every level of practice.

### Case No. 2: Illness as Rebellion in an Over-ordered Family

Miss VH is 23 years of age. Since the age of 16 she has suffered from well-documented episodes of mania. All but her last hospitalization were to an organically orientated psychiatric unit, where a wide span of major tranquillizers and Lithium was tried, which may have quelled the acute crises, but seemed to have little prophylactic effect on her disability.

Her last admission was to a less organically orientated unit, but followed the same cacophonous pattern. On arrival she showed clinical signs of mania in her psychomotor acceleration, distractibility, emotional liability, prickliness, grandiose and discursive thinking, and so forth. However, the doctor sensed her underlying sadness and despair. He offered her his observation saying, 'It seems to me that underneath all this you're feeling really miserable and helpless'. She stayed silent for some time and her mania seemed to evaporate giving way to a rather sad and confused child. 'Yes', she replied, 'nobody ever listens to me at home, especially my father, so I get angry and they say, "Oh, she's getting ill again, we'd better call the doctor". And he's always on their side. He doesn't listen either, so I have to come into hospital again.' By inference it seemed that VH came from a household where anger and rebellion could not be expressed directly, only through illness – in this case mania. It emerged that VH is an only child, from a stable, professional and rather joyless marriage. Her father is a rigid, authoritarian, ex-military man whose need for order and obedience seemed indefatigable. Mother has learned to adapt through subdued compliance and stamina, but VH never managed this so successfully. Father's moralism and strictures with VH's social life indicated difficulties with his own sexual feelings, and possibly some incestuous impulses towards VH

It was only through acknowledging her very real anger, and frustration with her coerced dependence, that she was able to organize her emotional resources to deal with the problem realistically. In spite of her fear and pain she has now left home, is off her drugs and is forging her own identity slowly but surely. These substantial gains were demanding and difficult: she made good use of skilled professional guidance. Her manic 'illness' symbolized her battle for autonomy and has not returned.

### Case No. 3: A Desperate Struggle for Recognition in Infancy

Baby Kevin F. was aged five months on admission. His birth and first three months had been physically uneventful. For two months, however, he had been restless and posseted all his feeds, so that he had lost weight dramatically. On admission he was evidently very ill; his weight was on the third percentile, he was extremely frail and dehydrated, as attested by his sunken fontanelle, dry tongue and raised blood urea. His history was against congenital pyloric stenosis, and barium studies failed to show a hiatus hernia. In physical terms his diagnosis was one of rumination syndrome – he had no physical lesion, but was bringing back his food for self-gratification and to evoke contact with others.

The family and emotional diagnosis was more difficult and complex. His parents were an intelligent and ambitious couple, and this was their first child. Mother was an insecure and prickly woman, who escaped the conflictual relationship with her short-tempered father by getting married to a man who was very much like him. Mr and Mrs F. thus lived in a state of competitive discord, and Mrs F. harbours extensive grievances against men because she feels they will control her and usurp her independence. She had been doing well in her career as a teacher, and became pregnant ambivalently with pressure from her husband. Because of her feelings about the men in her life, she secretly hoped for a baby girl with whom she could develop an alliance of women.

With the birth of Kevin she felt bitterly disappointed, and found herself unable to give him the maternal and nurturing responses that were necessary. Kevin was fed, bathed and bedded efficiently, but was never played with or enjoyed. He would sit in this pristine cot wanting to explore or be loved, but mother sat silently and sullenly doing *The Times* crossword puzzle. Kevin's progress in hospital was dramatic. He was played with, chatted to and smiled at by the nurses, and his feeding difficulties soon settled, with the attendant improvement in weight. Mrs F. recognized her lack of nurturing, where it came from, and how it led to Kevin's severe illness. Fortunately, Mr and Mrs F. were able to embark on, and co-operate with, a mixture of individual and marital therapy, which brought about a greater fulfilment in their marriage, and a disappearance of Kevin's desperate strategies to be loved and related to.

## Case No. 4: Illness as an Escape Mechanism

Mr G. K. is aged 53 years. He had been physically healthy all his life until a number of apparently physical crises were brought to the attention of his general practitioner, and then the medical and casualty departments of the local hospital. Over several months he had a number of alarming attacks, consisting of tightness in the chest, a feeling of impending suffocation, paraesthesiae in the arms and hands and prostrating weakness and dizziness. Suspected cardiac and respiratory disease was never confirmed, but he continued to be subject to these crises, with the consequent hospitalizations and investigations. The only positive physical finding was a persistent mild idiopathic hypertension (BP 170/110). Eventually the recognition of these episodes as panic attacks led to an exploration of his underlying problems.

Mr G. K. is a Greek Cypriot but has spent most of his adult life in this country, has married an English woman and now has three teenage children. Early on in his life Mr G. K. decided that he must be strong, ignore his own feelings but look after other people, whom he needed to perceive as less strong than himself. He learned this life-role as a child because of his parents' own marital difficulties. Father was a large and unhappy man whose resentment with his lot was largely projected onto his wife and children via displays and acts of violence. These were exacerbated by his drinking and gambling, which gave mother an excuse to persecute him, thereby perpetuating the vicious circle. Although he might physically assault mother, he would stop short of this with his children. Mr G. K. learned, as a small boy, that he could rescue his mother by interposing himself between his parents. However, to do this he had to be able to deny his own fear of the situation. As a child of six years he learned that his mother's survival depended on his rescuing her with his bravado and fearlessness. This role was pursued relentlessly despite the circumstantial changes in his life. Father died and he came to England with his mother, where he soon met his future wife. Although his new family was under no real duress, he still felt the compulsion to be the never-failing rescuer and provider. He was a warm and caring man, but could only show this by working 'for the family' to the extremes of his physical endurance, and by taking on a firm patriarchal role in the belief that his family could never function autonomously without him. This hero at war was not an easy man to love at home; he and his wife insidiously became emotionally and sexually estranged.

It was the Turkish invasion of Cyprus that brought forward the collapse of this man's outdated and cumbersome defences. His home town was destroyed, and with it many friends and relatives who together formed so much of his emotional roots. His grief and hurt were enormous, but because of his lifelong bravado and denial of weakness or feeling he was unable to acknowledge these to himself, even less be comforted by others. In an effort to escape his feelings of impotence and loss, he worked at the expense of even more time and energy. Eventually this defence also became inadequate and led to his panic attacks. Although his taboo on verbal communication of distress made this initially impossible, the message in his panic attacks was quite clear. His pent-up feelings of loss, despair, fear and powerlessness were all evident in his cries, his choking and trembling. Here was powerful somatic communication, while his tongue had not yet permission to speak. Psychotherapy with this man has been brief and gratifying. Encouraging him to acknowledge, re-own and share his vulnerabilities and feelings has abolished his unwitting strategy of illness, and brought about much emotional growth in his family and marital life.

Medically it is noteworthy that he has reverted to being normotensive, and is now maintaining this without his hypotensive drugs. Such exploration and therapy of his somatic communications has hopefully freed him of the need to be ill in order to express and work through his distress. The absence of such intervention could have resulted in a much more real and physically damaging cardiovascular catastrophe.

## Conclusion

We are all an amalgam of what we consider to be creditable and discreditable qualities – what we wish to be, and what we fear we may be. Generally we are conditioned to thinking that 'good' qualities are those such as strength, autonomy, generosity and courage. However, there is a child-system of percepts and feelings in everyone which confronts us with our intense and primitive feelings of rage, destructiveness, infantile passivity and the wish to be taken care of. This infant part of ourselves remains active, but discouraged from expression by societal taboos. Some families, also, have more particular taboos with other feelings, such as fear and sadness. Because all these feelings are powerful but not allowed direct expression, they must be split off and expressed, covertly, leaving the rest of the apparent personality intact. Illnesses of many kinds offer such a system of strategy and communication; this not only applies to psychiatric and hysterical syndromes, but also to very tangible organic reactions such as duodenal ulceration and asthma. Although alternative skills are required to understand the language of illness, the results are often gratifying, and at times may even be lifesaving.

$$\Omega$$

**Reference**
Zigmond, D. *Update,* 1977, 15, 159.

**Bibliographical Note**
Nothing said about the relationship aspects of medicine would be complete without reference to the contribution of Michael Balint. His book *The Doctor, his Patient and the Illness* (Pitman Medical 1968) is now an established classic. I have also found the concepts of Transactional Analysis invaluable in formulating the developmental and transactional basis of illness as a form of communication. The following books provide an excellent introduction to this system of psychology:
Berne E, *Games People Play,* Penguin, Harmondsworth, Middx, 1967
Berne E. *What do You Say After You Say Hello?,* Corgi Books, London, 1975
Harris, T. *I'm OK – You're OK,* Pan, London, 1973
Steiner, C. *Scripts People Live,* Grove Press, London, 1974

Published in *Update* 1978

# Adjustment or Change?

## Radical Issues in Psychiatry

## Author's post-scripted foreword (March 2014)

'Adjustment or change?' was written in 1977 and is republished here, nearly four decades later, in its original form.

It is writing very much of its period: political debate was more sanguine and polarised, old fashioned socialism looked set for longevity (and the USSR for eternity). Vietnam was a fresh, sharp memory. Feminism was young, raw and accelerating. There was more righteous anger, optimism and political diversity.

Although this period-piece may now, in places, sound callow and strident, it still has important messages. Although theorists, politicians and planners are often now very mindful of the importance of social and environmental factors in the generation of illness, this is often not evident on the hospital ward-round, or in the doctor's consulting room. The contemporary practitioner is likely to confine his view to looking into two 'boxes': the patient (the locus of biomechanical breakdown) and the computer (for the abstracted data). Doctors now are likely to be less personally acquainted with a particular patient, their story, their social milieu and their physical environment. Doctor-patient interactions are now likely to be even more myopically confined to the biomechanical, and devoid of the kind of personal influences that create a broader view of growth and healing.

This article, for all its gauche rhetoric, is probably more relevant now than in 1977. Equally arresting are these considerations: where in the NHS could Mrs E (Patient 2) get such undesignated therapy?, and: what mainstream medical journal would now risk publishing such feral dissent from the frontline?

I can well remember my surprise and confusion when, as a medical student, I discovered the irrelevance of medical technology in the epidemiological patterns of tuberculosis. Until that time I had assumed that technical advances in diagnosis and management had been central to its decline. Like many aspiring professionals, I had imagined and wished my power to be far greater than it was.

## The medical model and social perspectives

To find that the overwhelming bulk of tuberculosis was more dependent on our arrangements for living together than on mass radiography, Mantoux testing or streptomycin, brought me acute awareness of how distorting the hospital and individual centred models of medicine can be. I learned far more about diagnosis and management of individual pathology than about the social framework that led to overcrowding, cold, damp and malnutrition. Poverty was parcelled, with an apology of scientific correctness, into 'social classes V and VI'. True, I was training to be a doctor, not a political radical, but I wonder how many doctors continue to be similarly oblivious, or indifferent, to the fundamental social forces operative in patterns of 'illness'.

## Illness as a scapegoat

The concept of illness may very often be seen as a way of 'scapegoating' a part of a problem so that the presenting patient is labelled, treated and despatched, leaving the forces acting on him unexamined or unchallenged. Tuberculosis sanatoria may have contained some individual cases of consumption, but were no substitute for proper working or living conditions. In this respect, treating the designated patient alone, while ignoring the pathogenic influences acting on him, can be seen as a kind of sop, or parrying manoeuvre. It is similar to the unhappy or ill family, whose discord is clearly related to alienating and depressing housing, who are told: "The council can't find you a decent home, but they'll send a social worker to see you instead". The social worker's implicit brief here is to act as a decoy and tranquillizer, so that the immediate symptoms of disturbance can be averted, if not suppressed. Perhaps she will have the skill to transmute a housing problem into 'casework' or 'family therapy'; the important point is, however, that she cannot provide a new house, only social work skills.

In formulating and dealing with symptomatology within the conceptual framework of individual pathology, it is easy to make the assumption that the only fault lies within the patient, not in the world in which he lives. Studies in social medicine and statistics may provide a theoretical antidote to such projection, but the actual practice of medicine and other caring agencies continues to enact this conservative principle. So long as we describe certain people as being 'ill', rather than oppressed or injured, the rest of us can feel blameless and unquestioning of the status quo.

## Illness and psychiatry

Nowhere is this concept more relevant but concealed than in psychiatry. At the present time this is exhibited most floridly and distastefully in the USSR, but the West has its insidious counterpart, which is probably equally extensive. Such a view has been elaborated from different aspects by Reich, Szasz, Laing and Illich. For the general practitioner, the extrapolation of variety and quantity of psychotropic drug consumption, while 'psychiatric morbidity' continues to rise is perhaps a more vivid and understandable illustration of these principles. In my earliest experiences of general practice I felt like the bewildered King Canute, trying to turn back waves of symptomatized discontent, armed only with my knowledge of psychiatric labels, and my power to prescribe tricyclics and benzodiazepines.

## Doctors and patients

Likewise, when I first became a hospital psychiatrist I felt like a casualty officer in Northern Ireland; I had no idea what all the fighting was about but nevertheless I patched people up, hoped that was sufficient, and sent them on their way.

The following case probably has an all too familiar ring to most psychiatrists and general practitioners, and serves to illustrate some radical questions in contemporary psychiatry.

## Patient 1

*Mrs B is 30 years of age. She has three children under the age of five years and lives on the 13th floor of a council high-rise block with her husband, who works in a semi-skilled capacity at a car factory. Although the block of flats is only 10 years old, it has the usual stigmata of anonymous public contempt, desecration and fatigued indifference; peeling paintwork, ubiquitous grime, litter and dogs' faeces on the worn floor covering. Aerosoled on the concrete wall outside is an impotent, misspelt, rebellious slogan overtly advertising the National Front, but in reality attempting to purge an uncomfortable burden of blind anger. Mrs B's flat is crowded and has only a small balcony looking out onto a grim, grey, industrial landscape. She spends her day controlling or nurturing her children and either seeing her husband off to work or awaiting his return. The architecture of the flats makes no provision for children to play or mothers to meet, so she sees few other adults during the day. Even shopping is a major expedition because of the demands of her children. Consequently she rarely goes out, and her husband shops at weekends. She welcomes the regular visits by her health visitor if only because it gives her some adult conversation and the opportunity to be looked after for a while when, at almost every other point in her waking life (and sometimes in her dreams as well), she is looking after others.*

***The health visitor****. The health visitor was first allocated to her after the birth of her second child, when she was hospitalized with a 'puerperal depressive illness' and, almost as a matter of routine, was* *then considered as being 'at risk' with the mothering of her child. In spite of the pleasant and friendly manner of the health visitor, Mrs B feels ambivalent about her. Although she feels she ought to be grateful for the trouble she takes, she perceives dimly that she is being patronised, and that somehow this is irrelevant to her underlying problems, which continue unformulated and unresolved.*

*Marriage. When Mrs B married at the age of 23 she was impelled largely by romantic fantasies of uncompromised closeness and sharing. Her own parents' relationship had been ground down to a state of indifferent semi-tolerance by their banal and repetitive life, but she did not yet anticipate this for herself. She envisaged her own marriage as plucking her out of this situation, so that her life could become the kind of existence featured in popular women's journals – a state of serene and gratified selflessness earned by courting her family with the whiteness of her wash and lightness of her pastry. The reality has been predictably and bitterly disappointing. Early in their marriage Mr and Mrs B were aware of a sense of emptiness and malaise that they could not articulate, communicate or understand. Mrs B felt emotionally unnourished and discounted, while Mr B felt trapped and nagged at. She needed Valium for her 'anxiety state', and he needed alcohol for his night out with 'the boys'. The birth of their children has driven them even further apart emotionally but, paradoxically, the bonds of guilt between them have grown, so that they both feel doomed to endure their marriage as it is, come what may.*

*Mr B. Mr B is not an unkind man but is unable to understand what is wrong in his life. Due to his wife's unaccountable (to him) unhappiness, he escapes the endless circular rows at home by saying he has to work late, and finding solace in pubs, male friends and the occasional furtive sexual encounter. Perversely, however, these make things worse rather than better. They both feel increasingly resentful, guilty, inadequate and paranoid, so that their contact together always culminates in a stalemate of alienated conflict. Mr B "just cannot understand it". After all, he works extremely hard and feels he shares the money he earns as fairly as he can. He finds his work as a body-*

*welder monotoncus, exhausting and unrewarding. The works milieu is enormous, noisy and anonymous. He repeats the same task about 60 times daily and, in spite of the increased bargaining power of his union, he continues to feel disposable, unimportant and depersonalized. He has never seen the people who make important policy decisions ct his place of work, and his ultimate employers reside in distant boardrooms reified for him only by mediators, memoranda and rumour.*

*He is an intelligent man but the deprived background in which he grew up furnished him with neither the norms nor the educational facilities, ever to aspire to further education or professional training. Like so many others in his situation he feels alienated, frustrated and cheated, but is unable to understand the basis of this sensation. His private and stored resentments are sometimes discharged publicly in bargaining disputes, but even when these are resolved with apparent success his underlying sense of oppression remains. He continues to feel trapped and used, but his bills have to be paid and so he works for the money. To counter the industrial wilderness he endures every day, he hopes this year to buy a colour television and spend a couple of weeks in Majorca. Not surprisingly, when he returns home to find a harassed, unhappy and demanding wife, he fails to understand his part in all this. "What more can I do? I work hard and then I get this every evening ...", he ruminates with glum rhetoric.*

**Admission to the local psychiatric unit.** Their sense of mystified powerlessness is further endorsed by the local psychiatric unit, where Mrs B has been admitted on three occasions in the last five years: twice with a diagnosis of 'puerperal depressive illness', and once with an 'agitated depressive illness'. Both Mr and Mrs B now believe that she has a 'disease of her nerves', which is what her psychiatrist conveyed to them. In any case they both see her unhappy and 'awkward' behaviour at home as being due to her 'depression'. They conceive, vaguely, that Mrs B has a 'fault' inside her and that this, rather than her marital arrangements or the environment in which she must survive, is the root of her difficulties.

**Medical assessment**. Their general practitioner has also been sucked into this collusion. Like most of us, his training taught him to look at people's problems from a basis of 'illness', from which they could escape only by reliance on medical personnel and their techniques. His view is confirmed by the vast bulk of literature and secondary medical consultations. Consider this letter written to him about Mrs B by the consultant psychiatrist.

"... As you know, Mrs B was admitted here at your request following her increasing depression and agitation, which she had consulted you about in recent weeks. The pattern of this episode was similar to her previous bouts of depression, and was accompanied by early morning wakening and a loss of interest in almost everything, including her appetite. On admission here we found her to be markedly agitated and tearful, with a lot of self-demeaning ideas typical of depression ...

"She is a cooperative patient and she made an uneventful recovery on Imipramine 75 mg t.d.s., and a short course of ECT, as she has done previously ...

"There is, of course, the question of her children and, in view of her relapsing condition, you will remember that you kindly arranged for a health visitor to visit regularly, and we will try to arrange for one of our nurses to visit. Mr and Mrs B both understand the necessity for this. Mr B seems very supportive, though I understand he works very long hours...

"If she has another relapse it may be worthwhile trying her on Lithium, though I note she had kidney disease as a child. In the meantime she should continue her present dose of Imipramine, and I will see her as an outpatient in three weeks ... "

From the phenomenological viewpoint this is a competent medical assessment (except that there is evidence that she recovered from hospitalisation, not medication), but such a style of assessment and care is loaded with politically important assumptions. It conveys authoritatively to Mrs B, and all who are involved with her, that she is the victim of something wrong inside her, that only doctors can understand and alleviate. It conspires with the whole fabric and style of her life in duping her into the belief that she is powerless, and that her world is something she must adjust to, not question or change. There are probably hundreds of thousands of women like Mrs B in the UK today. Theoretically, each one may be viewed as suffering from an affective disorder. From an anthropological view, however, the overall pattern appears more as a concealed form of impotent rebellion and social control, with doctors performing a task similar to, but more technical than, that of policemen.

## A radical political view of psychiatry

Awareness of the kind of matrix I have described has led recently to many fundamental and articulate challenges to the present status and ethos of psychiatry. In the USA particularly Radical Psychiatry has a large following. Even those who dismiss their political tenets can still derive perspicacity from the Radical Psychiatrists' clear-headed analysis of the present confused impasse of psychiatry. It is worth noting, however, that not all radical critics of psychiatry are politically left wing. Thomas Szasz is an example.

Claude Steiner, a Radical Psychiatrist in California, started formulating his standpoint at the time of the Vietnam war. This was a time when overt psychiatric morbidity, together with drug abuse among the young, rose to a very high level. The potential abuses and paradoxes of psychiatry became clearly highlighted at this time. Steiner captured this dilemma with a vividness and resolve that arose painfully out of his involvement. He writes:

"Consider a seventeen-year-old American youngster during the Vietnam war. He is told that he must offer his life to destroy the enemy in Asia. He is told that this is good for him, for his brothers and sisters, for his country, and even for the enemy. He is taught that a man will defend his country without question, and that a man who hesitates or questions this principle is a coward who does not deserve to be called a human being. If he fails to understand that he is being oppressed and if he believes these lies, he will eventually come to think of himself as less than human for not wanting to defend his country. He will doubt his own opinions and experiences concerning the war. He will come to consider himself a coward; he will become disgusted with himself; he will cut himself off from his peers and will become depressed. He may lose interest in everyday activities; he may begin to speak about hopelessness and meaninglessness; he may start using drugs to give himself a temporary reprieve from his despair. If his shame and despair reach large enough proportions, he may attempt to destroy himself. He will see himself as no good and will believe himself in need of psychiatric attention.

"If he were to consult a 'neutral' therapist, he might be asked, 'What is wrong with you? Why are you depressed? Why do you hate your father? Why do you rebel against authority? Let's talk about it, and you'll feel better. Tell me about your childhood. Maybe the bad things that happened then make you sad now. Other boys your age aren't depressed about the war and killing. These are troubled times, but others are able to adjust to them. Why don't you? Tell me your dreams. Maybe we can find what is wrong with you. The army is bad, I know, but it has its good points. It might make a man out of you'.

"This young man may eventually feel better because of the friendly and warm attitude of the therapist, thus mystifying his true feelings about the war. He may 'pull himself together', his personality-trait disturbance (passive-aggressive, aggressive type) may improve, and he may wind up in a flag-wrapped box. His therapist will feel and will contend that he was neutral throughout the therapeutic intervention and that he did not attempt to influence the young man. But in truth he acted as a recruiting officer for the army, all the more effective for his disarming smile."

Driven by such experiences, the Radical Psychiatrists drew up their Manifesto, which was presented in 1969 at the Annual Conference of the American Psychiatric Association. Again I quote at length, as I cannot effectively paraphrase:

1. The practice of psychiatry has been usurped by the medical establishment. Political control of its public aspects has been seized by medicine, and the language of soul healing ... has been infiltrated with irrelevant medical concepts and terms.

   "Psychiatry must return to its non-medical origins since most psychiatric conditions are in no way the province of medicine. All persons competent in soul healing should be known as psychiatrists. Psychiatrists should repudiate the use of medically derived words such as 'patient', 'illness', 'diagnosis', 'treatment'. Medical psychiatrists' unique con-tribution to psychiatry is as experts on neurology and, with much needed additional work, on drugs."

2. Extended individual psychotherapy is an elitist, outmoded, as well as non-productive, form of psychiatric help. It concentrates the talents of a few on a few. It silently colludes with the notion that people's difficulties have their sources within them while implying that everything is well with the

world. It promotes oppression by shrouding its consequences with shame and secrecy. It further mystifies by attempting to pass as an ideal human relationship when it is, in fact, artificial in the extreme.

> "People's troubles have their source not within them, but in their alienated relationships, in their exploitation, in polluted environments, in war, and in the profit motive. Psychiatrists should encourage bilateral, open discussion and discourage secrecy and shame in relation to deviant behaviour and thoughts."

3. By remaining 'neutral' in an oppressive situation, psychiatry, especially in the public sector, has become an enforcer of establishment values and laws. Adjustment to prevailing conditions is the avowed goal of most psychiatric treatment. Persons who deviate from the world's madness are given fraudulent diagnostic tests which generate diagnostic labels which lead to 'treatment' which is, in fact, a series of graded repressive procedures such as 'drug management', hospitalization, shock therapy, perhaps lobotomy. All these forms of 'treatment' are perversions of legitimate medical methods that have been put at the service of the establishment by the medical profession. Treatment is forced on persons who would, if let alone, not seek it.

> "Psychological tests and the diagnostic labels they generate, especially schizophrenia, must be disavowed as meaningless mystifications, the real function of which is to distance psychiatrists from people and to insult people into conformity. Medicine must cease making available drugs, hospitals and other legitimate medical procedures for the purpose of overt or subtle law enforcement and must examine how drug companies are dictating treatment procedures through their advertising. Psychiatry must cease playing a part in the oppression of women by refusing to

promote adjustment to their oppression. All psychiatric help should be by contract; that is, people should choose when, what, and with whom they want to change. Psychiatrists should become advocates of the people, should refuse to participate in the pacification of the oppressed, and should encourage people's struggles for liberation ..."

## An example of radical psychiatric therapy

### Patient 2

*Mrs E was initially referred to a gynaecologist because of her secondary amenorrhea. He did not feel that her amenorrhea was of great significance, but he became alarmed by her behavioural symptomatology. An urgent psychiatric assessment revealed to me the distressed and bizarre pattern of her present life. Apart from her amenorrhea, she had a marked appetite disturbance, so that she would either starve or gorge herself for periods of weeks, leading to a marked fluctuation in her weight. When gorging herself she would eat packs of butter and sometimes even scraps of food from the dustbin. Her comment about herself during these times was, "I'm fat and gross and disgusting, but I feel so empty; I've got to get something inside me". Her sexual needs were similarly cyclical. When overeating she would be sexually compulsive, insatiable and demanding. When starving herself, her disinclination for sex was so great that she would spend the night in a sleeping bag within her marital bed. In the background was her misery and depression and the 'escape hatch' of recurrently contemplated suicide should things get too bad. Mrs E was not 'acutely ill' insofar as she had received miscellaneous kinds of psychiatric help since a severe marital disruption six years before. Her husband had left her for a few months, leaving behind a trail of lies, veiled threats and innuendoes. She said of that time, "I think I died then. She (the other woman) represented everything I could never be. But it was the lies that hurt me most. Somehow I still think he hates me, although I don't know... ".*

It was the custom in the department in which I was working for a committee of psychotherapists to discuss suitability and allocation of all referred cases requiring psychotherapy. They were fascinated but dismayed by what I brought them. Their prevailing view was that her symptomatology represented a severe disturbance, with regression back to an early oral stage of development, with its accompanying psychotic component. Nothing short of extensive individual psychoanalytic psychotherapy, they held, would have any chance of helping her. This would only be possible within the context of private psychoanalysis (which she could afford) or one of the few NHS inpatient psychotherapy units.

**Marital problems and family background.** By the time the committee's assessment was made, I had a joint interview with Mr and Mrs E. From what I heard and observed, I felt that her overt pathology was quite as much a function of the dynamics of the marriage as Mrs E's intrapsychic difficulties per se. Mrs E had compromised herself for Mr E ever since the beginning of their relationship and, furthermore, her marriage closely resembled her parents'. Early on she supported her husband while he went to art college and, although he had become successful in his work, this pattern had largely continued, so that the bulk of the chores had been carried by Mrs E. She had been oppressed into believing that she was the lesser of the two partners and therefore must subjugate her needs to those of her husband and his work. Her own family had expected her to heed and tend to other people's needs before her own, and she had continued to relate to people in this way. Like many women, she received extremely little gratification for herself directly but was expected to compensate for this by such vicarious gratification as she could eke out of her nurturing role with Mr E and their small son. Ironically, she had come to see both of them in the same light: domineering, demanding and more important and powerful than herself. The resentment and anger that she felt thus came from a thwarted and one-down position. To compound her problems she felt mystified about her feelings, and thus assumed that her 'illness' was due to some fault in her alone.

**Therapy.** Mr and Mrs E declined the individual psychoanalytic approach that had been suggested and by this time viewed her symptomatology as being a product of their marriage, and had come to a point of wanting to do something about this. I agreed to work with them with the following explicitly agreed formulations and strategies:

That Mrs E's 'illness' had arisen because of her muted resentment, and represented her need to have her feelings understood, expressed and cared for. It also signalled her need to have as much space and autonomy as other members of her family.

Much of her sense of passivity arose from the inequality of power in their relationship. Mrs E was either not doing what she wanted, or doing what she did not want, far more often than Mr E.

Her bewilderment had many roots in her husband's mystifying and deceptive behaviour. (Due to his own family background, he had developed a great fear of closeness and a need to 'hide' what was going on in himself.)

Mrs E's part in overcoming these problems was to:
- clarify for herself what she did and did not want
- learn to ask directly for what she wanted
- make it clear to Mr E when she was doing anything that she did not want to do
- spend a certain amount of time each day doing something that was not at all accountable to others in the family, but was personally gratifying to her.

Mr E's part was to:
- really listen to his wife (which involved looking at her)
- accept her having her feelings, without trying to parry or rationalise them away
- nurture her more, and share much of the domestic work
- demystify himself by honestly owning and communicating his thoughts and feelings when she asked him to do so.

*My part in this programme was to remain as impartial as possible, to clarify and interpret, to mediate, to make practical suggestions and to protect them at times of emotional stress. I also undertook to provide alternative medical care if this failed.*

## Outcome and discussion.

*Six months after we had embarked on this contractual therapy, Mrs E was symptomatically clear of her presenting complaints. She spoke with an assurance and warmth that was not evident before. There had been times in therapy where the marriage had looked extremely tenuous, but overall its foundations and communications had become firmer, surer and more equally acknowledged and shared. Most gratifyingly they seemed able to resolve their problems without me.*

Such a method of therapy lies outside the medical model and its conventional psychiatric derivatives. Paradoxically, conventional psychiatric therapy ran the risk of driving Mrs E further into the system of thoughts and feelings that was central to her distress. Even classical psychoanalytic psychotherapy would have attempted to label and treat her individually without much emphasis on the real forces that were acting on her in the 'here' and 'now'. The psychoanalytic model would probably formulate her problem as "a narcissistic woman of passive-aggressive type, with weak ego-defences who has regressed or become fixated to an early oral infantile stage, with the mobilization of much archaic and hysterical material. Such material might lead to a psychotic transference reaction in psychotherapy, which should thus be avoided". To Mrs E this would have been as mystifying and alienating as a prescription for Imipramine. More importantly, it would have confirmed for her yet again that there was something wrong with her (although she would never quite understand what 'it' was), that she was powerless, and must continue to be confused in the world in which she found herself.

Ω

## Acknowledgement

Grateful acknowledgement is made to Grove Press and Claude Steiner for permission to reproduce material from *Readings in Radical Psychiatry*.

## Reference

Steiner, C. (ed.), *Readings in Radical Psychiatry*, Grove Press, New York, 1975.

## Further reading

Illich, I., *The Medical Nemesis, Calder* and Boyars, London, 1974.
Steiner, C. *Scripts People Live*, Grove Press, New York, 1974.
Szasz, T. *The Myth of Mental Illness*, Paladin, London, 1972.
Szasz, T, *Ideology and Insanity*, Calder and Boyars, London, 1973.
Szasz, T. *The Manufacture of Madness*, Routledge and Kagan Paul, London, 1971.
Wycoff, H. Love, *Therapy and Politics*, Grove Press. New York, 1976.

Published in *Update* 1978, 105

# The Elements of Psychotherapy

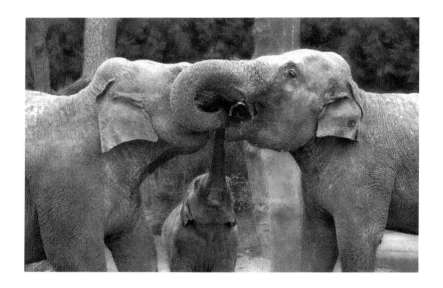

*'... Much will be gained if we succeed in transforming your hysterical misery into common unhappiness. With a mental life that has been restored to health, you will be better armed against that unhappiness.'*

(Freud, 1895, *Studies on Hysteria*).

Psychotherapy is a subtle activity, often opaque to outsiders. One definition might be: it is the deliberate and structured use of a professional relationship, enabling an individual to explore, discover and express aspects of themselves that otherwise would remain hidden and troublesome. Certain things follow: this expanded awareness and expressivity can then bring about a fuller, freer, better adapted self and its relationship with others. Put another way, psychotherapy is getting help to understand and express oneself more clearly and fully, so that we are empowered to grow beyond self-limiting or self-defeating patterns. Liberation from such internal traps and tangles, enables us to make choices that are more realistically gratifying and creatively responsive.

These definitions, although probably acceptable to most psychotherapists, are likely to arouse either confusion or scepticism in many medical practitioners. Pragmatically, what can it achieve, and how? When is it most likely to work, and in which form? What is its relevance to medical practice? This article offers some introductory answers to these questions.

## Psychopathology

Before the elements of psychotherapy can be understood, it is necessary to survey some of the principles of 'psychopathology': the theory of what goes wrong for individuals, and why.

The basics of these are:
- As infants and small children we are all highly vulnerable, in much need of attention and protection. We probably have a rich, sometimes violent fantasy life, and are unable for some

years to subject this to reality-testing (Bowlby, 1971, 1975, 1981; Klein, quoted in Segal, 1964; Piaget, 1952).

• It follows that the infant and young child are crucially dependent on caring figures for stability, safety, reality-testing and love. Consequently, if these are not forthcoming, the person will grow up with an impairment of his image of self and others. These determine our ability to relate trustingly, realistically and positively; to develop our own creativity and to healthily integrate our most primitive impulses or feelings (Bowlby, 1971, 1975, 1981; Balint, 1968; Winnicott, 1965). The latter requires an inwardly directed capacity for reality-testing (Rosen, 1962; Schiff, 1975).

• Some feelings and impulses are very threatening to the conscious self and its sense of integrity. This may lead to 'ego-defence mechanisms', which are involuntary attempts to ward off destabilising internal conflict or distress (Freud, 1936). When excessive, these defence mechanisms may themselves cause problems: 'presenting symptoms', ranging from recurrent relationship difficulties to mental and physical illness (Freud, 1963).

• In suitable and motivated individuals, such dysfunctional patterns may be ameliorated or resolved by professional help. This happens by:

• Perceiving and understanding the origin and current consequences of such patterns. This is a large part of historical *insight*.

• Experiencing, within the therapeutic relationship, an encouragement, consistency or caring which was lacking in early original experiences. This can enable *healing*.

• Acknowledging, experiencing and expressing feelings and impulses that have become fearsome and forbidden for the individual. This unlocking can free the individual for *growth*.

• Recognizing the distinction between archaic yearnings, frustrations and impulses, and present reality. This kind of operational insight will help an individual navigate the lifelong psychological tasks of *immunity, growth* and *repair* (Perls *et al.,* 1973; Berne, 1961).

## The tool of talking

It is sometimes claimed, particularly by those whose outlook is mechanistic, that 'talking can't do any good', or 'you can't change a person's make-up'. In a sense these claims are true, in that words cannot have the same predictable impact on another person, as can a surgical procedure or a drug when the doctor necessarily assumes control over the patient's internal processes. Physical medical treatment is unilateral and hence more controllable than the bilateral process of psychotherapy, where the *dialogue* is at the very centre of its effect. The patient is here far from being a passive recipient; he is an active synthesizer, and ultimately the effectiveness of what is given depends on what he does with it.

Given these limitations, verbal communication can still be immensely valuable when used skilfully and appositely. Its benefits are various and multiple. It can be an antidote to isolation, a way of externalizing internal confusion and thus gaining clarity or a different perspective, a method of de-pressurizing built-up feeling systems and – perhaps most important – a way of forming a *common language* with another person. This latter is an important step to creating a compassionate understanding and acceptance, both of the self and others. Such a common language can only develop, however, when there is a *therapeutic rapport*: this itself implies the conscious wish to develop capacities for trust, discovery and sharing. Some aspects involved in this process are depicted in figure 1 (Luft, 1966).

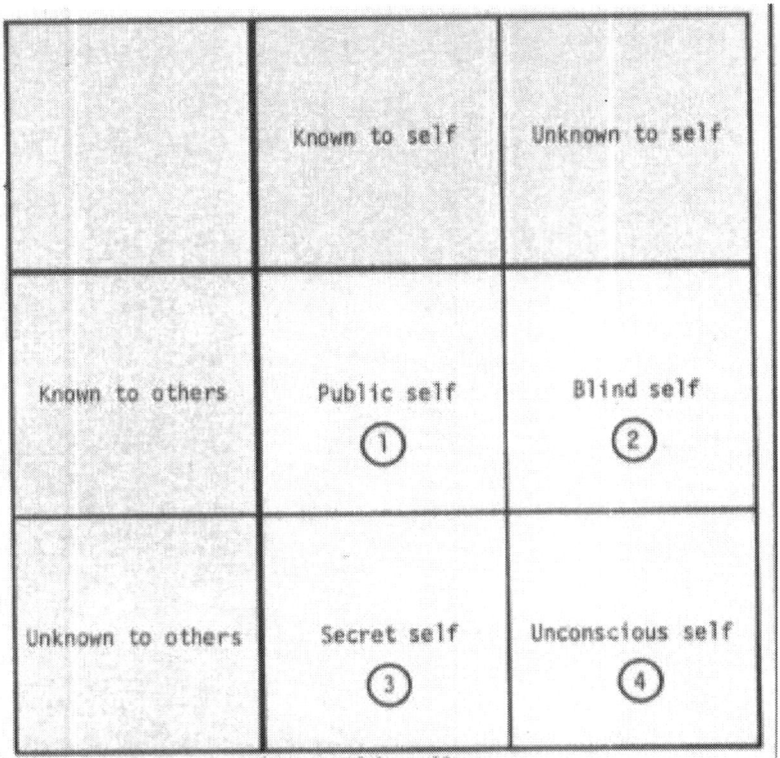

| | Known to self | Unknown to self |
|---|---|---|
| Known to others | Public self ① | Blind self ② |
| Unknown to others | Secret self ③ | Unconscious self ④ |

FIG. 1.—*Operational parts of the self*

It can be seen that different styles or levels of psychotherapy can act to bring about different kinds of integration of parts of the self:

A depressed and isolated man, unhappy with his loneliness, is unaware of the way he is critical of those who approach him. Other members of a therapy group confront him with this, and he begins to see his contribution to his problem.
*Integration of (1)* ⟷*(2)*.

A woman who is ambivalent about her sexual relationships begins tentatively to talk to her therapist about the misty but intense sexual longings she used to have for her father, about which she still feels guilty and afraid. *Integration of (3)* ⟷*(1)*.

A middle-aged man, prone to depressive episodes when he feels rejected, tells of a dream, which the therapist thinks indicates his lifelong searching for his father who died when the patient was a boy; the patient denied missing or thinking about him much prior to the dream. *Integration of (4)* ←→ *(3)* ←→ *(1)*.

Why do we need to integrate these different parts? In general it can be said that:

It is not possible to have mastery of those parts of ourselves of which we are unaware.

Relegating distressing and unresolved parts of ourselves to secrecy is likely to seriously limit our capacity for intimate and authentic attachments, and may 'leak out' to produce symptoms.

It is only possible to be competent and responsive social beings if we have a fairly clear idea of how other people see us.

Of course, the mere awareness, or expression, of these unintegrated parts of the self does not of itself bring about the required change or integration, but they are essential prerequisites. In much the same way, a map may help us plan a journey, but it cannot bring about the travelling for us. The actual 'travelling' in psychotherapy is a complex matter, involving many different components of resource and motivation, in both patient and therapist.

Almost all psychotherapeutic interventions are some type of *support, confrontation* or *interpretation*. Each of these may be a powerful facilitator when used correctly, but may be damaging when untimely or poorly attuned.

**Figure 2** – *The therapeutic triad*

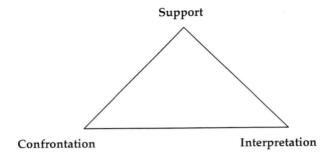

Support

Confrontation                                    Interpretation

## Support

Support interventions are those that accept the patient as he is, without the pressure for greater awareness or change. It creates what Winnicott (1965) termed 'the facilitating environment'; a *safe base* from which the patient may begin the more difficult task of exploring and expressing material which has not previously been verbalized or shared. It is a paradox of the human condition that often we cannot change the way we operate until we have really accepted ourselves as we are. As a consequence, the therapist must at first accept the patient as he is and support him in his present *modus vivendi*, before other endeavours are undertaken. For this reason many therapists would agree that skilful support is the most basic element in this triad; often, an individual will find his own resources and understanding merely with such help. This is particularly true of those reacting immediately to loss and other crises, and thus is particularly pertinent to the work of the general practitioner. The style of therapy derived from Carl Rogers (1961) and counselling holds that 'unconditional positive regard' is the most important facilitator in therapy. However, for more severe difficulties such as prolonged grief reactions, or longstanding personality disturbance, a therapy with other components of the triad is called for.

## Interpretation

Interpretation helps a patient to make new sense of communicated experience by deliberately introducing associations with previously unlinked experiences and images. In general, it is true to say that there are no 'right' or 'wrong' interpretations, only those that a patient can use within the therapeutic rapport. Thus, an interpretation that may be 'correct' to the therapist but cannot be assimilated by the patient is edifying only to the former and, if asserted dogmatically, will damage the development of rapport. In this sense interpretations should not be 'made' or 'given', but 'offered' tentatively and experimentally. When interpretations are successful they lead to a *deepening of rapport* (Malan, 1979), where the patient feels an increase both in his own understanding and the sense of his being understood, so that he feels safe to explore and share more (Menninger, 1958). Often the most gratifying and facilitating examples of interpretation are also the simplest.

The following two examples illustrate some of these principles:

## Example 1

*A young woman had been admitted to hospital four times in five years with episodes of mania. Her treatment had consisted mainly of custody and suppression of her symptoms with drugs, evidently with limited and transient effect. On her last admission she exhibited her usual pattern of grandiose thinking and hyperactivity, but the doctor was aware of her eyes glistening. After spending a while with her, he said gently: 'underneath all this activity and bravado, I get the sense that really you're feeling very sad and helpless'. She collapsed and sobbed for several minutes, confirming the doctor's intuition of concealed feelings underlying her 'manic defence'. Later, albeit with pain and difficulty, she developed a sufficient therapeutic alliance with the doctor to explore some of the unarticulated emotional problems generating her episodic illness.*

### Example 2

*A woman in her early forties was convicted of a shoplifting offence and referred for psychotherapy. Six months before her offence she had had a hysterectomy. She was late for her initial interview and the male therapist found her to be 'sexually provocative'; he then made an interpretation to the effect that she had wanted to redress her sexual loss by stealing, first from the shop, and now from him (his time and his penis). She curtly denied understanding of either the remark or its relevance, and did not attend further appointments.*

This complex interpretation may have been psychoanalytically 'correct', but was untimely and unwieldy: it could not be incorporated into the fragile rapport between patient and therapist, which had only just begun. This woman did not feel sufficiently understood and accepted as she was to be able to use such a comment, which was experienced by her as an attack or derogation.

### Confrontation

Confrontation is a term used to describe the therapist's action when he directly draws attention to an aspect of a patient's behaviour, without offering an explanation. Its aim is to enhance *awareness* of behaviour; the way in which he operates and how this may affect others. Generally, attention is focused on what is currently happening. Therefore group and family therapy often utilise this type of intervention because of the richness of interplay between its members, who will act as both confronter and confronted. The therapist's role is then to keep the confrontation within a scope of intensity and relevance that will be tolerable and therapeutic. If a patient is to consider seriously and assimilate the subject of confrontation, he must first feel an adequate sense of care and safety in the therapeutic setting, otherwise he will merely feel attacked. This will lead to an escalation of his defences, rather than the reverse.

**Example 3**

*A middle-aged man complained bitterly and with hurt about his estrangement from his son, who he described as secretive and surly. The therapist noticed his own sense of irritation and exasperation with the patient, who continually, but without apparent awareness, talked across the therapist, and made inaccurate assumptions about him. The therapist gently but firmly pointed this out, adding that this pattern was possibly also true with the son, leading to the painful impasse he had described. Because the man had a trusting rapport with the therapist, he was able to acknowledge and explore this pattern.*

Confrontation is a prominent component of the newer, humanistic therapies such as Encounter, Gestalt and Transactional Analysis. These can be potent catalysts to awareness of present functioning. However, this potency has the capacity to harm, by engendering too much material too quickly for the patient to handle. This caveat leads to the 'Rule of the Therapeutic Triad', which may be stated as: 'For rapport in psychotherapy to be maintained and beneficial, interpretation or confrontation should not exceed the support that is offered to the patient'.

**Transference**

It has already been outlined how our internal world-image and self-image is fundamentally influenced by our early experiences. All of us, more or less consciously, act from and act-out the kind of adjustments and decisions we made in infancy and early childhood. It follows that we transfer onto others our expectations and fears deriving from that period. If these early experiences were generally good and satisfactorily resolved, this will lead to healthy growth and adjustment. For those who were not so fortunate, the result will be recurrent and continuing difficulties with relationships, and expression and gratification of the self. In such cases it is important that the patient is able to understand what he is *projecting* onto others that hampers him, so that he may be able to grow beyond these ancient repetitions. This field of archaic projections is termed *transference* in psychotherapy and, in the more analytic therapies, is considered the most important diagnostic and therapeutic tool. In these 'deeper' therapies, it is thought to be necessary for the patient to:

Experience, in the present, the kind of fears, expectations and fantasies he had as a child and which he now projects onto the therapist (*Evolution* of transference).

With the help of the therapist, to understand their historical roots and present way of operating (*Analysis* of transference).

Slowly abandon these methods of functioning, by finding newer and more productive ways of relating to the therapist (*Resolution* of transference).

The analysis, or interpretation, of transference may be depicted by another triangle.

**Figure 3.** *The triangle of transference*

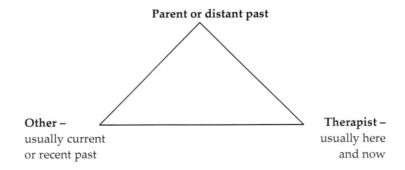

Figure 3 illustrates a scheme whereby the influence of the past may be understood in terms of both the therapy and the patient's current life-situation. For the fullest understanding, links are perceived between all three; at other times more partial insight may be gained by linking any two of the three.

### Example 3 (continued)

*After the middle-aged man understood how he was warding off the therapist, he began to see how he was also doing this with his son (O-T link). The therapist then asked him how he felt when he behaved like this, and then whether he could remember this same feeling when he was very young. The patient then became eager to talk about his fear of domination by others – even his son – and how he attempted to counter this by pre-empting and defining others. He then went on to talk of his relationship with his father and older brother, who he felt exerted a bullying alliance against him. He talked of his recurrent feelings of fear, humiliation and resentment. From this account he began to see how his experiences of the past were being re-enacted both with his son and the therapist (O-P and O-T links), and began to feel less bewildered and powerless in the face of his feelings.*

### Applicability of psychotherapy

Psychotherapy in its different forms may be helpful for a wide spectrum of disturbance or distress: from disabling life-crises, to chronically unsatisfactory patterns of adjustment or relationships. Always, though, the following are essential for any success:

• That the individual recognizes that he is not merely a victim of circumstances or faulty biological mechanism, but that he, in some way, is now an *active agent* in his pattern of distress.

• That he is willing, at least consciously, to pursue the possibility that reflecting on himself and sharing himself, in a professional setting, may lead to a newer and more worthwhile kind of integration and understanding. This is a complex issue, as there are frequently unconscious forces working against conscious motivation – the patient's 'resistance' – when, paradoxically, the distressed mode of functioning is equated with familiarity and security, and is therefore resistant to real examination or change.

- The patient must be able and willing to tolerate the frustration and pain that often accompanies 'the therapeutic process'. Self-disclosure and acknowledgement of long-buried parts of the self is often difficult and requires considerable investment and courage. It is here that the skill and personal qualities of the therapist can ameliorate the situation. It is also important that the patient understands the metaphorical nature of the relationship; for the care and attention he receives, and the feelings or impulses he has toward the therapist, are at the same time authentic but ritualized within the framework and boundaries of the setting. The patient must have the intent and capacity to 'talk-out', and not 'act-out', his difficulties.

It is the therapist's empathic and professional skills that can elicit, maintain and guide these capacities in the patient. When this happens, there is said to be a strong *therapeutic alliance* between patient and therapist, and they may create a *common language* that unifies the patient's experience of himself and the therapist's experience and understanding of him. The ability to pursue this at the beginning of therapy is usually a favourable prognostic sign, and also indicates the formation of a safe-base from which the patient may experience and work out his 'negative transference' towards the therapist – his covert and archaic fear, envy, anger or resentment – which may underlie his inability to make trusting or intimate relationships.

Many authors have drawn attention to the caution that should be applied in using psychotherapy in those suffering from severe mental illness, such as psychotic or obsessive-compulsive syndromes, or in personalities with poor social control. It is probably true, however, that these criteria apply equally to these more disabled people, as to the more common (and more easily identified-with) neurotic (Rosen, 1962); that, if a therapeutic alliance can be forged and a common language created (that requires special skill and experience), then the patient may grow away from his disturbed impasse.

## Psychotherapy and medicine

Psychotherapy and medicine work from very different assumptions: the former works from the position that the patient must develop his own resources, clarification and self-definition, while the medical model works from the opposite pole; the doctor provides the resources (treatment) and definition (diagnosis). The medical patient may present the problem, but it is soon converted into the language of the doctor who then commands the dialogue (Zigmond, 1982). Psychotherapy, in searching for a common language, cannot therefore be so rigidly defined in its process or outcome; because it has its roots in personal and evolving dialogue, it cannot be 'given' or 'prescribed', and it is probably fundamentally misleading to refer to it as a 'treatment': this word usually implies a passive patient who is cured by an active doctor.

In spite of these apparent incongruities, psychotherapeutic insight and technique has a definite place in helping the medical doctor to understand his own and the patient's behaviour and the meaning of patients' symptoms, particularly when these are not readily diagnosed and treated by conventional means (Zigmond, 1977; Balint, 1956). There are evident limits as to how much psychotherapy a doctor can competently and ethically introduce into his medical practice; he would be unwise, for example, to attempt to help a patient with recurrent relationship difficulties to work through primitive anxieties and conflicts, although exceptionally this is possible. He is, however, well-placed to recognize his patient's anxieties and help him to verbalize them, which is, in itself, often perceived by the patient as an act of great understanding and comfort. This is particularly so at times of crisis and loss, as the following example illustrates.

## Example 4

*A 70-year-old man, Mr F, consulted his doctor, complaining that he woke at night 'feeling like my body is on fire, and I get this terrible itching all over, so that I just can't stop scratching'. Routine physical examination and questioning confirmed that the cause was most unlikely to be organic, and the doctor explained this. The doctor, in simple terms, went on to explain that sometimes it is difficult to express or resolve certain kinds of feelings and thoughts. These then upset the body, causing the kind of symptoms of which Mr F complained. The doctor asked Mr F if this made any sense to him and, if so, whether he had any idea of the kind of thoughts and feelings that were troubling him. Mr F replied that his trouble had started soon after his wife had died, of cancer, three months previously, and he wondered if this had anything to do with it. The doctor maintained a warm and attentive silence, which encouraged Mr F to say, 'It's stupid, I know, to be so upset after this time; I should be over it by now', which the doctor softly countered by reassuring him that such a basic loss often leaves a very long wake of disturbed feelings – that none of us ever completely leaves behind the hurt or the sadness from such a loss. At this point Mr F cried, and then talked about his sense of emptiness, and also his hidden regrets. The doctor then asked him if he was also angry that his wife had been taken away, or had abandoned him, leaving him alone – that although it is not 'rational', all of us can feel angry when we lose someone precious. Yes, Mr F agreed, he had at first been angry with the hospital, then himself, for her death; he knew it didn't make sense, but he still felt resentful. The doctor asked if he had talked with anyone about these feelings; 'No, doctor, not like this. People have their own lives to lead. I don't like to bother them'.*

*After another few minutes Mr F could see that his feelings were inevitable and important; they could only be conjured out of mind by the development of disturbance elsewhere, i.e. his skin. He found, too, that he could begin to share his feelings; his parting remark was simple but deeply felt: 'Thank you so much for listening to me, doctor. It's good to know there's somebody who understands how I feel'.*

## Comment: integrating the elements of psychotherapy

The example of Mr F illustrates how some of the elements of psychotherapy may be brought to bear in situations other than intensive psychotherapy programmes. He represented a problem familiar to many doctors who attempt to provide some form of holistic care, and it is arguable that such basic psychotherapeutic skills should be part of their clinical repertoire.

Mr F did not need the kind of prolonged psychotherapy required to help longstanding personality or relationship difficulties, but rather psychotherapeutically enlightened practice. The doctor first of all created a situation, a 'facilitating environment', where a therapeutic alliance evolved. Mr F felt sufficiently supported and trusting to reveal his 'secret self'. The doctor had then gone on to interpret his somatic defence, which enabled Mr F to share his underlying grief and resentment. Because the doctor had shown care and understanding to the vulnerable part of Mr F, the lonely widower would now probably adopt a more tolerant and understanding attitude to his own 'unreasonable' feelings This acceptance could then free him, to heal and find a new equilibrium. It is also important that the doctor was prudent in the use of his interpretations; he refrained from attempting to explore the patient's deeper unconscious where, perhaps, there had been hostile feelings to his wife when she was alive, and for which he now felt guilty. If this were true, it would become manifest later, and to raise this issue in an untimely and premature way would do more harm than good; it would seriously undermine their nascent therapeutic alliance. In this respect one of the most important elements of psychotherapy, as in medicine, is knowing when and where to stop.

$$\Omega$$

## References

Balint, M. (1956) *The Doctor, His Patient and the Illness* Pitman, London.

Balint, M. (1968) *The Basic Fault.* Tavistock, London.

Berne. E. (1961) *Transactional Analysis in Psychotherapy* Evergreen, New York.

Bowlby, J. (1971, 1975, 1981) *Attachment and Loss, Vols. 1, 2 and 3.* Hogarth Press, London.

Freud. A. (1936) *The Ego and Mechanisms of Defence* Hogarth Press, London.

Freud. S. (1963) *The Complete Psychological Works. Vols. 15 and 16.* Hogarth Press, London.

Luft, J. (1966) *Group Processes: An Introduction to Group Dynamics* Palo Alto National Press, Palo Alto.

Malan, D. H. (1979) *Individual Psychotherapy and the Science of Psychodynamic* Butterworth, Sevenoaks.

Menninger, K. (1958) *The Theory of Psychoanalytic Technique* Basic Books, New York.

Perls, F., Hefferline, R.F. and Goodman, P. (1973) *Gestalt Therapy* Penguin, London.

Piaget, J. (1952) *The Origins of Intelligence in Children* New York International Universities Press, New York.

Rogers, C.R. (1961) *Client Centred Therapy* Houghton Mifflin, Boston.

Rosen, J. (1962) *Direct Psychoanalytic Psychiatry* Grune and Strattas, New York.

Schiff, J. (1975) *Cathexis Reader* Harper and Row, New York.

Segal. H. (1964) *An introduction to the Work of Melanie Klein* Heinemann. London.

Winnicott, D. W. (1965) *The Maturational Process and the Facilitating Environment* Hogarth Press, London.

Zigmond, D. (1982) *The Psychosomatic Approach* April: 699-709
Zigmond, D. *The Psychosomatic Mosaic* The Practitioner, April: 711-720
Zigmond, D. (1977) *Scientific Psychiatry: Progress or Regress?* Update, October: 675-679

## Further reading

Brown, D. and Pedder, J. (1979) *Introduction to Psychotherapy* Tavistock, London.
Kovel, J. (1976) *A Complete Guide to Therapy* Pantheon.
Storr, A. (1979) *The Art of Psychotherapy* Heinemann Medical. London.

Publ. in The Practitioner 1280, *Psychopathology* Vol. 225, Sept. 1981

# A Psychosomatic Approach

*'I have never yet seen a case of psychological ulcerative colitis!'*

A physician's retort to a psychiatrist at a case conference

The very term 'psychosomatic' produces difficulties. It attempts to capture patterns of physical distress or dysfunction which are not simply caused by physical determinants. The structure of the word itself indicates an outlook in which mind and body are considered *together*. However, Western theory and practice of medicine is so thoroughly rooted in Newtonian scientific thought, a system which we rarely question, that the psychosomatic approach continues to evoke mystification, confusion and denial. The foregoing quotation perhaps typifies these reactions in a doctor adopting a defensive attitude to a psychosomatic viewpoint. This series of two articles explores and clarifies some basics of the psychosomatic approach; they are not intended to be authoritative statements on the subject. They offer an outline as to how different kinds of medical practice tackle this problem, and how both patients and doctors perceive, and act upon, different parts of this problem at different times.

## The somatic approach

To understand our difficulties with the psychosomatic* viewpoint, we need first to survey briefly the roots and assumptions of our present medical practice. Medicine and medical psychiatry are based on the disciplines of the (Newtonian) physical sciences and their underlying philosophies of dualism and determinism. Dualism, explicated in the writing of Descartes, Malebranche and Geulinx (Russell, 1961), holds that the world is composed of two separate substances, matter and mind, which are independent but synchronous in activity; the two modes are governed by their own laws and run parallel courses (fig. 1).

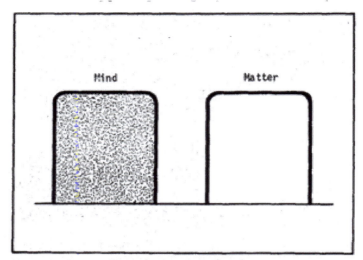

*FIG. 1.—Philosophical dualism. Mind and matter separate.*

Newtonian physics, and the consequent school of scientific determinism, takes these assumptions ever further. There is an axiom here that only outwardly observable events (matter) are valid and `real'. Mind or experience are subsumed under the dictates and laws of this observable world in such a way that the subjective world ceases to be of importance, and is regarded as an artefact or interference.

This scientific determinism is the root and prevalent philosophy in our present Western technological culture, where the bulk of our endeavours incline to engineering, that is, the direct alteration and control of physical structures. Medical practice, deriving from this outlook, is based on the assumption that distress can only be alleviated by changing behavioural or physical manifestations of that distress. Antacids for dyspepsia, tranquillizers for anxiety, and behaviour therapy for sexual dysfunction are clinical examples of this engineering philosophy. The experience of distress, it is held, will yield to control of its physical determinants; there is no need to explore or amplify the experience itself, as the experience is only a reflection of disturbed underlying mechanism.

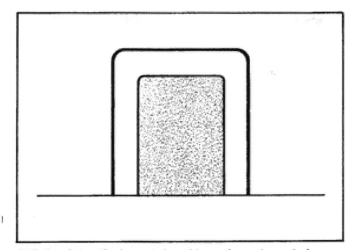

*FIG. 2.—Scientific determinism. Matter determines mind (somatic approach).*

In clinical practice this approach may be termed 'somatic', and an essential component of this system is the concept of physical causation (fig. 2). This defines events as being hierarchical in operation, so that one happening is rigidly determined by its material antecedent. Such a somatic-causational frame of reference is highly effective, even mandatory, in certain clinical situations; for example, when attending the patient with a perforated duodenal ulcer. At other times, however, it may be simplistic to the point of exclusion and distortion.

An example of this might be the unhappy asthmatic child whose disease is said to be caused by house-dust mite allergy; even if the allergy is dealt with, he may still remain wheezy. And then if the wheezing is controlled, he may well succumb to some other form of illness. Such problems are common in primary medical care, when simple physical diagnoses are evidently inadequate to explain the patient who suffers from a changing mosaic of apparently unrelated complaints, or the family which seems prone to perennial illness (Balint, 1957).

## Monism

What is lacking in the latter situation is a *holistic* approach that deals with the person, his experiences and environment in a less piecemeal, and more global, manner. Philosophically this alternative approach has been termed 'monism' and is represented in our culture by the philosophical writings of Spinoza and Bergson. Here there is no division of the world into mind and matter; there is only one substance which is experienced differently: internally as mind and externally as matter (fig. 3). The differences are due to the different positions of those undergoing the experiences, not the nature of events *per se.*

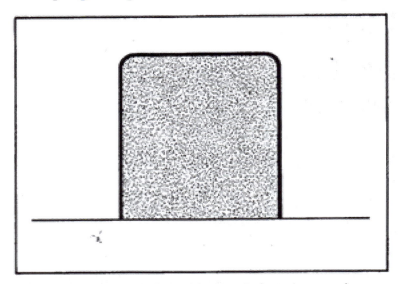

FIG. 3.—*Monism or holism. Matter-mind coexistent and indivisible (Psychosomatic approach).*

It is sometimes claimed that such an approach is unscientific but, in fact, it accords with the development of physics since Heisenberg (Russell, 1959) and Einstein (Einstein and Infeld, 1938). Relativity physics, for example, demonstrates that events and structures which appear to have a definite order or design to one observer, will show a different pattern to a differently placed observer. Consequently, the concept of causation breaks down, as one event does not necessarily precede another unless the frames of reference of the observers are similar. Physics overcomes this by fusing space and time which were previously conceived as inviolable and distinct. By analogy, a holistic approach integrates mind and body in the same way that relativity physics has fused space and time.

Within this model it can be seen that there is not a simple causational (hierarchical) relationship between mind and body; they are merely different aspects of the organism. A change in the body is bound to be accompanied by a shift in mental equilibrium and vice versa. The two are co-existent and indivisible. While the deterministic approach looks for a causal relationship between mind and body, the holistic approach observes changes in the whole organism. An example of this can be illustrated by the two different views on an anxious person with ulcerative colitis. The somatic approach will conceive of the anxiety and colonic inflammation as being 'caused by' disturbances in neurotransmitters, inflammatory mediators etc. The psychosomatic approach will view the experience of anxiety and the signs of colitis as being manifestations of disturbance within the whole person and his environmental field; the inflamed colon and the experience of anxiety being the small part of the disturbance, which both patient and doctor are aware of at the present time.

There are important theoretical and practical difficulties which arise from the traditional scientific method, and what can be contained within it. In the world of biology, science, as elsewhere, is confined to the outward and material manifestations of life. The inner experience, or mind, remains unobserved and thus outside strict scientific assessment of formulation. The nearest that such methods can get to the mind is through such signals as words and behaviour, from which we assume the inner experience. It follows that the somatic approach fits most comfortably within the scientific compass, while the psychosomatic method flows outside in many directions. The validity of the psychosomatic framework is, therefore, difficult to appraise objectively; as I shall suggest in the next article, it may only be practically effective if it has subjective meaning, particularly where the patient is concerned. This may account for the many confusingly inconclusive or negative studies which have been scientifically designed to discern components of 'anxiety' or 'depression' in illness, or the efficacy of psychotherapy in their relief. In these studies the unmeasurable variables are subtle and possibly innumerable, so that studies of complex clinical problems necessarily reduce them to a somatic distillate; the truly psychological (experiential) component having evaporated in the process.

It is crucial to note that there is no 'right' or 'wrong' approach. By analogy, relativity physics has not indiscriminately supplanted Newtonian physics. The two systems have different areas of operation and different yields. Sometimes the somatic approach is entirely satisfactory for the task at hand, at other times the psychosomatic approach will be more effective. Inappropriate use of the somatic approach leads to practice that is too simplified, unnecessarily intrusive or controlling, and alienating. On the other hand, when the psychosomatic approach is used indiscriminately it can lead to practice that is dangerously unfocused or inactive. It will be indicated later how there are often subtle factors of dependency, both in the patient and his doctor, which largely decide which kind of model is used in any particular medical situation.

## East and West

At this point it is interesting to observe that different cultures have traditionally conceived the world differently, leading to contrasting types of medical practice. The West, which is increasingly influenced by a materialist-determinist philosophy and its consequent technology, has produced a pattern of medical practice which is strongly somatic in its bias; we consume an ever-increasing quantity of drugs to allay our discomfort or distress. Grief, despair, madness, or sexual disinclination, are all easily slotted into syndromes for which a prescription is found. The pursuit of the 'biochemical cause' of, for example, cancer and schizophrenia is to our technological culture what the Holy Grail was to early Christian societies. The results of such endeavours are often not dissimilar. Eastern and pre-industrial cultures are traditionally more monistic or psychosomatic in their approach; mind and body are not analytically dislocated as they are in the West. It is believed, therefore, that any attention to the body will change the mind, while calming the mind is bound to reduce disturbance in the body. The repertoire of resulting practices, which is extremely varied and often incomprehensible to those of us familiar only with Western practice, includes massage, yoga, incantation, exorcism, dietary rituals and acupuncture. At present many people are turning to these Eastern practices, which may reflect a disillusionment with the overgrowth of our medical technology and other cultural trends, experienced as controlling and depersonalising (Illich, 1976).

Even the world of non-organic psychiatry is subject to this division. Traditional Western therapies evolved from a scientific-deterministic framework. Psychoanalysis, ultimately has its roots in Freud's training as a neurologist, and behaviour therapy is based on learning theory. In both of these, the model of disturbance and therapy incorporates the notion of a determining cause. Also, they tend to be applied within a highly defined mode of experience; the latter with overt behaviour patterns, the former with verbal communications. Some of the new humanistic therapies have attempted to incorporate Eastern monism. Gestalt (Perls *et al*, 1951) and bioenergetic therapy (Lowen, 1976), for example, regard bodily and mental experiences as being correlative and interchangeable. In these therapies there is equal attention paid to all forms of experience, sensation and behaviour. It is noteworthy, also, that the former types of therapy have found a place in the current realm of medical practice, while the latter have not yet found a comparable assimilation.

## The responsibility spectrum

Illness, as usually conceived, is separate from the self as experienced in our conscious thoughts and feelings. It is something that 'happens to', or 'attacks', the self through organisms, accidents or fate. It is not usually considered as the expression or function of the self. The complex of intention, thought and feeling (the self) is thought to be quite different from the world of the body, much as a person and the house he lives in are thought to be distinct. This, of course, is the dualistic approach.

The doctor's conception of illness, and its relationship to the self, often veers even further towards the scientific-deterministic view, which sees a person as being controlled and defined by his body through genetics, chemical transmitters and the like. The quintessence of this approach is found in 'organic psychiatry', which considers mental and behavioural aspects of a person to be 'caused' by an underlying physical matrix. The fact that this matrix is often not well substantiated or defined does not detract from the influence of this model in practice (Zigmond, 1977).

It can be seen that these two approaches see illness as 'ego-dystonic', that is, having no connection with conscious volition, feeling or responsibility of the self. Illness becomes a fault in the machinery of the body; such mechanisms being dictated by the impersonal forces of physics and chemistry. The person is merely a passive and powerless onlooker to his internal processes. Changing such processes, if possible, is seen as coming from the outside, through powerful agencies which manipulate the physical and chemical mechanisms. Alleviation of illness thus becomes the responsibility of the medical attendant, not the patient. When a person goes to a doctor as a patient he largely disowns and encapsulates his distressing experience, and expects the doctor to define it and take it away (Zigmond, 1977). Often, of course, this system is efficient and mandatory; a man with renal colic cannot be expected to make his own diagnosis and relieve his own pain. At other times, however, the issue is less clear-cut. Perhaps most primary medical consultations do not involve structural disease, but rather disturbances of function and bodily experience, which are related to conflicting and unexpressed feeling. Tension headaches, 'needing a tonic', nonspecific musculoskeletal and abdominal discomforts make up a large part, if not the bulk, of the primary doctor's work. Such complaints sometimes yield to suggestion and physical intervention alone. More often, however, this application of the Medical Model serves only to parry the distress syndrome for short periods of time. My next article will explore how application of other non-deterministic models may make more substantial therapeutic inroads into these clinical situations.

If a person's distress is conceived by that person as an expression of inner conflict or turmoil, he is unlikely to think of himself as ill, merely distressed. In this instance the complaint is 'ego-syntonic' ; the bodily disturbance and the self are perceived as a unit. The sufferer sees his experience as being his own responsibility; he may wish that someone (for instance a doctor) could assume responsibility for taking away his discomfort, but in reality he knows that this is not possible. If such a person asks for help it is for compassion, suggestions or new understanding, not magical exorcism. Naturally, it is uncommon for a person to contact his doctor from the outset with these notions, although he may acquire them through consultation.

Such a process of identification is called 'gaining insight', and marks a shift in the patient's thought and feeling process, from a dualistic/deterministic to a monistic/holistic approach to his distress. This change implies also a shift in ownership and responsibility of distress from the doctor back to the patient. It is an important intention of psychotherapy for psychosomatic complaints; in this area the aim of psychotherapy is to help the patient 'identify with' his symptoms so that they are seen as a reflection of feelings, needs or conflicts that are not being dealt with successfully in other ways. Such holistic awareness confers a personal and creative meaning on symptoms; they become the body's signal of disequilibrium pushing into awareness, and providing the opportunity for exploration, expression or resolution. Understandably, many people are not able or willing to make this kind of reclamation as it involves feelings or conflict that are painful to acknowledge. Those who do so may only be able to make this transition with much support and guidance.

How a person experiences, conceives and communicates physical distress and how the helper intervenes may be represented as in the table, below. Generally, traditional medical disciplines and skills operate best at positions (1) and (2) on the spectrum. Here the concept of illness is dealt with as an alien or malevolent intrusion into the self. Position (4) is juxtaposed to these in regarding illness as an expressive syndrome. Position (3)— `it's just your nerves'—is an interesting midway point; in return for the patient assuming partial responsibility for his dilemma, the doctor offers him a metaphorical structure upon which to hang this responsibility. A patient's 'nerves' imply an immutable and constitutional quality, and cannot be cured by the doctor as can an illness; nevertheless the patient may expect some kind of soothing or tranquillization of the metaphorical structure.

| The psychosomatic-responsibility spectrum | | | |
|---|---|---|---|
| **Somatic** | | | **Psychosomatic** |
| Physical illness ① | Mental illness ② | 'Nerves' ③ | ④ Reactive physical discomfort/disturbance |
| **Responsibility** Predominantly doctors | | 50% doctor, 50% patient | Predominantly patients |
| **Psychological dynamic** Encapsulation + internal projection to actual physical structure | Encapsulation + internal projection to assumed physical structure | Encapsulation + internal projection to metaphorical physical structure | Ownership and conscious conflict/distress |
| **Language** Physical structures | Psychological structures | 'Nerves' | Distress described in ordinary language |
| **Implied philosophy** Determinism | | Dualism | Monism/Holism |
| **Nature of help** Biological Engineering = 'doing to' | | Support + social engineering | Empathy = 'Being with' + understanding experience working through |
| **Intention of help** Cure = destruction of illness via outside agency | | Enhanced coping mechanisms 'learning to live with' disability | Growth = increased understanding. Resolving conflicts/relationship difficulties, thereby abandoning illness as an expressive and communicative mode |
| **Perceived relationship to the 'self'** External and attacking the self | | Internal and compromising the self | Coexisting with and expressing the self |

## A clinical example

Let us take a simple and common clinical example to illustrate some of the features of this spectrum.

*Mr A is a healthy young man who presents with cervical-occipital headaches for which no significant structural disease can be found. If he communicates his symptoms in wholly physical terms, and is accepted and dealt with at this level by the doctor, then both are functioning in position (1). The symptom is thought of as an excrescence; an autonomous disease focus to be cured or suppressed with drugs, while leaving Mr A himself immune from challenge or examination. The doctor calls Mr A's complaint 'fibrositis', and Mr A is pleased with this utterance as the mystifying nomenclature has taken his complaint away from him, and placed it in the province of medical science. The doctor has assumed responsibility for its* definition and removal, and Mr A need not now worry about the meaning or nature of his bodily sensations.

Suppose, now, that the doctor expands his questioning and elicits that Mr A feels worried, wakes early in the morning, is sexually disinterested and often feels like weeping, but does not yield to this. He cannot, or will not, disclose to the doctor why this should be so and the doctor does not pursue the meaning for the patient of this disturbed behaviour or experience, as he feels that he has reached his diagnosis of 'depressive illness with somatic manifestations' (position (2)). The phenomenon is now encapsulated into a framework that implies a physical causation for the distress, though less tangibly or specifically than in position (1). However, the doctor's tone and language convey authority and a technical understanding of the patient's experience, which both lie beyond the patient's sphere of influence. The doctor, in treating 'depressive illness', has assumed the bulk of the responsibility for the distress. The patient's expected role is to remain cooperative, that is, to do what the doctor suggests.

Another doctor (or the same doctor on another day!) may not wish to assume this kind of responsibility. He may, too, be less convinced of the cogency of 'mental illness' as a workable diagnostic tool. He wants Mr A to assume responsibility for his plight, so he says 'Well Mr A, I've examined you and listened to your story and I'm quite sure that there's nothing seriously physically wrong with you to cause your headaches. I think we can put it down to your nerves. After all, you've always been a worrying type and you've also been under a lot of strain recently. Perhaps you need to take some time off work. These tablets might help, too, to relax your nerves'. There is an interesting shift in this consultation. At the beginning of the interview, doctor and patient conferred at position (1), but now the doctor has moved to position (3). He is willing to remain responsive to Mr A, but does not wish to assume total responsibility for his condition. If Mr A is responsive to this proposal, the consultation will move to a gratifying completion. Mr A will feel that he understands his complaint a little better, and the doctor may feel that he has shared his clinical responsibility rather more, thereby reducing his own burden.

But Mr A may not be amenable to such a move. He may deny he is a worrier, though his friends and family clearly experience him as such. Or he may say (angrily) 'Yes, I am a worrier but that's got nothing to do with these headaches, they're terrible, you know'(!) Assuming the doctor has been tactful and competent, Mr A's communication to him now implies something like 'I don't wish to explore the nature or meaning of my discomfort, and I don't want to take any responsibility for it'. If the doctor does not respect this defence, and persists in operating from position (3), it is likely that he and the patient will swiftly reach an unworkable impasse. The situation is akin to the child who does not want to eat what is offered; the feeding adult may 'know' correctly or mistakenly that it is 'good for' the child, but until the child himself is willing to take it, all attempts at feeding will be met by various forms of sabotage. Overt refusal, hiding the food in the cheek or napkin, or vomiting it back, all have their analogues in the medical consultation and the more complex task of psychotherapy. In the above example it is likely that the doctor will retreat back to position (1), confirming his act with a prescription as a token of his (albeit ambivalent) medical responsibility.

If Mr A responded readily to the doctor's suggestion of 'nerves', and showed an interest in how his complaint was associated with his feelings and relationships, the doctor may, if he has the time and interest, venture to position (4). If successful, Mr A will not be content merely to accept the label that he is a 'worrier' who suffers from 'bad nerves' but will want to integrate, understand and modify these mechanisms. He may see the doctor as a friend, a counsellor, a refuge in times of discomfort, but he does not expect technological magic or panaceas. In philosophical language he is perceiving himself `monistically' and his distress as an expression of himself, for which he, ultimately has responsibility. Naturally, such a position can seem frightening and lonely; it is often far more comforting to experience oneself dualistically, and have someone else take care of our distress *and difficult feelings, while denying that there is a deeper or more extensive problem.*

It is interesting to observe how shifts in the spectrum may often work in the reverse way to these illustrations. In this case the patient will attempt to understand and integrate his illness holistically, while the doctor persists with a deterministic approach so that he can, without being undermined, assume his potent caretaking role (Zigmond, 1977, 1981, 1982).

*I remember a previously healthy man aged 80 years who developed lobar pneumonia soon after his wife died; 'I think I got this because of the wife going', he said to the doctor, 'I feel so lost I just don't want to carry on'. 'That's nothing to do with it', retorted the doctor authoritatively, but not unkindly, 'your pneumonia is caused by the pneumococcus germ'. True, the old man needed antibiotics, but perhaps his diagnosis was also correct, and could have been advantageously pursued. In such instances it is likely that it is the doctor, not the patient, who is unable to integrate certain kinds of feeling; perhaps this doctor was uncomfortable about his own feelings of grief or loss.*

In many medical consultations we are faced with this spectrum and options for changing our position. However, one of the rules of clinical communication is that consultation can only begin and go on with any viability if doctor and patient are operating from the same position and model. Likewise, there has to be accordance between patient and doctor for any shift to be beneficial; as the adage points out 'You can take a horse to the water, but you can't make him drink'. Reaching this common language and understanding is the central process in creating a therapeutic rapport. The route to such dialogue, as we have seen, is inevitably complicated by the distortions and resistances of both patient and doctor.

Mr A represented what Michael Balint (Balint, 1957) termed 'unorganized (non-structural) illness'. My next article explores how these principles may be applied to organized (structural) illness.

Ω

Figures (1), (2) and (3) are modified from Bertrand Russell's 'Wisdom of The West'. Rathhone 1959.

### Note
*The terms 'psychosomatic' and 'somatic' are used in a particular way in this text which may not be in accordance with other writers. Some literature implies that psychosomatic illness is 'caused by' the mind and its conflicts. This article uses the word in a different sense, so that mind and body may be seen as equivalents and not necessarily as cause and effect.*

### References
Balint, M. (1957) *The Doctor, His Patient and the Illness*. Pitman, London

Bergson. H. (1911) *Creative Evolution*. Macmillan. London

Einstein, A. and Infield, L. (1938) *The Evolution of Physics*. Cambridge University Press, Cambridge

Illich, 1. (1976) *Limits of Medicine, Medical Nemesis; The Expropriation of Health*. Penguin, London

Lowen, A. (1976) *Bioenergetics*. Penguin, London

Perls, F., Hefferline, R., Goodman, P. (1951): *Gestalt Therapy*. Julian Press, New York.

Russell, B. (1977) *An ABC of Relativity*. Allen & Unwin, London

Russell, B. (1961) *A History of Western Philosophy*. Allen & Unwin, London

Spinoza, B. de. (1955) *Ethics*. Dover, New York

Zigmond, D. (1977): *Update*, 15, 675

Zigmond, D. (1977): *Update*, 15, 903

Zigmond, D. (1981): *Update*, 23, 1811

Zigmond, D. (1982): *Update*, 24, 281

Publ. In The Practitioner Vol. 226, April 1982

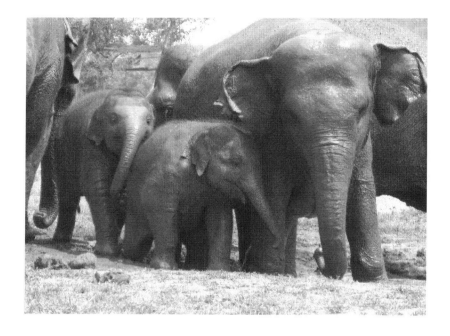

# The Psychosomatic Mosaic

*'It is the theory that determines what is observed.'*

Albert Einstein

It is, perhaps, a universal wish to find, and relate to, an orderly universe, and yet the advancing edge of science always produces more that is questionable than answered. Medical theory and practice do not escape this principle. Whether it is cancer or the common cold, the mysteries of illness continue to outflank our organizing concepts. We find 'causational agents' – carcinogens or viruses – to explain disease and yet they remain partial explanations. Why does Mr H., who smoked only 15 cigarettes a day develop lung cancer, while his brother who smoked 40 remain clear? Why does Timothy develop a cold and not his four brothers and sisters? The traditional sciences, usually, have no substantial answers to such simple questions.

## Levels of organizing concepts in illness

The quotation from Einstein is not just a philosophical principle. Our theories determine the configuration, content and outlook not only of scientific activities, but also our *personal* methods of experiencing and responding to the world. In medical practice this leads to professionally self-validating views and models of illness which are confined to the physical and deterministic. Analyses of illness are thus conventionally expressed in terms of anatomy, physiology, chemistry and the like.

There are, however, many other possible levels or approaches to illness, but they do not fit into this traditional mould.

*Figure 1* illustrates how we may conceive illness from the level of subatomic physics to political theory.

*Figure 1*

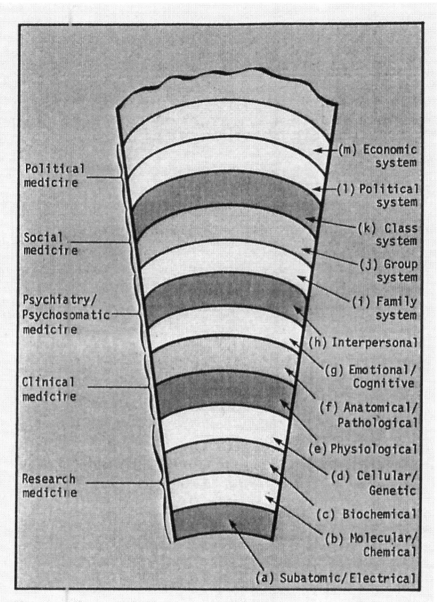

*Levels of organizing concepts in illness*

It is important to note that, although formulations at different levels may be dissimilar, they are not exclusive of one another; they are merely different levels, or angles, of observation and analysis. Much confusion has arisen because of our tendency to attempt to reduce our diagnostic and therapeutic formulations to only one, or a few, levels of organizing concepts.

Ascribing a man's duodenal ulcer to acid hypersecretion rather than his unresolved and repressed infantile hostility, may thus tell us more of a doctor's inclination, training and frame of reference than of the cause of the patient's illness. Our models derive as much from our psychology, as the world which we are attempting to define or influence.

Lord Kelvin, a once-eminent physicist, remarked 'If it works, it is true', and it is this pragmatic principle which should define the level and manner in which we operate in any particular clinical circumstance. Nevertheless, most doctors operate predominantly at levels (e) and (f), this being largely a reflection of the social definition of their role, and also how they see themselves; the image of potent biological engineer has its roots both in private fantasy and public expectation. Other levels of formulation and intervention thus tend, in practice, to be disregarded, avoided or dismissed, even though at times they may 'work'.

The reasons for such exclusion are both practical and complexly psychological. In practice, doctors often do not have the time, the expertise or the interest to pursue these other levels. Also the patient may neither expect nor want his doctor to perform anything beyond the traditional medical services. Yet deeper psychological issues define the pattern just as much. The doctor's fear of powerful feelings underlying the manifestations of illness, or his wish to exercise command over both his patient and what his patient brings him, are common examples. So, too, is the patient's wish to divorce his physical disturbance from its matrix of internal or relationship conflict; the man whose psoriasis gets worse when his wife goes on holiday alone, might be an example of this.

To illustrate how these principles may be employed in both diagnostic and therapeutic ways, a case history of a young asthmatic girl will be described. The letters in brackets correspond to the levels of organizing concepts in the figure. The ways in which the doctor might focus his attention and organizing concepts at different levels are also illustrated. Because of the author's interest, levels (g), (h), (i) and (j) are examined in greater detail. Levels (k), (l) and (m) are not considered to be in the scope of this article.

## A 'simple' case of childhood asthma

*Carol F, aged six years, was seen by her doctor at home because of her increasing wheeziness of one week's duration. This had become more severe, despite the competent use of antispasmodic, and later, antibiotic drugs. By the time of his visit Carol showed signs of marked bronchospasm and respiratory embarrassment ((e), (f)) and Mrs F was both agitated and anxious about her daughter's condition ((g)). Shortly before his home-visit, Dr V received a telephone call from Mr F. asking for a visit; the doctor felt Mr F.'s tone to be unduly threatening and accusatory, as if, somehow, Mr F blamed the doctor for Carol being ill. Dr V bore this with resigned stoicism and, by the time of his visit, had decided that Carol should be admitted to hospital, which he later arranged.*

*Carol had always been prone to chestiness; as an infant she had frequently been slightly wheezy and catarrhal, and Dr V.. had repeatedly treated this, with transient benefit, with the usual medicines ((c), (f)). He elicited the fact that Mr F's family had been prone to asthma, as had Mr F as a child, so he thought that Carol's complaint was partly genetic in origin (d). Dr V confirmed this hypothesis when Carol also developed flexural eczema, a sign of `atopic allergy', thus also showing a hypersensitivity component to her* *illness. Her increased wheeziness when the pollen-count was high in summer was another manifestation of this (d). In the winter, too, Carol would have more trouble with her breathing and this was thought to be an allergic sequel to infections of her respiratory tract (d). Dr V had noticed how Carol was a 'very good' but quiet and introspective child (g) but he had explored this only so far as to say to Mrs F, 'Do you think Carol is worried about anything?'; to which Mrs F responded by turning to the little girl and asking rhetorically, 'I don't think so, dear. You're not worried, are you?'. Carol, duly hypnotized, nodded a whimsical 'No' to the avuncular Dr V, who asked no more.*

*Dr V is a practical doctor who has little time to pursue modern thinking of prostaglandin activity or immunological aspects of the globulins in the role of asthma ((b), (c)). He is vaguely aware of the efforts of medical research workers in this area and recently was interested by an article which suggested that changes in the ionosphere could affect the electrical activity of cell membranes in vivo, thereby precipitating certain types of episodic illness (a). Dr V cannot make any use of these theories in his clinical work, though sometimes he wonders how these facts will be incorporated into future patterns of practice.*

*Dr V's observations about Carol's compliance and sensitivity were easily made. She is a slight, pale child who looks unduly timid and worried, and talks with submissive reticence. Indeed, in his dealings with her, Dr V had noticed how she rarely spoke for herself, even when perfectly able, her mother quickly interposing herself between Carol and the doctor, and then commandeering the dialogue (h). He thought this might be due, simply, to the effect of her recurrent illness and mother's ensuing anxiety.*

*Carol developed this attack of asthma, her worst ever, just as she was due to start at primary school; a fact which Carol and her mother were keenly aware of, but which had escaped the notice of Dr V. Had Dr V been attentive to this, he might have correctly supposed that Carol was 'anxious' about this important development in her life (g).*

*And yet Carol's two other siblings, Brian (eight years) and Sue (nine years), never showed anxiety of this kind, so why should Carol?*

## Parental history

*For many years Mrs F had seen Dr V for protean and ill-defined somatic complaints, which had little to suggest structural disease, but which he nevertheless, at first, investigated. Eventually he concluded that Mrs F's complaints were 'functional' in nature. He experienced Mrs F as an anxious, taut and frightened woman, who seemed to radiate a sense of fear, urgency and wanting. In her visits to the doctor she would always refer these feelings back to her presenting physical complaints. On a few occasions Dr V had said something like, 'I can't find anything physically wrong with you. I think it must be your nerves. Is anything in particular upsetting you at the moment?'. At this suggestion she seemed uncomfortable, perhaps affronted, and with a blank look she would shift uneasily in her chair, foreclosing the interview by asking for 'a tonic' or repeat prescription.*

*Mr F, by contrast, rarely attended the surgery and, when he did, it was usually for a tangible medical complaint which the doctor could quickly and easily deal with. On several occasions, though, he had come with his wife, to amplify her complaint and underline her conviction that 'something must be wrong, and that Dr V must do something about it (h). At these times the doctor felt pressurized, and usually escaped from the corner into which he was being forced by arranging a hospital referral, which he knew to be unnecessary. Dr V is vaguely aware, therefore, that there may be important tensions in Carol's family which could be contributing to her illness. But within the context of his brief clinical encounters with them, he has been unable to define or use these patterns to either diagnostic or therapeutic advantage.*

*Let us look in greater detail at the members of Carol's family and the patterns that emerge at levels (g), (h) and (i).*

*Mrs F had always hoped for different things from her marriage. She herself is illegitimate, and was reared in a variety of institutions* and by foster parents. So far as she knows, her own mother became pregnant at the age of 16 years, by an American sailor, at the end of the Second World War. The relationship lasted only a few months and, although the mother had wanted to keep her infant, her own wishes had been swept aside by the wave of her family's shock and indignation. As a child Mrs F was often treated kindly by her caretakers, but she was unable either to understand or predict what was happening to her, and developed a submissive wariness in her attachments.

By the time she was five years old she came to the conclusion that there must be something wrong with her, for her mother and father to have abandoned her. Failing to understand the complex reasons for the fragmented pattern of her care, it seemed to her that any satisfaction of her need for stability and love was sooner or later countered by unaccountable and sudden loss. At first she would openly show her anger and sadness over such losses, but eventually she thought it best to conceal her hurt, initially from other people, but later from her own conscious awareness.

As an adult Mrs F seems to cope 'normally' although, as we have seen, Dr V has noticed her hypochondriasis and tension. But to Mrs F, her life and relationships seem much more tenuous than an outside observer might suppose. Despite her apparent social integration, she describes her life as 'like hanging on to the edge of a cliff'; in her dreams this is reflected by a 'terrible vision of falling into nothingness'. Her relationships are accompanied with much inner anxiety, in which Mrs F has a vague but ominous sense of imminent catastrophe. Socially, however, she seems merely to be rather tense and circumspect.

Mr F's childhood was very different, yet equally decisive. As the last (and probably accidental) birth in a family of eight children, he had a stable, but harsh, family experiences. By the time he was born, his mother was weary and his father resentful of the added responsibility brought about by his birth. It was not only food and money which were in short supply for the little boy but love, patience

143

and attention. Mr F's father had a bullying and vitriolic streak and, by the time Mr F was a toddler, his father was using the boy as a vent for his frustrations. But Mr F was a resilient child and, rather than succumb to his father's dominance and sadism, he devised precocious strategies of avoidance and independence. As a schoolboy he looked to his friends for support and identification, and at the age of 15 years resolutely left his family for the Merchant Navy.

Some would consider it coincidence that Mrs F married a sailor. Psychoanalytic theory might postulate that she was trying to reclaim the father who had abandoned her. Transactional analytic theory would maintain that she did so to maintain a homeostatic system, where she could repeat the conditioned patterns of her childhood as this, paradoxically, represents security; the world she has experienced and knows how to handle. Whatever the explanatory theory, Mrs F is beset with the same feelings of insecurity and impotent wanting that she experienced as a child. Mr F is a dutiful, though patriarchal, husband and father, a good provider and a source of reliable practical support when at home. But he avoids the finer nuances of trust and closeness, and Mrs F is mute in the face of her need for such emotional nourishment. As she confided once to an interviewing psychologist: `He's so good really, and he isn't often home; I couldn't really criticize him... I'd be afraid to rock the boat …(!)'.

When her children were infants, Mrs F found herself more serene, secure and satisfied than at any other period of her life. She felt a sense of attachment and belonging, which she wished could go on forever. For all their demands and inevitable episodes of difficult behaviour, her babies would continue to want her and love her as a mother. She sensed in herself a streak of resentment and sadness as her two older children became more independent and looked to other adults and children for their sense of belonging. Mrs F did not want to be abandoned with finality, and so Carol, as the youngest child, became special and precious for her mother; both a repository for her vulnerable feelings and a buffer against her own loneliness and fears of abandonment.

*Although Carol had not yet the command of words or concepts to articulate her dilemma, she knew that mother was somehow frail and in need of protection. She sensed a danger in growing apart from mother, as if mother would collapse or stop loving her. Confronted by this wordless threat, Carol complied with what she sensed as her mother's demands. She became a rather clinging child, disinclined to contact with other children. When other children played in the street, Carol would rather keep her mother company indoors. Her physical illnesses could be seen as a somatic expression of her own, her mother's, and perhaps the whole family's conflicts. Her asthma both reinforced the bond between the child and her mother, and expressed the anger which she felt towards her mother for controlling and burdening her as she did. Carol often felt overwhelmed by what she experienced as her mother's needs, and sometimes in her fantasies, in an effort to be free, she would harm her mother or even make her disappear. Such strong images would usually bring in their wake intense feelings of fear and guilt because of what, in fantasy, she had brought about. Carol's asthma then seemed to her like a containment or punishment. In psychodynamic and interpersonal senses, her illnesses expressed and enacted the cycle of love, hate and reparation; her need to love and belong, her need to be separate and destroy, and her need to undo her destructive impulses.*

*Carol's illness has other significant functions within the family. It allows Carol to express the feelings of fear or helplessness for others, who can then disown such feelings in themselves and act in a responding and caretaking capacity. In this way Carol may be considered as a kind of siphon or amplifier for the unacknowledged, unspoken but important and persistent feelings of others.*

*Mrs F's covert emotional life has already been discussed, but what about Mr F? Perhaps Carol's illness might serve as a way for him to express both his tenderness and his frustration, which is so hard for him to share directly with his wife. Carol, as a constant focus of attention, creates a route by which Mr and Mrs F can both communicate and avoid one another; they talk a lot about Carol, but little about themselves. Carol thus becomes both a shared concern and a buffer between them. If they were deprived of Carol's sick-role, the difficulties between them would emerge more sharply and inescapably.*

*For Brian and Sue, too, Carol's illness has its functions. So long as mother's attachment needs are channelled into her care and concern for Carol, they are not discouraged from making other relationships outside the home and eventually growing apart from their mother. Should Carol become well, the mother's fear of separation would be transferred to them with greater intensity.*

*Table I* summarizes a psychodynamic analysis of Carol's illness.

| | |
|---|---|
| **Carol** | (1) Keeps mother loving and safe in the only way she knows how |
| | (2) Expresses anger and also reparation for her guilt from her fantasized anger |
| | (3) Makes mother and father seem closer together |
| **Mrs F** | (1) Keeps Carol close and special for her where Mr F has disappointed her |
| | (2) Helps her avoid issues of abandonment and aloneness |
| | (3) Allows Carol to express her own (Mrs F's) (unexpressed) vulnerability, fear and impotence |
| **Mr F** | (1) Allows him to show care and concern where this is difficult in other situations |
| | (2) Produces a common problem through which he can relate to Mrs F |
| **Brian and Sue** | (1) Deflects mother's oversolicitousness, thereby enabling them to be more autonomous |
| | (2) Makes mother and father seem closer together |
| **The marital system** | (1) Makes for a common bond between Mr and Mrs F when this would otherwise be lacking |
| | (2) Deflects feelings of neglect, resentment and uncertainty about marriage which would otherwise have to be encountered |
| **The family system** | Produces cohesion by: |
| | (1) Facilitating bond between Mr and Mrs F |
| | (2) Projecting otherwise disturbing difficulties and feelings into one family member thus leaving the others feeling unthreatened and unencumbered |

*Table 1:*
*Relational and psychological factors in the patient's illness*

This table contains hypotheses which are inferential rather than directly observable, and this is generally true of psychological and psychodynamic formulations. How do we know if they might be true? There are two main methods which can be used.

*Empirical and deductive method* – Our hypothesis will make sense of otherwise disconnected facts, and predict usefully what might happen in future.

*Deepening of rapport* – Our interpretations, if skilfully conveyed to the patient, will lead to an increased thoughtfulness and increased disclosure and trust on the part of the patient in a manner which may bring about greater integration of split-off impulses and feelings, leading to change in symptomatology or behaviour. This will be examined further in the next section.

This empirical-deductive method of assessing psychological factors in illness is usefully illustrated in Carol's case. After hospitalization her asthma became much less severe, but she became seriously school-phobic and was referred to a child-psychiatrist, where the problem was eventually tackled in a family-therapy context. Her school phobia dissolved over a period of months, probably hastened by father's decision to change his job to that of a shore-bound ship's pilot. Although Carol's asthma became quiescent, and her school phobia resolved, her parents continued to attend the hospital for marital therapy, as problems were now emerging between them which they recognized as being theirs, not Carol's. This would be a likely prediction of the above formulation, and reinforces the notion of Carol's illness being the function, in part, of other family processes.

## Level of rapport and the nature of diagnosis

If, as suggested, Carol's illnesses reflected unresolved conflicts and tensions at an intrapsychic and interpersonal level, how is an attending doctor to make use of this notion? As we saw, Dr V had noticed Carol's introspective submissiveness, the mother's overprotectiveness and hypochondriasis, and the father's rather truculent but protective attitude. He made a cursory attempt to understand the situation better by, for example, asking Carol `Are you worried about anything?', but this was met by mother's resistance in the form of denial. Perhaps the doctor's question was experienced by Carol and her mother as being too bold to yield candid exploration.

Psychological examination has intricacies similar to the physical examination and untimely questioning evokes a similar response to the sudden production of a doctor's cold hand on a frightened patient's abdomen. The doctor's shifting from a physical to a psychological frame of reference may have been too abrupt for the patient to adjust to and assimilate. It is now well established that response and compliance to taking prescribed drugs are significantly influenced by the size, shape and colour of the tablet or capsule. This principle is likely to be even more important in what we offer the patient verbally. How we offer an interpretation is perhaps more important than its content.

Dr V could, perhaps, have gone some way to bridging the gulf between his observations (Carol's passivity, Mother's anxiety) and the presenting complaint (Carol's asthma, Mother's hypochondriasis) by phrasing his question differently. With Mrs F, for example, he could say: 'I've listened to your story, and by examining you I can tell you that there is no serious disease causing your headaches. From experience we know that in many people the pain is due to tension in the body. With all of us, if we have strong or mixed-up feelings which we can't put into words or get rid of, then these feelings get stuck in different parts of our body, to cause tightness or pain. Sometimes I've thought that you look as though you have a lot of worry which you can't express or let out, so I wonder if you think this could apply to you?'

This form of question is more likely to be considered by Mrs F than the more direct, 'Are you worried about anything?', as it demonstrates the doctor's serious recognition of Mrs F's pain, and also offers her an explanatory link between her dualistic,* and his monistic,* frame of reference. If Mrs F were to pursue his suggestion, there follows a change in the level of rapport. Referring back to figure 1 we can see that her presenting complaint (headaches) is at level (f) – organ symptomatology – while the doctor's suggestion is at level (g), (h) or (i), depending on whether she chooses to focus on, for example, her own feelings (g), her anxieties about Carol (h) or the difficulties in the F family as a whole (i). If the level of rapport changes to one of the other levels, the diagnostic formulation will also change, as shown in table 2.

| Level of rapport = level of organising concept of illness (see fig.) | Type of diagnostic formulation |
| --- | --- |
| (f) Organ pathology and symptomatology | 'Functional headache' 'Atypical migraine' |
| (g) Emotional/cognitive | 'Anxiety neurosis' 'Obsessional ruminations over loss etc' |
| (h) Interpersonal | Extended symbiotic attachment of mother and daughter |
| (i) Family system | Complex family tensions projected into somatic breakdown in two family members |

*Table 2: Level of rapport and type of diagnostic formulation*

In the F family the level of rapport presented itself, and remained for some time, at level (f) so that Dr V. was dealing with Carol's asthma and eczema, and Mrs F's headaches, in a physical and dualistic manner, by conventional drug prescription. Communication between patient and doctor was confined to the events and language of organ disturbance and, consequently, diagnosis was in physical syndromes.

When Carol was first referred to the child psychiatrist because of her school phobia, she was initially seen individually and their communication was focused on Carol's fear of her angry feelings and the fantasies which she had of what would happen to mother, were she to leave her at home by going to school. The diagnosis now became that of the neurotic anxieties of the little girl.

The decision to take the F family into therapy changed the level of rapport again. The communicated problems led to a diagnosis of Carol's anxieties within a matrix of unexpressed marital tensions, whereby the mother's fear of Carol's separating from her reflected a displacement of the anger and hurt she felt towards her husband in this respect, and, reciprocally, Mr F's fear of closeness and the demands he felt which more substantial commitment would lead to.

All these observations and inferences are part of 'the psychosomatic mosaic'; no one part expresses the whole on its own and each part, ultimately, only makes sense with reference to its place among the others. Equally important, no one part 'causes' the rest of the picture to be formed, although it is true that at times one part of the mosaic will become more prominent and demand separate and complete attention. Carol's severe asthma attack needed immediate physical attention (level (f)) and an interpretation of her repressed anger (level (g)) at the time might be 'correct', but would certainly be untimely. Eventually, however, such an intervention made a substantial contribution to the holistic approach to her care.

The F family represent a fairly unusual example of illness in which the psychosomatic mosaic can be seen in a fairly whole form, albeit retrospectively, and after much professional time had been spent in broadening the rapport in a number of different contexts. More often the doctor is familiar only with one or a few pieces of the mosaic, perhaps because he is too busy and has neither the inclination nor the training to seek, or assemble, the other pieces. Usually such elaborate endeavour is not asked for, or needed, by the patient and would thus become an unnecessary professional burden or intrusion.

Sometimes, as illustrated by the case of Mr A in my article *A Psychosomatic Approach*, the doctor may wish to broaden the pattern of communication which the patient brings in somatic form, although the patient may steadfastly hold to his physical symptoms. Clinically we might label such a patient `hypochondriacal' or suffering from a 'depressive illness with somatic manifestations'. In psychodynamic terms the patient is employing a somatic defence whereby conflicts or impulses which are intolerable to the conscious mind or the patient's *modus vivendi* are split off and expressed by the body, leaving the conscious 'self' clear and unthreatened.

At times such a defence represents an acceptable and efficient working compromise between the self which is known, and the self which is forbidden. In these instances a doctor's zealous attempts to complete the mosaic would be fraught with difficulty; premature removal of defences is likely to be followed by a decompensation of the underlying psychopathology. Like inflammatory tissue, such defences are primarily protective and only secondarily pathogenic. A woman whose feeling of a lump in the throat, for example, is a defence against her unconscious wish to scream at and assault the dying mother she cares for, might be managed best along wholly physical lines; unmasking the conflict might be more than she can bear.

On the other hand, Carol F perhaps represented the opposite pole; the somatic defence was progressively decompensating and dangerous, but the underlying material was accessible and, with skilled help, could be worked through advantageously.

The question of when and how to expand our rapport and diagnostic image of patients is probably as important as the more traditional and familiar medical practices. The skills which we need, to be sensitive to such nuances, are as intricate, and at times as important, as any the doctor has learned in his conventional training.

*For the special sense in which the words 'dualistic' and 'monistic' are used the reader is referred to the previous article 'A Psychosomatic Approach'.

Publ. in *The Practitioner* Vol. 226, April 1982

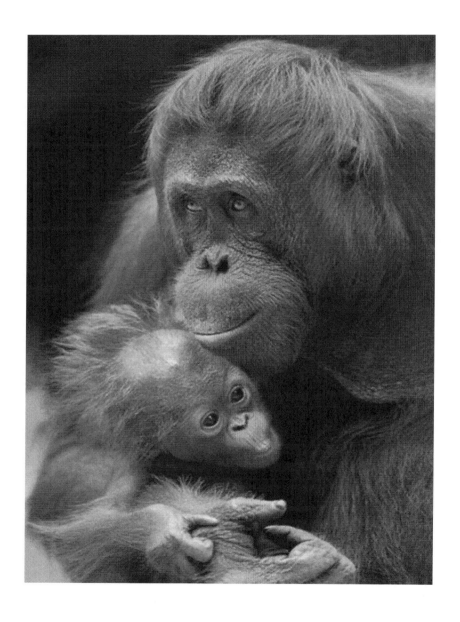

# Mother, Magic or Medicine?

## The psychology of the placebo

*"Physicians must discover the weaknesses of the human mind, and even condescend to humour them, or they will never be called in to cure the infirmities of the body..."*
Charles Caleb Colton, *Lacon* (1825)

It is not surprising that most contemporary observers and practitioners of medicine assume that drug treatment in medical and psychiatric practice is a kind of "pharmacological engineering". A sample of any text or medical dialogue concerned with this subject is likely to support the notion of the doctor in his role of engineer; his diagnosis locates or defines a malfunction in the body, and his medical treatment is applied as a specific chemical remedy. The practice that follows is guided by purely technical considerations— finding the most specific drug for the problem, working out its route, dose and timing. Explanations as to how drugs work are similarly inclined— replacing depleted chemicals, neutralizing acids, altering proliferation patterns in certain types of cell, inhibiting or catalyzing specific chemical interactions—are common concepts used.

And yet while doctors and medical researchers work painstakingly to refine such scientific theory and its application, the patients themselves often have quite a different way of experiencing the doctor and his medicines. For example, the evidence that most drugs prescribed outside a supervised hospital setting are not taken at all, or not as prescribed (Parkin *et al.*, 1976; Pearson, 1982) strongly implies that the doctor's "scientific" endeavours have quite a different meaning, or lack of meaning, for the patient. For all the technical talk amongst doctors of pharmacokinetics, serum concentrations, drug half-life and so on, if there is such a discrepancy between what a doctor assumes and intends and what a patient does, the questions arise "what is this activity, who is it for, and why does it exist?" For the doctor, prescribing in the prescribed manner has a number of functions. It helps him pass the time with the patient in a way that offers him the security of familiarity, and confers on him the mantle of "physician"; a cloak of potency, authority and legitimacy. It legitimatizes, too, his activities with his colleagues and gives him an identified place among them— they act in a similar way and so he is part of their group. It helps him feel helpful, even if this is not the help that is really needed; there are many studies suggesting this is often the case. The act of prescription may also provide the doctor with the comforting illusion that he is controlling or "managing" the patient's problem.

The foregoing indicates a little of why, for psychological reasons, the doctor may have his own compulsive need to prescribe. The main emphasis of this paper, however, deals with the complementary pattern—the psychology of the patient's need for drugs—which is equally fascinating and important. It is well established that placebos can have a positive therapeutic effect in a very wide range of disease processes in any bodily system (Doongaji *et al.*, 1978). Placebo response to severe injury pain (Beecher, 1955) and angina (Benson and McCalle, 1979) are now classic studies. Severe mental disturbance in those labelled "chronic schizophrenic" often responds to placebos (Silverstone and Turner, 1974).

Some of the fragments of placebo psychology can be deduced from further research. A positive response depends upon an expectation of successful treatment (Lesse, 1962), a trusting and positive attitude to the administering doctors (Black, 1966), and the social status of the "healer" (Silverstone and Turner, 1974). In this latter study, patients with a demonstrated peptic ulcer responded symptomatically to a placebo given by a doctor (70%) but much less with a nurse (25%) The deeper and symbolic meaning of the placebo – which this article discusses later—has received less attention. Among the most interesting studies is that of Balint (1970) who studied, over a period of some years, repeat prescriptions in general practice. He concluded that the repeat prescription often represented less of a treatment than a diagnosis—that the patient was wanting protection and reassurance from the doctor, but not direct contact with him. Such patients were emotionally needy but afraid of a more direct or intimate contact, and so settled for this ritualized "dose of doctor" which represented a symbolic "something" that was "good, reliable, unchanging and always available". Clearly this need is similar, if not the same, to those needs of security and protection that run throughout our infancy and early childhood, and Balint here equated the drug's symbolic protection and goodness with mother, or earlier, the breast. Certainly Balint's notion was supported by the observation of protest, rage or crisis of some kind when the doctor attempted to stop or change the drug, usually with "clinically sound" reasons—the drug for the patient was not a mere "pharmacological agent", it was a symbol of caring, security and regard; its withdrawal seemed threatening to the patient, far beyond any possible medical implications.

Doctors' training generally does not involve recognition of these important principles, and certainly the skills by which they may be marshalled and used therapeutically have received little attention. The "rational", physical, components of prescribing have been pursued as a legitimate clinical study at the expense of those "irrational", psychological, determinants which, as we have seen, may be decisive, for better or worse. This indifference, or implicit contempt for the placebo, seems to have coincided with the "pharmaceutical explosion" in the 1950s (Doongaji *et al.*, 1978). It seems that the world of medical therapeutics reflected in miniature much wider social processes – a consuming and increasingly exclusive interest in technology, at the expense of psychological and social needs that have been with us since our beginnings. The consequences of over-investment in technology and attention only to the manifest, at the expense of more radical but hidden human needs, is an increasingly pervasive theme in our culture.

The following three cases go back to the "irrational" in treatment for their guiding principles. At first sight it might be easy to discuss them as in some sense "unscientific" or "quackery", but, on closer inspection, the skilful use of such situations and transactions involves some kind of applied science of the early mind.

## Case No 1: A bridge over troubled waters

*A 62-year-old woman, Mrs F, was knocked off her moped by a car emerging from a side-turning, driven by a young man, rapidly and without due observation. Mrs F was not seriously injured, but suffered painful bruising and lacerations. More troublesome for her were her symptoms of dizziness, shakiness, headaches and loss of confidence which the first doctor (Dr E) told her was "the shock coming out in you", and for which he prescribed a tranquillizer. A fortnight later she returned to see a second doctor (Dr G) saying she felt worse; she still had the same symptoms, but now she felt "unsteady and tired all the time". Dr G asked about the kind of thoughts and feelings she had toward the young driver, which led Mrs F to talk tentatively of her anger and resentment, which she had not previously expressed; "he was so kind and polite and apologetic . . . and I was too shocked at the time to say anything . . .".*

*But there was more to her resentment and sense of injury, which Dr G intuited from the little he knew of her. She had recently been made redundant from work, after 20 years with the same employers; they had themselves been "bought-out" by a younger and more aggressive company, which had decided to streamline the old order. At the same time, her husband had recently become ill with angina, following soon after his retirement. Her three children in recent years had married, moved away and become increasingly involved with their young families. In short, she was facing a period of rapid change and loss where the old order, and her familiar roles, were no longer viable or valued. Dr G had acknowledged and shared this dilemma with her, for brief periods, when she had seen him on two previous occasions. On this occasion, behind the miscellany of her physical complaints, Dr G was touched by the tears which kept welling up in Mrs F's eyes, only to be quickly dabbed away with self-disparaging apology. After an intimate pause of a few seconds the doctor said softly "I imagine your whole life at present is a bit like riding your moped. Trying to retain your balance and sense of direction while larger more powerful cars pass you by, often blindly, not aware of your vulnerability. It must have seemed like the last straw when that young man knocked you down. . . Perhaps it's unavoidable that you have strong feelings about this; if that's so, I think you'll need to face and talk about your feelings, rather than take tranquillizers to pretend they're not there."*

*Mrs F sat and cried for about a minute. Dr G was attentive but silent. This time she did not wipe away her tears, either literally or with apologies. "You've been a great help doctor, helping me express my feelings like that. You're right, they are my feelings and I do feel better just talking about them. I don't want a drug that 'gets into my system' —what about a good old-fashioned tonic?" Dr G's response, a prescription for a multivitamin syrup, was accompanied by his comment: "I think you will feel stronger and more able to cope with this. Come and see me next week."*

*Mrs F did indeed feel much better with her "tonic". "I know I have to get my confidence back myself, doctor, but that red medicine does me a power of good. I'd like it for just another week and then I think I'll be all right."*

*Her request complied with, her prediction proved correct.*

## Comment

What had Dr G done that was different from the first doctor, and can we deduce any scientific principles, even if in embryonic form, to account for his effectiveness?

Dr E had attempted to label and rapidly dispose of Mrs F's feelings by didactic reassurance and tranquillizers. He diagnosed "shock" without, in any way discovering what this shock had meant to her, and thus his verbal help could extend only to sympathy, not empathy. Dr G, however, had entered into her world a little, and understood something of her distress before making any attempt to change it. His intervention, when it came, was an empathic act; Mrs F felt validated and accompanied by Dr G in her hurt and despair. With Dr E, on the contrary, she had felt alone, alienated and discounted. Dr G had offered her, in a symbolic, brief but skilled form, an embracing and protective presence—those elements of successful parenting that all children need successfully, to pass through the many hurts and crises of childhood.

In the words of Guntrip (1964) "we do not grow out of childhood, we grow over it" and it is this Child within us that re-awakens and cries out in times of stress. Dr G sensed that it was not enough to give Mrs F adult reassurance, he had to somehow establish a dialogue with her inner Child, before the panic could be calmed. He knew also that her request for a "good old-fashioned tonic" was Mrs F's primitive need for a symbol of the doctor's concern, protection and understanding which she could take with her, and literally ingest, when he was no longer with her. Balint (1957) talked of patients taking "a dose of doctor" to describe the device of extending, symbolically, the therapeutic relationship. The following two cases explore this theme further.

## Case No 2 A balm for grief

*Mr D was 78 years old when his wife died. She had suffered a stroke two years previously, which had left her chairbound, dysphasic and dependent on her husband for all her domestic needs and the little contact she had with the outside world. Mr D provided this with great compassion, fortitude and humour, despite his own age and frailty. Her intense dependence on Mr D led to a strength of feeling and an intimacy between the two old people that had previously only existed*

*50 years before, at the beginning of their marriage. When she died, Mr D, despite his tears of grief, acted with the same courage and independence as before. Two weeks later, after he had completed all the funeral arrangements, he developed shingles on his chest wall and sought Dr E's advice. The doctor, after explaining the medical nature of the problem and offering a sympathetic warning to Mr D that he would probably experience several weeks of pain, sat back in his chair saying reflectively to Mr D "These must be hard times for you. I'm sorry I can't offer you more." The old man sat silently and sadly for a short while, looking at the floor. Raising his eyes to Dr E he said "I feel there's a big hole inside me—like somebody has taken something away." "Yes," the doctor concurred, "I think losing those we love does leave holes in us which we can never really fill in. Sometimes, though, with time, good new things can grow around the holes." Mr D smiled wistfully at his doctor before leaving with his prescription. "I think the talk with you is my best medicine, doctor. I don't feel so alone now."*

*Long after any specific medication could affect Mr D's shingles, he was continuing to want "something to rub into my skin" even though his skin was now clear and he had little in the way of residual pain. The doctor had at first resisted prescription, countering Mr D's request with a medical explanation of how it was impossible for a cream to now help his condition, which was largely resolved anyway. The old widower's eyes looked blankly at the doctor during his didactic effort, and then changed to an expression of hurt when he had finished. "I suppose you're right doctor but I feel ever so much better if I have something to rub in ... " Dr E now realized that it was not pharmacology that was required of him, but a kind of symbolic mothering. An inert cream, not recommended in any medical text, brought an expression of relief and seemingly inordinate gratitude from Mr D.*

*For three years the old man walked slowly round to see his doctor, to collect his prescription for his simple cream. He insisted on seeing the doctor personally; collection from the receptionist was not enough. The medical business of his consultations was perfunctory, the important transactions concerned the sharing, if only briefly, his world and feelings.*

*Mr D died alone, asleep in his bed, unexpectedly one night. Dr E was summoned by the neighbours to certify his death. Beside his bed were his dentures and spectacles, a glass of water, and a large pot of cream he had collected from his doctor two days earlier.*

## Comment

Mr D, like Mrs F, was facing a dramatic and painful change in his life. While more concretely-minded sceptics might claim that his outbreak of shingles was coincidental to his wife's death, it seems clear that the "treatment" Mr D wanted from his doctor was of some kind of representation of the doctor's understanding and permissive presence. Dr E had empathised with his aloneness and the grief and hurt that were expressed more by his body than by his words. The cream, for Mr D, was a way for him to have continuous, if symbolic, access to the palliative and nurturing presence of his doctor. The familiar religious symbols of Holy Bread and Water may confer on the believing recipient a sense of purification, forgiveness or strength; the clinical situation here is probably analogous, Mr D receiving from his cream a sense of caring attachment.

Many writers and researchers have stressed the importance of touch in the mental and physical development of the young child (Spitz, 1945; Harlow and Harlow, 1966) and the continuing health of the adult (Berne, 1961). Healing or palliative procedures based upon touch have a long history, and are still prevalent in Eastern medical practice. For the distressed infant, the touch of a protective adult is probably the most effective nonspecific remedy. Even as we grow older touch remains among the most potent and direct antidotes to pain, panic and distress. Mr D's choice of a "touching" medicine— "something to rub into my skin"—probably indicated a wish for this most basic of comforts, as a balm for the most basic of pains; the loss of a loved person.

## Case No 3 Mother's milk

*When Mr S, a solitary man of 40 years, became the centre of an angry cacophony in Dr T's waiting room, the doctor became apprehensive, but was not surprised. Mr S, he knew, had a lifelong tendency to violent outbursts, though never before with the doctor or his staff. Most previous contacts with the doctor had been for fairly simple requests, and on these occasions Mr S had had a rather submissive, faltering and lost manner; Dr T had the fleeting mental image of a small boy searching for a (his?) father. Dr T could recall other times when Mr S had come for "tonics" or hypnotics; the preceding events had usually followed a similar pattern: he would react impulsively and sometimes violently to a real or imagined slight or rejection, to be followed by a period of remorse, confusion and despair. Predictably, he was often unemployed, had spent several short periods in prison, and lived alone, as no partner could tolerate his periodic and explosive violent tantrums. After such episodes Mr S would seek help from his doctor, and would bring with him an air of injured dejection and deflation. It was at these times, in a rather piecemeal way, that Dr T learned something of the life of this hurting and hurt man. Mr S had suffered from the most elementary and early of hurts—the loss of both parents before he could remember. An accidental and illegitimate conception, he had spent his childhood from infancy in a variety of threadbare orphanages and, later, borstals. As far back as he could remember, he had been haunted by the fact of his early rejection, and had developed a primitive and only partially conscious notion of others as being untrustworthy and hurtful; a notion which he would spuriously validate for himself by provocation. Ten years previously, following a depressive reaction to one of his destructively cathartic episodes, a local psychiatrist had referred him to a unit specializing in a therapeutic community approach to "psychopaths". To Mr S's further sense of injury, he was rejected for* having "insufficient insight or motivation to make use of the group-therapy approach."

The affray occurring in the waiting room at first involved only the receptionist. Dr T had no appointments left that morning except for "genuine medical emergencies", which did not seem to apply to Mr S, as the receptionist tried patiently to explain to him while offering an appointment that afternoon. The receptionist's positive efforts were rapidly swept away by a rage in Mr S that could not be reasoned with. "I DON'T CARE," he bellowed, "I'VE GOT TO SEE THE F_____ DOCTOR NOW." The doctor, his more routine and polite consultation quickly terminated, and realizing he was dealing with an emergency (even if not "genuinely medical"), entered the waiting room, much to the relief of his rather frightened and confused reception-ist. "You seem to be very upset about something, and if you wait for only about half an hour I'll have some time for you . . ." While saying this the doctor looked directly at Mr S while putting a hand firmly but comfortingly on his shoulder; he felt Mr S instantly stiffen at his first touch, and then yield a second later, as if he suddenly found a sense of trust and acceptance in his doctor.

"I have this terrible feeling doctor, I'm afraid I'll explode, go mad and kill somebody . . . I'm afraid of what I may do . . . I didn't know who else to tell." The doctor, asking Mr S to describe recent events, established that he was reacting, again, to an event which Mr S interpreted as being a personal slight and rejection. It was, in reality, more likely to be the inflexible, but impersonal, bureaucracy of the Social Security Office. After talking for some minutes of the variety and threatening intensity of his feelings, Mr S sat back in his chair exhausted, lost and on the point of tears. Pausing deliberately, Dr T then said quietly: "You know, I imagine that all these feelings you have are the same ones you had when you were a little boy and you felt unloved and that something bad was going to happen to you. I think at those times life really did hurt you in a way you couldn't understand, and all those experiences have led you to thinking that the same kind of things are happening to you now, even when they're not ... and then *you get all those old feelings crowding in on you. That desperate and unhappy little boy in you wakes up, and cries out, and starts fighting for his life . . ."*

*"That's true, that's exactly how I feel . .. But what can I do, doctor?" replied an attentive and thoughtful Mr S.*

*"Well, what would the 'grown-up you' want to say to the 'little boy you', knowing what he does?"*

*"I see what you mean ... I've never thought about it like that ... I think I'd like to say to him `You really had it rough and I feel sorry for you ... but you're the past and I mustn't let you run my life now' ... But how can I do that, doctor, I mean when I get upset I just see red and get mad and lose control of myself. I just can't help it ..." Mr S pleaded.*

*Dr T was insistent, if kindly, in his disagreement of this last statement. ''Well, I don't agree that you can't control your actions. You can, but I understand that it's very hard for you and that you may need some help. I have an idea to help you, but it will only work if you want it to, and if you follow my instructions carefully. Will you do that?" he asked, looking at Mr S steadily.*

*"Yes, I will . .. I do want to try something. . ."*

*"What I suggest to you is simple but you must do it properly for it to work. When you feel the beginning of one of your strong feelings of panic or anger you must sit down quietly somewhere and suck one of the tablets I'm going to give you. Suck it and don't swallow it whole; you'll find it has a soothing effect as it goes down, first in your throat and then in your chest and stomach. When you're sitting there I want you to think about what we've been saying, and to have an imaginary talk with that little boy inside you. The tablet will calm you when you're doing this." At this point Dr T reached forward to touch the hand of Mr S briefly but significantly. "I'll give you 40 tablets to begin with and I want you to come and see me at the end of the week to let me know how you are."*

*Dr T's prescription was simple but thoughtfully chosen — a more uncommon antacid/antiflatulent tablet with a pleasant milky flavour.*

*Mr S two weeks later claimed that "those tablets have really done the trick. I know that if I've got them with me and do what you say then I won't get so upset or 'blank out' ... " He returned every few weeks to collect some more tablets and to talk with the doctor who would reinforce Mr S's new patterns and help him, in a piecemeal kind of way, with the thoughts and internal dialogues Mr S discovered, often while sucking. Two years later Dr T's unusual therapy had proved its underlying psychological theory. Mr S had not been radically transformed as a personality but he had sustained those important controls which enabled him to hold a single job for longer than at any previous time and remain free of the kind of violent outbursts that had been his previous hallmark. The price of this was a limited psychological dependence on his doctor and his antacid tablets.*

## Comment and Conclusion

There are a number of principles and metaphors we may use to describe and explain how this doctor made effective and sophisticated use of the most basic therapeutic tools.

He recognized that the disturbance in Mr S was occurring at an early child, even infantile, level of his mind, and that his communications had to be made accordingly. Reasoning, threatening or bargaining with Mr S's "grown up" part had been tried many times before and never with success. On the hypothesis that the outwardly aggressive Mr S harboured an inwardly frightened child reacting to some fantasized danger, Dr T knew that he must quickly make an alliance or rapport in a way that was both age and feeling appropriate. The careful choice of touch, simple words and eye- contact were designed to engender feelings of security and inclusion in Mr S, who was previously feeling alienated and turbulent.

It was not enough for Mr S to be "tranquillized" in this way only while receiving Dr T's attentions. His life had to be lived outside the consulting room, and Dr T had to find a way of helping his patient take with him an internalized representation of the doctor, which he would re-evoke at crucial times of stress and threat. Common notions of hypnotism usually call to mind formal procedures of trance-formation, but hypnotic suggestions may be made in ways far more various and subtle, as much recent work indicates (Brander and Grindler, 1975). Dr T's deliberate emphasis of certain words, pausing at certain times and touching Mr S when he wished to make a particular impact, were all ways of "anchoring" his message, of making a lasting hypnotic-association and imprint (Brandler and Grindler, 1979).

Long after the infant has drawn nourishment from his mother's breast, he continues to draw a sense of comfort and security from the use of his mouth, particularly when sucking. The persistence of this need into adulthood is often masked, channelled and ritualized, but remains ubiquitous. Dr T used this most natural of tranquillizers very directly in his choice of a white, sweet "sucking" medicine, and in doing so also took the opportunity to reinforce and anchor his earlier (hypnotic) suggestion.

As we grow into early childhood we have, increasingly, to learn to live without mother's omnipresence and undivided attention. This difficult process of separation is often accompanied by various manifestations of fear, protest and anger on the child's part, and he may often turn to an inanimate object as a source of solace. Teddy-bears, dummies, blankets are all familiar "transitional objects" (Winnicott, 1958), helping the child face the unknown outside world. The child confers on the object special powers that once belonged only to mother. This need, too, persists into adulthood and is likely to become more intense in periods of stress and loss, where those much earlier feelings of peril and aloneness are reawakened. All three cases described illustrate the process where the doctor's medicine had become a kind of transitional object. Mr D (Case No 2) faced his last years accompanied, not by a loved-one by his side, but by a tub of cream into which he projected loving qualities; a rather sad substitute, perhaps, but one which brought him great comfort.

In the film *The Wizard of Oz* the young heroine, Dorothy, believing in the Wizard's powers, finds resources and courage in herself with which to confront the Wicked Witch of the West. She does not know, at first, that the Wizard is only an ordinary man with no more power than she; it is her belief in him which enables her to face those things she would have previously fled from. These principles, too, lay behind the successful placebo-effect in all three cases, and are well substantiated by experimental evidence (Lesse, 1962; Black, 1966; Silverstone and Turner, 1974).

The last principle I wish to outline is quite as important in practice. In the cases described, the practitioners entered into their patients' mental world, in an intuitive and empathic manner, before confidently prescribing the placebo. Recent investigators (Balint and Norell, 1972) described what they termed 'The Flash' in the medical interview where the doctor, leaving behind the usual protocol and ritual, is freer to understand the inner and existential dilemma behind his patient's presenting complaints. While this often seems an essential component of successful placebo prescription so, too, is the skilled application of principles of how the child's mind develops (developmental psychology), and how this "child-residue" is manifest and operating in the adult (psychodynamics and psychopathology). This is particularly so when dealing with the kind of character problems illustrated by Mr S. The other two cases, depicting some kind of life crisis amidst periods of rapid change and loss, but against a background of otherwise stable personality structure, are undoubtedly easier to deal with but involve similar qualities of interest, flexibility, dexterity and genuineness from the practitioner. It is interesting to note that these seem to be the most important elements of effective psychotherapy generally (Truax *et al.*, 1966). Some practitioners might object that such endeavours are too time consuming to be practical. It is noteworthy, however, that even the relatively complex but crucial interview with Mr S took a little over 25 minutes. Dr T would probably have spent more time and energy dealing with the repercussions, had he refused to see his desperate but accessible patient.

Others might balk at the very idea of placebos, all too frequently used ineffectively and crudely as an act of blind, simplistic reassurance or, worse, a cynical and deceptive "quick trick" to get rid of a "troublesome" patient, under the guise of being helpful. However the intention and (lack of) scientific basis lying beneath such patterns of practice are quite different from the three cases described, where the process of diagnosis and selection was of quite a different order; they should not be confused.

In an age obsessed with increasingly complex technological activity and accompanying official (often vacuous) slogans such as "The Treatment of the Mentally Ill in the Community" it is often a valuable challenge to re-examine and develop those more intimate and human skills that, despite protean fashions in technology, remain a cornerstone of practice. Healing involves far more than physical engineering. The placebo effect serves well as an example.

$$\Omega$$

## References

Balint, M. (1957) *The Doctor, his Patient and the Illness.* London: Pitman.
-- (1970) *Treatment or Diagnosis. A Study of Repeat Prescriptions in General Practice.* London: Tavistock.
--& Norrell, J. S. (eds., 1972) *Six Minutes for the Patient.* London: Tavistock Publications.
Bandler, R. & Grindler, J. (1975) *The Structure of Magic I & II.* Science & Behaviour Books.
-- (1979) *Frogs into Princes.* Utah: Real People Press.
Beecher, H. (1955) The powerful placebo. *Journal of the American Medical Association,* 159, 1602-1606.
Benson, H. & McCallie, D. P. Jr. (1979) Angina pectoris and the placebo effect. *New England Journal of Medicine,* 300, 1424-1429.
Berne, E. (1961) *Transactional Analysis in Psychotherapy.* New York: Grove Press.
Black, A. A. (1966) Factors predisposing to a placebo response in new patients with anxiety states. *British Journal of Psychiatry,* 112, 557-567.
Doongaji, D. R., Vahia, V. N., Bharucha, M. P. (1978) On placebo responses and placebo responders. A review of psychological, psycho-pharmacological and psychophysiological factors I & II. *Journal of the Postgraduate Medical Association,* 24, 91-97; 147-157.
Guntrip, H. (1964) *Healing the Sick Mind.* London: Allen & Unwin.
Harlow, H. F. & Harlow, M. K. (1966) Learning to love. *American Scientist,* 54, 244-272.
Lesse, S. (1962) Placebo reactions in psychotherapy. *Diseases of the Nervous System,* 23, 313-319.
Pearson, R. M. (1982) Who is taking their tablets? *British Medical Journal,* 285, 757-758.
Parkin, D. M., Henney, C. R., Quirk, J. & Crooks, J. (1976) Deviation from prescribed drug treatment after discharge from hospital. *British Medical Journal,* 2, 686688.
Silverston, T. & Turner, P. (1974) *Drug Treatment in Psychiatry.* London: Routledge & Kegan Paul.
Spitz, R. (1945) Hospitalism. Genesis of psychiatric conditions in early childhood. *Psychoanalytic Study of the Child,* 1, 53-74.

Truax, C. B., Wargo, D. G., Frank, J. D. *et al.* (1966) Therapist empathy, genuineness and warmth and patient therapeutic outcome. *Journal of Consulting Psychology,* 22, 331-334.
Winnicott, D. W. (1958) *Collected Papers.* London: Tavistock Publications.

Publ. in *British Journal of Holistic Medicine*, December 1984

# Physician Heal Thyself

## The Paradox of the Wounded Healer

The 'caring professions' suffer from higher levels of psychological morbidity, suicide and marital breakdown than many other social groups. The reasons for these excesses are explored. A model taken from transactional analysis is used to describe the *malignant symbiosis* that may develop between doctor and patient as the result of the doctor's background, upbringing and medical training. Suggestions are made as to how the re-thinking of medical attitudes towards patients, but even more so towards doctors themselves, might help to prevent the syndrome of the 'wounded healer'. The integration of the 'masculine' and 'feminine' aspects of the doctor's make-up is essential in this regard.

*'The stoical scheme of supplying our wants by lopping off our desires, is like cutting off our feet, when we want shoes.'*

Jonathan Swift, Thoughts on Various Subjects (1711)

Those who care for others, out of vocation or compulsion, often have difficulties in caring for themselves. Doctors are notoriously 'bad' patients, and the doctor who is required to help a sick colleague is likely to be himself confused and distressed by the complex tangle of feelings and distorted communications that follow. In the last two decades there have been many interesting, though ominous, studies on the morbidity and troubles of doctors. Perhaps the most striking data concern suicide statistics. All the studies concur in demonstrating a rate of suicide among doctors that is at least double that of the rest of the population (Rose and Rostow, 1973; Editorial, 1974). It is significantly higher than comparable economic and 'non-helping' professional classes. Among hospital doctors, the highest rate is found amongst psychiatrists, followed by physicians, surgeons and, finally, paediatricians (Blackley *et al.*, 1968; Rich and Pitts, 1980). Studies from the USA imply that psychiatrists, overall, are more likely to commit suicide than their patients.

In concurrence with suicide, the rate of drug abuse and marital breakdown amongst doctors is similarly high (A'Brook *et al.*, 1967; Vincent *et al.*, 1969; Editorial, 1970; Vaillant *et al.*, 1970; Emschwiller, 1973). Quite as important, though less easy to measure, is the common tragedy of 'marital dry-rot'. By this I mean the marriage that has atrophied in terms of emotional closeness, intimacy, and enriched sharing. As with the dry-rotted timber, the outward form may remain, but the underlying strength and substance has eroded – collapse or crumbling is a matter of time. *McCall's Magazine*, with its own brand of journalistic prophylaxis, warned its readers in an article entitled' Never Marry a Doctor' that 'Physicians are poor husbands, poor fathers, absent companions, prima donnas and about as useless in bed as an electric blanket when the power is cut off'.

Other studies are equally illuminating in filling the pattern. Doctors are more likely to break down than others, but usually do so in ways that are private and socially obedient; the formal diagnoses describing the doctor's difficulties are expressed in terms of *neurotic depression* rather than *schizophrenia* or *personality disorder* (Duffy and Litin, 1964; Editorial, 1967; Murray, 1977). They are less likely to be convicted of crimes of violence, burglary and causing an affray. Clearly, even in illness and distress, the doctor's exemplary persona remains intact. Doctors' frequent but concealed alcoholism repeats this theme (Vaillant *et al.*, 1972). Typically the problems will be borne and hidden by his colleagues and family, but the wider community will be left in peace.

## Humanising the data

What can we infer from such statistics? It seems that doctors, together with others in the caring professions, are relatively incapable of acknowledging or allowing themselves the frailties they may look after so assiduously in others. When it comes to a crisis in our own lives, there are many doctors who prefer to be seen dead (literally) than in any way compromised, dependent or weak. Our armour of assumed omniscience and omnipotence has taken years to develop and is hard to discard. Many of us have developed a compulsive persona of exemplary independence, strength and rationality which we are both ashamed of and afraid to relinquish. Regression is for patients, not doctors. Both the structure and nature of many medical transactions and rituals create the illusion, and then conserve, the doctor's executive and emotional power. The medical model itself, with its didactic style of defining health, normality, sanity, pathology and therapy, is clearly a major vehicle in this authoritarian circus (Zigmond, 1976; 1977).

Clearly, it is not only as individuals that we suffer and perpetuate this dilemma. We collude together to minimise, conceal or deny these problems. The ethos of the stiff-upper-lip and coping-at-all costs is learned (by imitation and taboo) early in our training. It is ubiquitous, and played extremely hard, particularly in hospitals. How many of us have allowed ourselves to be openly depressed and comforted by a colleague? We are much more likely to maintain a stoical and inscrutable front and urge others to do likewise – unless they are patients, of course.

From my own experience, and from what other doctors have told me in psychotherapy, workshops or friendships, I can only deduce that there is a tacit and severe conspiracy of silence regarding this painful area. Traditionally, and still prevalently, the lack of emotional rapport and support within the caring professions is paradoxical but gross. Our expectations of ourselves and others to remain strong and intact, whatever the conditions, are unyielding, and frequently far exceed the conduct required for humane and competent clinical practice. Default from this Spartan code is allowed only in ritualized and contained settings. Publicly and manically it surfaces in the beer-saturated mess party. With more secrecy and restraint – commonly if the doctor is a psychiatrist – it appears in the framework of psychotherapy which can, in any case, be claimed as 'part of his training'. However, in many ways what he is doing is stealing away to a special place where, in total privacy, someone will listen to, and accept, the vulnerable, dependent and sometimes violent parts of himself. He is paying someone to respond to him as a permissive and feeling person. It is remarkable and ironic how other groups who claim no expertise or particular concern about human suffering, such as ourselves, cope with it so much better in their own groups. The emotional support, accommodation and latitude that people allow one another in shops, industrial organisations and so forth, frequently outstrip our equivalent performance and attitudes within the caring professions. The following account illustrates the tragic nature of such collusive and defensive responses.

## The case of Dr X

*Dr X was a junior hospital psychiatrist who started his first post in this specialty at the same time as myself. He had only just arrived in this country from the Middle East, had no family or friends here, and was resident in the hospital. As a late recruit to medicine he was in his mid-thirties, despite his junior status. His manner at work was tense, obsessional, earnest and very introverted. He seemed an extremely lonely man, who spent his off-duty time either studying or impassively watching television in the Doctors' Mess.*

*Over the months he became increasingly capricious, prickly and withdrawn. Nursing staff became uneasy with his odd and irascible behaviour with patients. On one occasion he sprinkled a patient with water while chanting from the Koran, explaining to an attendant nurse that 'the patient's being would be made pure'. This was followed by his writing a long, untrue and defamatory account about another doctor in a patient's case notes. Largely to satisfy the nursing staff's insecurity, it was decided that Dr X's clinical responsibility should be undertaken by another doctor. However, this was done in an oblique manner, so that Dr X was not confronted directly with the concern that was felt about him, and he continued official tenure of his post. This strategy seemed designed to 'paper over the cracks' so that no one needed to encounter the alienated and unstable Dr X until his contract had expired.*

*At this point I asked to see Dr Y, the senior consultant at the hospital. Although inexperienced, I was clear in my view that this approach was not only confusing and jeopardising to patient care, but that Dr X's increasing paranoia and depression required more in the way of concern, compassion and confrontation. I said that, for fear of encountering him in this way, Dr X was being treated with duplicity, and this fed into his sense of mistrust, powerlessness and alienation. It would be far better, I suggested, openly to acknowledge his painful and serious difficulties, to relieve him of his work in a decisive and kindly-parental way, and find him help outside the hospital. Dr Y's response was authoritarian, defensive and dismissive. I was made to feel that such a breach of conspiracy of silence was inept, impudent and unethical. I was sent on my way. Dr X, soon after, died from a suicidal overdose while still an employee of the hospital. It is doubtful that this man would have died amidst these circumstances in any other than a 'caring' profession. He would have received help.*

## Doctors' dilemmas

Doctors in clinical practice are confronted by some of the most private, primitive and powerful experiences that can be shared with another. Consider the following perennial situations that many of us become seasoned to:

Mr A has cancer and he does not know. What should I say? Shall I tell him, or if not he, his wife?

Mrs B's condition warrants my exploring her vagina and rectum.

Mr D has had ulcerative colitis for 10 years. I think he should now have his colon removed and be left with a life-long ileostomy.

I will not resuscitate Mr E. The probable quality of his future existence seems unworthwhile to me.

I don't understand Mrs F's sexual problem. I shall ask her about her masturbatory fantasies.

Although Mrs G. denies any problem, does not want treatment and has committed no crime, I postulate a mental illness, which puts her at risk. I will have her taken to an institution and treated against her will.

Each of these cameos is dramatic or devastating for the patient, but paradoxically commonplace for the doctor. Being crucial and decisive for our patients, our licensed tools and protocols are correspondingly powerful and dangerous. In consequence we can only use them legitimately if we are, or at least seem to be:

- strong
- patient
- worldly
- sagacious
- unselfish
- responsible
- impressively knowledgeable
- highly ethical and scrupulous
- uncorrupted by power, aggression, sexuality and greed
- always intact and alert to the most demanding and diverse situations.

Conversely in the face of such demands we cannot be:

- demanding for ourselves when others need us
- unable to face what is there
- uncomprehending
- self-indulgent
- indecisive
- ignorant
- weak.

Such formidable requirements tend to involve 'blocking-out', or at least controlling to an extreme degree, natural feelings and actions that would otherwise emerge. Disgust, fear or overwhelming sadness may be spontaneous, healthy and authentic reactions to situations that are unsavoury, offensive or tragic. The doctor's armour of detachment and continence is necessary – at least in part – if he is to get on with the job. The desensitising effect in doctors by constant exposure to pain, distress, tragedy and horror has yet to be studied in depth, but I believe it frequently to lead to a kind of emotional anaesthesia or woodenness. It may be impossible to remain a vulnerable, feeling or spontaneous person when subject to years of these kinds of demands and controls. Perhaps doctors become hardened and petrified in the same way as professional soldiers. The effect it has on intimate relationships is then, predictable, for, above all, intimacy derives from spontaneity, emotional expressiveness and accessibility. It is not possible to be close to someone who is relentlessly sensible and responsible. They may seem more, but are really less, than human.

## Transactional analysis; an organising language

I want here to divert briefly, and present in an extremely simplified form, the concept of 'ego-states' from transactional analysis, as my further points can be illustrated more succinctly using this language.

An ego-state is a system of thinking, feeling and behaving, all of which are interlinked. We all have three ego-states, although in each of us the content and strength of each ego-state will be different. The three ego-states are called *Parent, Adult* and *Child*. The content of the Child is largely complete by the time we are eight years old; Parent and Adult by adolescence.

The Parent develops from what we are *taught* by actual parents and other influential adults. It derives not only from what we are told explicitly, but also from what we observe them doing. The Parent is thus the seat of both *nurturing* and *controlling* impulses and behaviour, whether to ourselves or others. Subjectively our Parent feels protective or critical, and has the conviction of *knowing* what is correct and ethical, even when we might be mistaken. Generally, when we are in our Parent, we feel secure, and relate from a one-up position of 'right' and strength.

The Child, reciprocally, is the world of experiences and derivative thoughts and feelings that we had as children and re-experience and re-enact now. It has all the qualities of the unfettered natural child, as well as the child that has learned to adapt to survive amidst more powerful grown-ups. The Natural Child is fun-loving, pleasure-seeking, pain-hating, emotionally labile, demanding, impulsive, spontaneous, creative, curious, sexual, unashamed, greedy and loving. This part of us believes in magic, and may feel either omnipotent or completely helpless, just as we all did as small children. It is the part of us that shares and experiences with vividness and immediacy, and is thus the spring of our capacity for vitality and intimacy. As children, however, we had both to be socialised and to learn strategies of living with those we are dependent upon, and these dependent patterns of compliance or rebellion make up the Adapted Child. We relate here from a feeling of being 'one down', by justification, appeasement, rebellion or struggle.

The Adult is the reality principle in the personality. It is capable of observing, assessing, storing and patterning information in an objective way. It can turn these logical powers externally to the outside world, or internally to monitor and mediate between the other two ego-states. In many ways the Adult may be seen to function like a computer. For simplicity we can represent these personality functions diagrammatically (Figure la).

Fig. 1a—The three ego states. P = Parent—controlling, critical, nurturing, "one-up". A = Adult—Problem solving, logical, objective. C = Child—spontaneous, feeling, needy, creative, vulnerable, adapting to others, "one-down".

## The doctor's personality

In the preceding sections I have reviewed both how doctors take better care of others' needs than their own, and how the nature of their work calls on them to be uncompromisingly 'grown-up' in their conduct. Using the ego-state model it seems that doctors' personality structure and function is confined largely to the Parent and Adult. We may spend our lives looking after those who are sick or compromised, and consider ourselves expert in knowing what is 'good for' others. Many of us pride ourselves on our accurate observation, fund of factual knowledge and problem-solving ability. What we are often out of touch with is our Child. The world of chaos, irrationality, strong feelings, spontaneity and vulnerability is kept strongly in check, if not denied and defended against, by our Parent and Adult ego systems. Such armour may at first serve as a protection, but such security is bought at the price of inaccessibility and shutting out the joy and intimacy that keeps us vital. A diagram of this process is illustrated in Figure 1b.

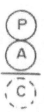

FIG. 1b—The doctor's personality. Strong Parent and Adult but blocked or atrophied Child.

## Symbiosis – helping the needy and needing the helpless

When we deny powerful needs or impulses in ourselves, we will either be intolerant or compulsively solicitous of these attributes in others. If it is the latter, then we can professionalize this problem by working in one of the caring professions. In this area we have licence to seek out and look after the part in other people that we disown or suppress in ourselves. Our needs may then be fulfilled, in an illusory and vicarious way, through a state of mutual dependence. Such an interlocked relationship may be diagrammed as in Figure 2, and may be termed 'symbiotic'. Symbiosis may be thought of as 'benign' when our own needs are peripheral to 'helping the needy'. Conversely, 'malignant' symbiosis is enacted when our own needs become more central, and we are then 'needing the helpless'.

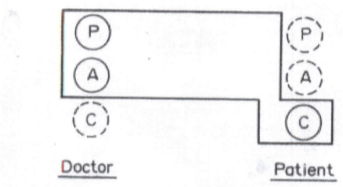

FIG. 2—Symbiosis in the doctor–patient relationship.

There is a tacit contract here, where the doctor's part reads:

- 'I will be strong if you will be weak.
- I will be sane/sober/logical/continent if you will be mad/drunk/confused/miscreant.
- I will support, guide and protect you so long as you are helpless and obedient.
- I will not express my feelings or difficulties, so you must have and enact them for me'.

Reciprocally, the patient's role in such a collusion reads:

'If you will be my Grown-up then I will make you feel potent, clever and important (or, not infrequently, the opposite). To make sure that is so, I will be passive, aimless and dependent'.

Such dependence upon our patients for our sense of power, self-esteem, worthiness and vicarious expression of locked-up feeling is often not conscious. In the semi-conscious or deeply unconscious mind there are frequently complexes of guilt, and the need for reparation, stemming from our earliest experiences where, in a primitive and irrational manner, we created inordinate notions of the damage we might have done or might still do. Compulsive and malignantly symbiotic patterns of help then represent a ritualistic undoing of the feared damage, but it is an impotent undoing which is never finished and must be repeated endlessly. In the short term this kind of 'helpfulness' may be harmless. The long-term effects, however, may be similar to many other relationships which are based upon rigidity and a radically unequal power distribution. Because attachment and gratification of both partners depends on a rigid status quo where no growth is possible, a sense of entrapment, waste and resentment is likely to evolve. In the interim, it may account for many harried, irritated and depressed doctors who are uncomprehendingly or unconsciously dependent on their patients' dependence. The end point of this process is the unnecessarily infantilised or institutionalised patient and the seriously damaged, or prematurely dead, doctor.

## The making and breaking of doctors

The factors that motivate us to become doctors are often those which later lead to the kind of stoical and compulsive unhappiness I have outlined. In this section I shall discuss briefly the kind of family and social backgrounds that make a radical and pervasive contribution to these difficulties.

Altruism, caring and empathic concern for others in distress are clearly ingredients of the most humane and proficient practice, and involve only benign symbiotic attachments, which is a necessary, if temporary, arrangement while dealing with distress and disability. It is the malignant symbiotic patterns that stem from the doctor's personal difficulties and lead, via his defences of workaholism, perfectionism and stoicism, to the even greater difficulties I have reviewed. In a general sense such doctors are likely to have grown up with the notion that it is forbidden, disadvantageous or damaging for them to express their feelings, make demands or be vulnerable, although they may be permissible or even expected in others. The reasons for this can, of course, vary from implicit social class mores to particular family circumstances. As an example of the latter, the following case history serves as an example:

## The case of George

*George is a physician in his mid-forties. He sought help originally when things were clearly going wrong in his life. In spite of his outward success, good professional standing and apparently stable family life, he experiences his existence in terms of deadness, hollowness, edginess, joylessness and inauthenticity. Clinically his problems might be described in terms of 'anxiety', 'depression' and an underlying 'obsessive-compulsive personality'. In more ordinary terms he is a man who works inordinately hard, is never satisfied with the work he has done, fears (unrealistically) any criticism from his colleagues or patients, and finds it almost impossible to assert himself or differentiate himself from others' expectations and wishes. His way of relating is thus usually either appeasing or reparative, but in being so, he accumulates much in the way of resentment with others (for their dominance), self-hatred and poor self-esteem (for his acquiescence) and alienation (from his inauthenticity). These consequences are expressed at home, where he becomes depressed, irritable and demanding, and periodically explosive with anger. His attempt to escape his passive-aggressive cycles via alcohol merely amplifies his problems of guilt, remorse, liability and despairing confusion. The effect on his marriage is seriously damaging and needs no further elaboration here.*

*George was born shortly before the outbreak of the Second World War. It is possible that his parents were never really happy together. Soon after his birth, his father was conscripted into the forces and saw little of his wife or son in the next six years. Even after the war the pattern continued in a similar way, as father was often away from home travelling in his work. George's mother was an unhappy and lonely woman who sought from her little boy not just the love expected from a son, but also the unavailable love she craved from an absent or unloving husband. During her lonely war years she took the boy into her bed, and when he was old enough to 'understand' she confided in him about her unhappiness with father.*

*By the time he was six years old, George had formed the decision that mother's stability, love and happiness depended upon his ministering to her. Family triangulations and oedipal conflicts are difficult to resolve even in less exceptional circumstances, but for George there was the added misery of inexorable and increasing alienation from father. Hardly surprisingly, father experienced the intense bond between his wife and son as an alliance against him, and indeed it was true that the closeness of these two depended on keeping father 'bad' or distant. The dilemma of the little boy was that he had to suppress his own feelings and needs and subsume these to another's, but that in doing so he necessarily drove father away or invoked his hostility. 'I just couldn't do the right thing; I couldn't make them happy' George recalls tearfully some forty years later, and it was certainly true that the task this little boy saw for himself was quite beyond his resources or understanding, or powers of influence. And yet he felt responsible and had to keep trying to find a solution.*

*He cannot remember now when he decided to become a doctor, but he does remember some of the thoughts that went with the decision. He would imbue himself with the powers of healing, but, in so doing, people would be genuinely grateful and thankful. Unlike his family (where he felt compelled to 'heal' his mother but felt bound to fail and instead collect feelings of guilt, fear and inadequacy) as a grown-up healer – a doctor – he would be potent, respected and unassailable.*

*Little George's compensatory and reparative fantasy has had very different consequences in grown-up reality. Not only did he not make mother and father happy or loving but, inevitably, some of his patients didn't get better. Often they seemed ungrateful, and occasionally they blamed him even when he knew it wasn't his fault. He responded with the same mixture of guilt, resentment and fear he had as a young boy, and tried harder. The characters and backcloth changed, but the theme has remained the same. George's malignant symbiosis with his patients can be seen as his attempt to solve archaic, and probably insoluble, problems within his family, but also, by identification with his patients, to get for himself the love, care and acceptance that were lacking for him. He compulsively gives to others what he has yearned for himself. In the long term, however, this route becomes a cul-de-sac, offering no real satisfaction or resolution. George's symptoms have signalled as much, and it has only been since he has been tackling and expressing his needs, wants and hurts more directly, and for himself, that he has begun to leave them behind. He has realised that charity must begin at home.*

George's difficulties and their origins are, in my experience, fairly typical of the common syndrome of the *Wounded Healer*. Others have remarked on how doctors and psychotherapists tended to have had significantly depressed mothers eg Storr, 1979) which led them not only to an empathic understanding of this in others, but also, less helpfully, to a compulsive need to sacrifice the self in 'helping'. Apart from the current of guilt that underlies this impasse, there are other components of this syndrome which damage and distort our self-esteem. In seeing our lives in terms of what we offer to others, often in a very confined and ritualistic form, we do not value ourselves for what we really are, but only what we *do*. Such a central dissatisfaction with ourselves may account for much of our motivation in seeking out the compromised parts of others. In this symbolic union, we imagine, we can allay our own loneliness and sense of incompleteness. The cruel and inescapable truth, however, is more often the reverse. It is only through loving ourselves that we can enact creatively an authentic and discriminating love of others.

We need also to consider the way in which our social and class backgrounds contribute to these patterns. Doctors have traditionally been recruited from the middle and upper classes, particularly those which have a strong parental ethic. There is a tendency for this section of society to pride itself on knowing best what is 'good for' other members of society. We take the *Times, Telegraph* or *Guardian;* our experience of the world (and often the world itself) is for organisation, edification and improvement – not enjoyment. It is not only doctors, of course, who emerge from this patriarchal mould. We produce a plethora of other parental types: lawyers, clergy, captains of industry and politicians. We are prepared early for these tasks. How many of us can remember being told prematurely to 'grow up', 'don't be silly' or 'to be more responsible' when we were not yet eight years old, and childhood with all its tumult and selfishness should have been our right? Later, this false and precocious acceleration into adulthood may have been compounded even further by education in public schools, with its essential ingredients of rules, responsibilities, hierarchies and titles. In such environments, our emotional life or private world is regarded as a hindrance or aberration, deflecting or subtracting from our more important public performance. We thus become more oriented to achievement than experience; what we *are* is important only in so far as it is expressed in what we *do*. The 'masculine' nature of such cultures has a particularly inhibiting effect on the feeling, vulnerable 'feminine' side of ourselves.

I remember at the age of eleven standing alone with my 'tuck-box' on the station platform, awaiting the steam train to take me to boarding school. I was fighting back the fear and the tears, and trying bravely to look grown-up. Like George, I developed this concealment over the years, to become a 'false self'. Ultimately, it has needed dismantling before I could excavate and pay attention to the buried Child within me. Here, too, charity has had to begin at home.

## Physician heal thyself – but how?

Official recognition of the disturbed doctor who may be a liability to his patient represents only a surface layer of a problem which, as I have outlined, is extensive and complex. Public concern about this problem has led, in recent years, to the implementation of the 'three wise men' whose task it was to assess, caution, make recommendations to, and sometimes discipline, the aberrant doctor. However, such a 'casualty department' approach, even if doing a little to protect the public, has little impact on the underlying and seemingly ubiquitous difficulties: these have their roots in deep-seated emotional problems and social mores.

The teaching of psychiatry via a medical-model didactic type of approach is now a well-established discipline conveyed to medical students. More recent, and less developed, is the introduction of the teaching of the psychology of the patient or the person who is ill. What is lacking in both of these approaches is any significant consideration of the doctor and his psychology and distress patterns. It is somehow assumed that these problems do not exist, or are insufficiently important to merit teaching time and expertise, or that somehow the doctor will muddle through successfully. Clearly, the facts indicate otherwise.

All creative acts can be interpreted in terms of some kind of psychopathology. Compensation, identification, projection, denial, escape and sublimation are some of the technical words we might use to describe the mechanisms lying behind many endeavours. The fact that a young person is prepared to spend many arduous years training to license himself for the lifelong task of involving himself with unknown persons' distress is, on the surface, a perverse choice and likely to be based, at least in part, on such covert forces. Yet it would be wrong to assume that these kinds of motivations need necessarily be problematic or pathological in practice. Very real gifts and predispositions for caring and empathy may arise from such factors in ourselves. Indeed, it is probably not possible to develop a humane and compassionate resonance with another unless we have some identification with them. We have to have faced similar pains, losses, conflicts or needs ourselves. The important point is that we are both aware, and in control, of these forces within us. By doing so we convert a liability into a gift.

Yet the medical educational establishments whose task it should be to help the medical student or young doctor successfully navigate these dilemmas and transitions fails to realise either the presence or significance of this task. By concentrating solely on the 'masculine', scientific, organisational and didactic aspects of the doctor's role, medical education falls short of being an 'education' and remains a 'training' – a constriction or moulding into the required role. What is lacking in this process is the more 'feminine', nurturing approach, where experience is accepted and understood at a more feeling level. It is only via this more candid and allowing attitude that the developing doctor will find himself in an environment where he can successfully engage and transcend what will otherwise become a series of impasses which become translated into the kinds of stoical, insensitive or malignantly symbiotic patterns of lifestyle and practice we have considered.

There are practical ways of achieving this. From the first day at the dissection table, medical teachers should consider it part of their task to encourage students to talk about their attitudes, feelings and problems. Clinical teachers should share with their students the difficulties they encounter in, for example, caring for the incurable, the inexorably dependent and the dying, or making mistakes! They might enlighten the students too, in discussing with them the human resources they have had to develop to deal creatively with these situations. Integrated into the curriculum, alongside the more formal and traditional teaching, there should be seminars or discussion groups where personal disclosure and interaction about these issues would be skilfully and sensitively encouraged. Many clinical teachers might, at first, be threatened by this requirement that they become humanistic as well as technical teachers. They might feel that self-disclosure would be undermining and would diminish their position of respect and authority. My own experience has been opposite to this. The teacher who can share his difficulties and humanity while remaining a master of his craft grows in the esteem of others and serves as a model as to how these things may be reconciled.

It is clear that many young and established doctors have needed, and will continue to need, professional help for the problems that are likely to emerge within them in the course of their careers. As I have demonstrated, this is to be expected as a natural consequence, at least sometimes, of the nature of ourselves and our work. It should carry no more stigma or alarm than the football player who needs physiotherapy to relieve his pain and heal him so he may again be competent for his task.

I have not said anything about the kind of social mores and public expectations of doctors, which feed into how the doctor feels he should be and compound his individual difficulties. This would require a separate article of equal length. However, I would anyway urge us to desist from this large and formidable task of analysis and intervention until we have our own house in order. We are, of course, already proudly 'expert' in defining what is wrong with others and what they should do.

Charity begins at home; physician heal thyself.

Ω

## References

A'Brook, M.F. Hailstone, J. D. & McLaughlin, E. J. (1967) Psychiatric illness in the medical profession. *British Journal of Psychiatry*, 113, 1013-1023.

Blackley, P.H., Disher, W. & Rodmer, G. (1968) Suicide by physicians. *Bulletin of Suicidology*, 1-18.

Duffy, J.C. & Litin, E.M. (1964) Psychiatric morbidity of physicians. *Journal of the American Medical Association*, 189, 989-992.

Editorial (1967) Emotional illness in physicians. *Medical Tribune* (March 29), 1.

— (1970) Drug abuse. Growing occupational hazard for doctors. *Hospital Physician*, 6, 60.

— (1974) Suicide among physicians. *Journal of the American Medical Association*, 228, 1149-1150.

Emschwiller, J. (1973) Doctors still drink too much and pop too many pills. *Medical Times*, 101, 58-61.

Murray, R.M. (1976) Characteristics and prognosis of alcoholic doctors. *British Medical Journal*, 2, 1537-1539. [Not referenced in the article]

— (1977) Psychiatric illness in male doctors and controls: an analysis of Scottish hospitals in-patient data. *British Journal of Psychiatry*, 131, 1-10.

Rich, C.L. & Pitts, F.N. Jr. (1980) Suicide by psychiatrists: a study of the medical specialists among 18,730 consecutive deaths during a five year period 1967-72. *Journal of Clinical Psychiatry*, 41, 261-263.

Rose, K.D. & Rostow, I. (1973) Physicians who kill themselves. *Archives of General Psychiatry*, 29, 800-805.

Storr, A. (1979) *The Art of Psychotherapy*. London: Heinemann.

Valliant, G.E., Brighton, J.R. & McCarthur, C. (1970) Physicians' use of mood-altering drugs. *New England Journal of Medicine,* 283, 365-370.

Valliant, G.E., SobowallL, N.C. & McArthur, C. (1972) Some psychological vulnerabilities of physicians. *New England Journal of Medicine,* 287, 372-375.

Vincent, M.O., Robinson, E.A. & Lave, L. (1969) Physicians as patients. *Canadian Medical Association Journal,* 100, 403-412.

Zigmond, D. (1976) The medical model, its limitations and alternatives. *Hospital Update* (August), 424-427.

— (1977) Scientific psychiatry: progress or regress? *Update* (October), 675-679.

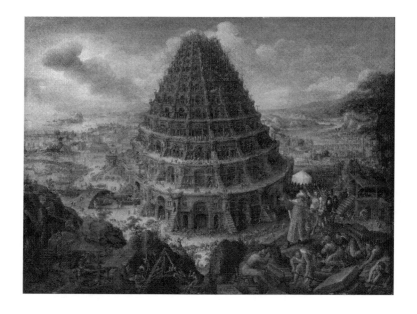

Master van Valckenborg the Elder – *The Tower of Babel* 1595

# Babel or Bible?

## Order, Chaos and Creativity in Psychotherapy

*The quest for certainty blocks the search for meaning.*
*Uncertainty is the very condition to impel Man to unfold his powers.*

Erich Fromm, *Man for Himself,* 1947

Several years ago, an intelligent and troubled friend of mine – I shall call her Carol – then in her mid-twenties, was sent to a psychiatrist because of worsening symptoms of depression. She remembers him as a kind, fatherly man who asked her a comprehensive range of questions to survey her symptoms, life and dilemmas. Before she left, he informed her of his view that her pattern of distress would be 'best treated by psychotherapy', and that he would make arrangements accordingly. Carol, although a bright and educated young woman, came from a background largely alien to matters psychological and introspective. Her parents, pragmatic Northerners from an industrial city, represented a culture and way of thinking very different from the psychodynamically sophisticated psychiatrist she encountered; she did not know what psychotherapy was and he, perhaps unwittingly, did not explore this gulf between them. It was several weeks before Carol received a standardised letter from the hospital, telling her of an appointment with Dr L, a psychotherapist, in four months' time.

By the time Carol went to see Dr L her most troublesome depressive symptoms had largely subsided, perhaps due to medication she had been prescribed. She was, however, left with a churning, ineffable dis-ease inside her, which became heightened on the day of her appointment; the fantasy of her imminent meeting with Dr L produced an added, tense composite of hope and fear. A long period of waiting in a neon lit and threadbare waiting area preceded the appearance of Dr L 'Miss Jackson? I am Doctor L. Will you follow me please', was Dr L's sparse greeting. His voice seemed uncompromisingly dry and neutral, Carol thought, as she was led along a corridor and into a small, bare room in which there were two easy chairs. Dr L closed the door behind them and silently gestured to one of the chairs, as he sat down himself. A period of silence followed which, for Carol, was unexpected and increasingly uneasy. Her previous encounters with her own doctor and the psychiatrist had been in some ways embarrassing and difficult, but reassuringly structured by the initiative they took in asking questions, and offering explanations and suggestions of various kinds; at those times she had felt encouraged by the elementary support and interest shown to her. Dr L, however, seemed quite different – with the silence growing laden and unnatural, Dr L's gaze felt paralysing to Carol, and, when he turned his eyes to the floor, she felt unaccountably abandoned and unsafe. She had wanted to ask him what she was expected to say or do, but became increasingly anxious that she might be breaking some kind of unspoken code by doing so, although part of her was aware of the irrationality of the notion, Dr L's silence and inaccessibility in the face of her mute need and fear, had turned him, in her mind's eye, into some kind of omniscient and unappeasable giant that she could not now approach directly.

Perhaps ten or fifteen minutes passed in this kind of ominous wilderness before Dr L, shifting slightly in his chair, spoke with dry rhetoric: 'I suppose you're rather angry, but don't know how to express it'. 'Angry, why should I be angry? I just feel rather confused ...' pleaded Carol, disoriented and frustrated, imagining that she had somehow missed her cue, that he demanded some kind of 'correct' response that she had not been able to fathom or, therefore, provide. 'Confusion can be an excellent way of avoiding strong feelings when they seem threatening', came Dr L's reply, authoritative and consummate. 'But I still don't know what you mean. Who am I angry with?' replied Carol, beginning to find some kind of clarity and confidence, perhaps because this silent and inscrutable man was now, at least, speaking to her. 'Perhaps with the hospital who kept you waiting for an appointment so long. And then, again, with me for keeping you outside (in the waiting area) – isn't that what happened in your family, that they kept you "waiting outside", when you were sent to boarding school?'

Carol was slightly taken aback by his knowledge of her; again her fantasies turned to his omniscience, and her sense of his having a secret cache of understanding about her, and a hidden agenda with her, to which she was denied access. Bewildered by these potent images, she retreated to the more tangible suggestion that he made: 'But I understand the NHS system; I know that there are waiting lists for all kinds of services, and that I can't blame anyone for that. Anyway, I have been feeling rather better lately...', said Carol with a mixture of appeasement and defiance. 'Perhaps so, but knowing about things doesn't necessarily make you less angry. Your "feeling better" might also be a way of avoiding angry feelings ,' countered Dr L didactically, but not unkindly.,

Carol felt impotent and at an impasse with Dr L, and the two again lapsed into a silence, as long and uncomfortable as the one which had preceded it.

'I don't think individual psychotherapy would be suitable for you, but I'll see what the possibilities are for a group that you might be able to attend', opined   Dr L: his magisterial manner indicating that their session and relationship were at an end.

Carol sensed, at that time, and a retrospective view indicates her correctness in this, that a group was not what she either needed or wanted. Carol's contact with the hospital was lost.

Carol was not 'damaged' in any obvious or dramatic way by the failure to develop any rapport with Dr L, but she reacted by developing a well-articulated suspiciousness of psychotherapy and its practitioners, which, at its sharper end, had a cynical and truculent edge. The blunter aspect revealed a wariness, more vulnerable and afraid. Her symptoms, so deeply rooted in her first and now current relationships, and her internal representations of these, continued a fluctuating but unresolved course. Only in recent times, after talking with me at length about her experience in particular, and the problematic nature of therapy and therapists in general, has she come to modify and destructure her mistrustful view.

Now, Carol is not the 'easiest' patient; often feeling threatened and hurt, she has developed a formidable capacity to distract by quips, intellectual commentaries and apparent 'insight' which, in fact, conceals from herself and others what she does not want revealed. These strategies were probably even more difficult to counter when Dr L saw her. But she maintains, and I believe her, that even ten years ago she might have been accessible to psychotherapy, had her interview been more geared to making contact rather than interpretations.

Let us shift our focus now from Carol to Dr L and construct a plausible, if hypothetical, understanding of what he was doing. The evidence, of course, is Carol's, but she is a reliable witness with a good memory and, most importantly, the pattern she describes is too frequent and significant for it to be glibly and technically dismissed, as merely a defensive manifestation of patients' difficulties; there is wisdom as much as hostility in the many bad (and good!) jokes about psychotherapists and analysts.

It seems that Dr L's style was prescriptive and didactic in its process. He presumed a well-defined and elaborated model by which to codify and 'understand' Carol's difficulty. So wedded was he to this model that it automatically led to a 'technique', which he immediately applied; rather than slowly establishing a dialogue, he confronted her from the outset by the paradox of non-contact. The purpose of this, presumably, was to deprive Carol of her usual props and strategies, and via the ensuing anxiety to 'make her aware' of her fear, hostility, manipulativeness, or whatever. We may assume that Dr L was working from a psychoanalytic base, where he preconceived Carol's depression as being a consequence of retroflected anger, and that this anger itself is a residuum of her earliest developmental tasks of separating herself from mother, and integrating 'good' and 'bad' objects and feelings. Carol sees now that this kind of understanding has value in making sense of her turbulence, but is certainly not the only, or even the most effective, way of doing so. Other family and social factors have been equally important in leading Carol to her present conflicts and impasse. Dr L seems not to have heeded this, however. It is likely that he was a therapist of precise and rigorous training and strong conviction, who 'knew' what her psychopathology was, and the only effective therapeutic stratagem to be applied; all else would be an avoidance or dilution of these central truths. He did not, first, need to make a relationship with Carol, where he could learn about Carol's world in her own language. The important task was that Carol should learn from him, that he should demonstrate quickly and clearly to her the issues she must necessarily confront. He did not require much time to do this; his training had made him skilful and dexterous, and many of his colleagues admired and reinforced his articulate commitment.

According to Hannah Segal (1979), Melanie Klein believed that 'things cannot be a bit like this and a bit like that. In matters of science, there can be no compromise...'. While this may be a necessarily pragmatic principle in a Court of Law, where `truth' must be clear-cut and accessible to bureaucratic process, it is liable to become absurd or sinister when applied to situations that are as complex as understanding human nature. Those scientists concerned with the most precise observations and formulations – physicists – have long ago given up the search for inviolable truths. Since Einstein and Heisenberg (Einstein & Infield 1938) 'truth' has become relativistic and pragmatic; sometimes it is convenient to consider `matter' as a wave-form, at other times a particle – the 'truth' is either, neither, or both of these. The skill of the physicist lies in the sophistication and knowledge behind his 'juggling' with the different models.

In the realm of understanding ourselves and our fellows, this relativistic principle is even more important than in physics; our models may have a relation to truth, but they are not themselves 'true' in an immutable sense. We can introduce an illustration (Figure 1) here to clarify this theme:

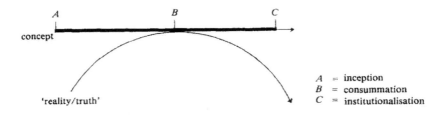

*Figure 1. Concept and reality* (The darker line, denoting 'concept', implies easier mental accessibility than the ultimately elusive, and fainter 'reality'.)

Notice here how the straight line 'concept' touches the curved 'reality' at only one point, *B*, but that further travelling along the concept departs increasingly from reality. Our psychological formulations often have this quality: we sketch a rudimentary idea, seeing a certain relation to reality, *A*; as we develop and refine the idea we reach an optimum point, *B*, of contact with reality, but further thinking along this line departs from it. The process of *A→B* is disciplined, creative and exploratory, but *B→C* is increasingly dogmatic, defensive and professionally solipsistic. It is part of the art of psychotherapy to know when 'point *B*' has been reached, or passed, and to consider another approach.

In academic and intellectual circles, ideas are often assessed by logical connection and coherence with other ideas. It is assumed that if a body of knowledge or theory is internally coherent, then it is somehow more true than one with internal discrepancies and contradictions. While such a philosophy has a certain aesthetic appeal, and may keep us in familiar territory, it is no test of the validity or usefulness of an idea. Eastern philosophies have long recognised the fruitfulness and wisdom in reconciling opposites and incongruents (ie Yin and Yang of Taoism). Another diagram (Figure 2) illustrates opposing concepts and their relation to reality. If we use this to survey psychotherapy, then concepts 1 and 2 would be closely related approaches, which are complementary and easily reconciled, unless they become institutionalised: an example of this would be Freudian and Kleinian Analytic approaches, both of which stress the importance of discovering or uncovering unconscious and archaic conflict.

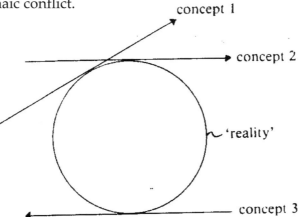

*Figure 2. Complementary and opposing concepts and their relation to 'reality'*

Concept 3, however, deals with aspects of reality in a way that is both juxtaposed and in the opposite direction; Glasser's Reality Therapy, which insists on personal responsibility in the present, and regards interpretation as likely to be an avoidance of this, represents such an opposing and incongruent concept. Although widely separated and having opposing vectors, concepts 2 and 3 come closer to resembling a circle than do concepts 1 and 2. Translated back to the realm of psychotherapy, we can see then that a therapist who discriminatingly chooses to work interpretatively from a Freudian base at one time, while at another will not do this but insists that the patient merely look at his actions and their consequences, is closer to the patient's reality (the circle) than the therapist whose eclecticism, for example, extends only to a choice of interpretative frameworks (concepts 1 and 2), or even more than the therapist who has only one conceptual system – his choice, then, is limited to how zealously to apply his technique. We can understand Dr L's professional behaviour as being an example of this.

'Scientific' studies in psychotherapy are concerned with the development of concepts from their inception (point *A* in Figure 1) to their consummation (point *B).* Tenacity to concepts beyond this point becomes an issue of institutionalisation or religious conviction, important phenomena which will be discussed later. The 'art' of psychotherapy may be thought of as the ability to draw different tangents at different times, to know when and how diverse forms of understanding and intervention may contact a patient's reality, and how these different lines may connect to make a whole (Figure 3).

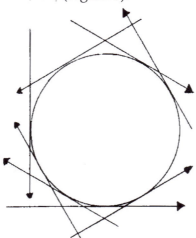

*Figure 3.    Holism or eclecticism*

Such 'holism', of course, can never be complete, for it would require an infinite number of integrated approaches. However, a large part of our task in being a `good-enough therapist' consists in having competent and fluent use of a wide variety of ways of understanding. To evoke another metaphor, understanding people who come to us is like musical composition. The composer who knows about only one instrument will be restricted in the sounds he can create. The more he is acquainted with different, sometimes 'opposite', instruments and the relationship between them, the richer and more creative the music. Of course, the composer is thoroughly trained in the use of one instrument first, but it is the transposition of this discipline to other, less familiar, instruments and the learning of the new discipline of 'orchestral holism', which leads to the desired sound. Eclecticism in psychotherapy is often disparaged by more doctrinaire practitioners as being unformed, undisciplined and unfocused. I would maintain a different position: as with the composer, we must first learn one approach thoroughly, and then the fresh task of orchestrating the diverse and the unfamiliar awaits us. Our unwillingness to make this transition may lead us to the limited arena of expert, but stereotyped, performances: we may even institutionalise our performance, and validate our endeavours by having contact only with those professionals who agree with us. As with Dr L, though, we may develop skills much respected by our ideological cohabitees, at the price of relating to our patients with freshness and creativity; Dr L almost certainly had more rapport with his colleagues than with Carol.

It is not the psychoanalytic base of Dr L's practice that is in question here, but the fact that he seemed unable to part from it. With considerable sophistication he had turned a 'base' – which allows departure from it – into a 'trap' that does not, and to which Carol could respond only by acquiescence or struggle.

Such reductionism has earned mental health professionals the title of 'shrinks' who, by inference, reduce patients' human complexity, so that it may become subordinate to the professionals' sphere of influence and explanation. In this regard, psychoanalysis offers to such practitioners the same opportunities and dangers as other 'convergent' modes that have developed well-defined and elaborated systems of language, explanatory theory and professional protocol, for example traditional psychiatry. By contrast, those approaches, which are 'looser', more divergent and have less linguistic or conceptual precision, eg Existential or Client-Centred Therapy, would seem freer from this dilemma (though confronted equally by others). As in the realm of physical medicine, techniques and tools that penetrate, define and disable, however briefly, offer their potency inextricably linked with their hazards. Such activities require special capacities of discrimination and responsibility.

There arises also the important distinction between 'training' and 'education'. 'Training', the more formal and didactic learning process, is almost certainly an important and elementary cornerstone in our development as therapists. The discipline involved in becoming thoroughly and systematically acquainted with one conceptual system is an essential requisite for later, more exploratory, ventures. Just as the infant needs a secure base in a consistent mother, to be able to leave her and relate to others and the vicissitudes of the wider world, perhaps therapists need a 'mother-model' which provides consistent familiarity, before the wider world of psychotherapy, with all its paradoxes, lacunae and frustrations can be confidently and creatively encountered. The process by which we venture away from the 'mother-model', and make new and unforeseen contacts and syntheses, is our task of 'education'. There are other interesting and enlightening images we may draw from this metaphor; just as some children have a fearful and insecure attachment to mother, and cannot tolerate separation to make other relationships, so there are therapists who need always to cling to the mother-model, and respond with many kinds of anger or fear if this is challenged. As the mother-child relationship becomes fixed, so does the therapist-model relationship become institutionalised (as in Figure 1). Dr L probably represented this kind of petrified developmental arrest.

By contrast, the therapist who is able to internalise a good and consistent mother-model, and confidently but discriminatingly move into new and different therapeutic systems, is like the child who values and trusts his mother, but knows there are other good things for him in the world beyond.

'The will to truth is merely the longing for a stable world', Nietzsche (1888) wrote, many years before such matters became psychologically and academically scrutinised. His maxim is particularly relevant to those of us constructing (some might wish to say 'discovering') truths which we then apply to others. Many of us, perplexed and frightened by chaos both within and without, hope that some doctrine – religious, psychological, philosophical or political – will free us from this tempestuous burden. In recent times, the previously castle-like refuge of religious doctrine has crumbled, leaving psychology and politics, in particular, as ideological havens from a world that can otherwise seem frighteningly outside of our control, purpose and understanding. There are other quasi-religious functions involved: the formation of groups of fellow-believers can imbue members with a sense of mission, enlightenment and righteousness, making outsiders appear in darkest error. Viewed in this way, we can see why the definition and possession of the 'Right Way' in psychotherapy can be such a quirky, often jealous and paranoid business. It accounts also for Carol's first round of experience in this psychotherapy-roulette; she was dealing with Dr L's credo.

From the end of our intra-uterine life onwards, it is a central and never-ending task for each of us to learn to live creatively in the constant shadow of uncertainty. At our beginning, the womb expels us, the 'ideal' mother disappears or disintegrates, younger children unaccountably appear to supplant us. At the other end of our lives, our internal resources become erratic and fail us, friends and loved ones die, often without warning. In the middle is the swirling mosaic of choices, dilemmas and unfinished projects that make up the lot of Man in a rapidly changing world.

The task of tolerating and using uncertainty, to open up new possibilities, lies at the heart of sanity, growth and intimate relationships. Whatever formal diagnosis we apply to those who come to us, much of what we deal with are manifestations of disruption in meeting this challenge; we cling to archaic adaptations, notions, feelings and formulae largely because, whatever distress they may cause, they are ways of being that are relatively certain, familiar and predictable. A crucial part of our role as therapists then, if the patient is willing, is to beckon him away from his private but painful base of distorted 'certainty' and, in measures he can tolerate, introduce him to a more unpredictable world in which there are many more possibilities, both in how he perceives himself and how he may relate to others. An important practical question arises from this: how can the therapist who is anxiously and rigidly attached to his mother-model, help the patient abandon his subjective but 'certain' fictions, and journey out into a more real, but more uncertain, world?

True, there are equally vital and opposing tasks in psychotherapy. In some situations, if only for short periods, we need to operate with clarity, authority and a large degree of certainty. Just as children, at times, need a parent who is uncompromising and unswerving, so, of course, do patients. The therapist who is unable to do this when it is needed, faces similar long and short-term consequences as the parent who is unable to set firm, clear boundaries and rules. In taking this stance, however, we must satisfy ourselves that it emerges from a substantially considered choice, rather than our own incapacity to encounter the alien and the uncontrollable. Cleverness, often the product of training, is frequently and ritualistically overvalued in our professional culture, and then consists of pursuing a concept or ideology to the limits of sophistication and elaboration, giving an illusion of mastery and command over the unfamiliar.

Wisdom, the more delicate child of education, contrasts with, and departs from, such cleverness, and invites us, instead, to enter less charted areas, where the incongruous, the uncertain and the ungovernable await us, and our willingness to acknowledge them. It is perhaps a hallmark of maturity and substance in all our endeavours, to be able to make this kind of transition.

$$\Omega$$

### References

Einstein, A. & Infield, L. (1938) *The Evolution of Physics*. Cambridge: Cambridge University Press.
Nietzsche, F. (1888) *The Will to Power*.
Segal, H. (1979) *Klein*. London: Fontana.

Publ. in *British Journal of Psychotherapy*, Vol. 2(4), 1986

# Three Types of Encounter in the Healing Arts

## Dialogue, Dialectic and Didacticism

Western Medical and Psychiatric practice, anchored to its theoretical base of scientific determinism, tends to interventions that are administrative and prescriptive. This is derived from, and reflected in, the way in which knowledge is constructed, and the use of language. While this pattern of practice often works well in acute, circumscribed physical syndromes, it is usually far less effective when dealing with other, more frequently encountered, patterns of distress. In such situations the doctor needs to develop alternative ways of meeting and understanding his patient, which implies change in the 'metabolism' of language and knowledge. The discipline and discrimination involved in orchestrating these various kinds of encounter may give us a fresh perspective of 'holism'. A clinical case is described and a model presented to illustrate and amplify these principles.

`To think justly, we must know what others mean: to know the value of our thoughts, we must try their effect on other minds.'

William Hazlitt (1826), *On People of Sense*

`Mystification is the principal semantic tool of the would-be leader; demystification, of the man who wants to be his own master. Rousseau, Marx, Freud mystified; Emerson, Mill, Adler demystified. It is perhaps one of the immutable tragedies of the human condition that while the demystifier influences individuals, the mystifier moves multitudes.'

Thomas Szasz (1973), *The Second Sin*

Distress foreshadows and reflects fear and uncertainty in us all, and with it, to greater or lesser extent, the wish for the potent and protective figure or formula that will illuminate our way and absolve us the burdens of confusion, pain and the unknown. In our largest social groups we enact this in our choice (or extinction of choice) of political leadership, or legal and religious institutions. On our own, or in our most intimate groups, we devise more personal and idiosyncratic beliefs, rituals and protocols to ward off the potential storms or deserts of uncertainty.

Medicine and the healing arts span both these realms. At the public level, the doctor's white coat, his portentous professional institutions, and quasi-militaristic career structure all serve, in large part, to convey a variety of images, notions and experiences that create a sense of authority, confidence and safety. At a more private level, the doctor's use of technical language, and the way in which he makes physical contact with a patient, have the same psychological and social aims of ritualizing control, management and predictability. Such behaviours work best when they are harnessed to visible and effective problem-solving, such as an acute surgical emergency, but the further we depart from this type of situation, the more problematic this style of approach may become.

There are many kinds of distress which come to many kinds of healers where this type of structured and prescriptive manner becomes, at best, cumbersome, ineffective and insensitive, or at worst, infantilizing, insulting, injurious, and even corrupt by way of engendering unwarranted helplessness or damage in the recipient. It is, perhaps, the doctor's most challenging and unending task of self- education to discriminate when, how and to what degree to structure, define and manage what a patient brings to him in order to confer authority and predictability on the situation, and when, rather, to abandon such predication so that new forms of knowledge and interchange may evolve, which themselves spawn their own kinds of diagnosis and healing.

To understand more fully the roots and ramifications of these issues, we need to look at how we build up 'knowledge' and how this is transmitted or changed by the use of language. Both of these 'elements' — cognition and linguistics — are mechanisms underlying the more observable 'compounds' of patterns of practice that will be considered. For this reason a brief theoretical diversion is offered here to underpin considerations of language and knowledge that run as developing themes through this paper. It will be seen that such apparently 'academic' notions have an important, even determining, relationship to the important issues of dependency, autonomy, responsibility and awareness that many regard as crucial factors in healing and the maintenance of health.

## Dialogue: the preliminary encounter

When any two individuals come together to relate and to communicate, each has his own 'framework of experience'. This comprises awareness of himself and the external world (percept); his ideas, theories or expectations concerning himself and the world (concept); and a feeling state accompanying these two (affect). Figure 1 illustrates this as a coherent system, the circle encompassing the triangle denotes the individual's framework of experience at the time of the interchange, expressed verbally in this kind of encounter in 'individual language', where each participant's utterances remain relatively uninfluenced by the other, and thus idiosyncratic.

In a 'dialogue', then, there is a free interchange of these components of experience, so that each will bring to the encounter elements of all three in his own manner, as a kind of exchange. Importantly, in the realm of dialogue, the experience and language of each participant remains autonomous of the other so that a 'free-trade' situation operates, as indicated in Figure 2. Note, also, that there is a distance between the two, which buffers each individual from any unwanted 'trespass', invasion or inclusion by the other.

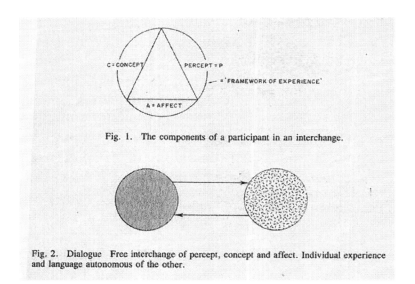

Fig. 1. The components of a participant in an interchange.

Fig. 2. Dialogue Free interchange of percept, concept and affect. Individual experience and language autonomous of the other.

There are, evidently, innumerable everyday examples of dialogue where individuals make contact in a manner that retains, intact and separate, the framework of experience of each participant. Let us look at how this operates in a typical and authentic medical situation.

## Situation 1:

Mrs G, a recently widowed woman of 60, consulted her doctor, Dr H, about pains in her chest, particularly on awakening in the small hours of the morning, when she would become frightened by the unknown-ness of her distress and her alone-ness in having to endure it. She described her mixture of physical sensations (percept), the limited sense she made of them (concept) and the feelings which accompanied them (affect), while Dr H attempted to structure what she communicated to him and what he observed (P) by referring these to both the organizing concepts he had learned in his medical training (C) and, rather less, the feeling that arose in him during the consultation (A). He elaborated this process by asking her some routine questions about her chest pains and emotional state, and performing a physical examination. In attempting to fit all this 'information' about Mrs G into his professionally learned organizing concepts (diagnoses), the doctor became aware of his difficulty in this regard; he was most concerned about her heart, although some features were not typical of this source. The other categories that came to his mind focused instead on Mrs G's oesophagus or mind; in regard to the latter she had described to him her fear, and she appeared rather sad and tense. Dr H shared the dilemma arising from their dialogue, by saying 'Well I'm not sure what's wrong with you, Mrs G, I can't find anything on examination, but I think you should have some tests done at the hospital to see if there's any problem that I can't detect here, but which may need attention. I'll ask Dr J to see you.'

Let us stand back from this situation and see what has emerged. Mrs G and her doctor are in a 'free-trade' situation where they exchange unorganized 'bits' of experience, feeling or conceptualization, each with a different emphasis. The patient's main concerns and communications are of her disturbed bodily sensations (P), and emotional state (A); her ideas about these (C) are primitive and poorly organised. The doctor's focus is an attempt to form an organizing diagnosis (C), from what he observed and hears (P); Dr H did not pay much attention to the feeling of protectiveness and sadness (A) aroused in him by Mrs G's presence, he was too busy attempting to subsume Mrs G's story and their encounter to a well-defined form of his own thought and language (a medical diagnosis) which would transform the 'dialogue' into a form of 'didacticism', a form of interchange to be considered presently. His failure to do so urged him to refer the unfinished dialogue to Dr J, who, he hoped, would complete the transformation.

## Didacticism: the organizing encounter

### Situation 2:

When Mrs G went for her appointment with Dr J she was aware that she was going to a 'specialist'; someone who had greater effectiveness than her own doctor in defining the nature of her problem and what should be done. By the time she encountered him, she was apprehensive lest she was not able to give a clear and precise account of her problems; she felt awkward, too, in confiding in a stranger, particularly those fantasies and fears that so disturbed her in the early hours of the morning. Dr J greeted her in a polite, but busy and professional manner, getting quickly to the point of his many questions, which seemed both more numerous, organized and difficult to interrupt than those of her own doctor. Perhaps to her relief, he did not dwell on her emotional turbulence on waking, and passed quickly on to the questions concerning her physical symptoms. Mrs G then underwent a number of physical investigations which, the doctor explained, would help him locate the source of her pain. Dr J was, perhaps even more than Dr H, invested in doing this with speed and finality; he had spent many arduous years learning the required skills, and his professional status depended on his being seen to exercise them. He may have been a little dismayed, then, that Mrs G's physical examination, radiography and cardiograph were unremarkable, as he now had less definitive material with which to make his decision. 'I think your pains are caused by mild angina which isn't yet serious, and so isn't reflected in any of the tests', he explained to her, before elaborating the physical meaning of this, and the treatment he was prescribing for her. Mrs G's complaint was not typical of the diagnosis he made, but her answers to his questions suggested it as a real possibility, and Dr J thought it was too important a diagnosis to be missed. He 'discharged Mrs G back to her doctor', therefore, thinking he had defined the nature of her complaint and initiated a 'policy of management'.

As before, let us distance ourselves a little more from this situation and look at the emergent patterns. Mrs G's mosaic of physical sensations, thoughts and feelings has been sampled by Dr J, who has reorganized and redefined them according to his own method of perception (the physical examination) and conception (his deductive process of making a medical diagnosis). His own feelings while doing this were not within his awareness, partly because they did not fit into this way of 'diagnosing' a patient's problems. Mrs G came to the doctor with `dis-ease' which she expressed in her own language, but could find no personal meaning for; she leaves him with `disease' which is now expressed in the doctor's language, and to which he confers a meaning, which he must explain to her. Her own framework of experience with regard to her symptoms has become engulfed by the doctor's concept.

A consequence of her suffering from 'disease' rather than 'dis-ease' is that she can do little about it, except obey the doctor's instructions. It is as if her dis-ease, which has become transformed into disease, is now the doctor's property, though unfortunately residing in her body; he knows about it, defines it in his language, 'treats' or 'manages' or 'cures' the affliction, which she accommodates as an involuntary host. This process of 'didacticism' is illustrated in Figure 3.

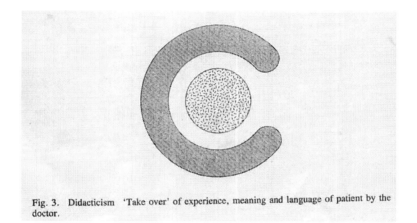

Fig. 3. Didacticism 'Take over' of experience, meaning and language of patient by the doctor.

Note that the 'Free-Trade' profile of the dialogue has changed into a 'take over', where one has 'engulfed' the other; the interchange now is not 'free', but organized and structured by one (the doctor), while the other (the patient), becomes a passive recipient. In the illustration, the patient is shown as being largely encompassed, which is true in a psychological and social sense as long as they are together, and is one of the most important features of this didactic approach. The patient here is protected and carried much as a kangaroo in its mother's pouch and, as in this analogy, it necessarily involves an abdication of autonomy, self-definition and self-determination on the part of one of the parties, while the other takes on these functions for the two of them. Didacticism is thus part of the way 'regression' and 'dependency' become organized professionally. Whether or not this is welcome, or ultimately advantageous to one, or other, or both parties is a complex issue which will be explored later. Clearly, if Mrs G, for example, was overcome with acute and severe chest pains and breathlessness, she would almost certainly welcome the opportunity to abdicate all responsibility for understanding or reacting to her experience while critically ill. On the other hand, the excessive or ill-timed use of didacticism will lead to unwarranted intrusion and control, with its later sequels of passivity, resentment and 'guerrilla warfare' of the psychological kind.

In Figure 3, which may illustrate Mrs G and Dr J, Mrs G is not totally encompassed, retains her own boundary and a space between the two. She still knows who she is, and can 'squeeze her way out' of this didactic arrangement if she so chooses. This is not so in extreme forms of didacticism. Within the healthcare field this would be illustrated by the critically ill patient in an intensive care unit who is physically encompassed by technology, or the institutionalized mentally ill who are contained and surrounded by a hospital environment. Such a situation is shown in Figure 4, and the analogy here could be made with the baby in utero; protection, enclosure and dependence are complete – there is little possibility here for the self's assertion or expression.

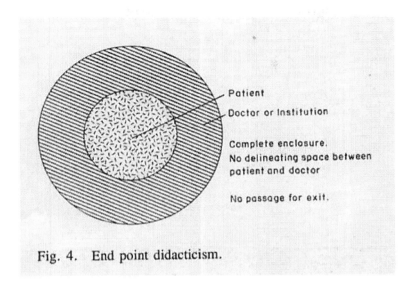

Fig. 4. End point didacticism.

## Dialectic: the intimate encounter

**Situation 3:**

Mrs G was at first comforted and reassured by Dr J's authoritative and knowledgeable manner and the many tests he performed to see what was wrong with her. Unfortunately, the tablets he gave her didn't seem to make any difference to her symptoms, and her own doctor at first responded by increasing the dose, again without effect.

The next time she saw Dr H, he seemed less busy than usual, and Mrs G felt under less pressure to produce a rapid précis of her experience, so as 'not to waste the doctor's time'. Dr H, partly due to the reduced demands on him, felt fresher and more receptive than he had been when Mrs G had previously seen him and, as she walked into his consulting room, he paid attention to a sudden feeling of sadness arising in him, a tugging sensation located in his chest, as if she had brought the feeling in with her. In the wake of this clear but unexpected visceral signal, he recalled the death of her husband, Harry, six months previously – an event which he had heard about indirectly, and which, for some reason, had previously eluded his focus. When she went on to talk of her thoracic discomfort, he asked her to elaborate it in her own words: 'it's like a knot here' (rubbing the front of her left chest), 'as if there's something there that's going to burst, and then I go dizzy and feel I can't breathe . . .'.

Dr H then asked: 'When you lie awake at night, what do you think about?'

Mrs G's eyes moistened briefly, as she quickly looked up into the corner of the room, simultaneously biting her lower lip:

'Oh, I don't know . . . silly things, you know. It's difficult to say . . .'

Although not finishing her sentence, she looked at Dr H deliberately and directly, a desolate but tacit gaze.

Dr H paused a couple of seconds, sat forward a little closer to her, saying gently and tentatively: 'As you're talking, I have the sense that you feel sadder and more full of grief than you've conveyed to anyone . . . I'm wondering, too, about how much you want to say to Harry, about his leaving you, about being left on your own'.

Mrs G now sat forward, allowing herself to lean on the doctor's desk and saying: 'Oh yes . . . you seem to understand that. There's so much of it inside of me, pulling my mind in different directions; but I've always been one to keep a brave face . . . my daughters tell me I've been "wonderful" the way I've coped, and I haven't wanted to tell them just how bad I've felt, how lonely I feel . . .', she shrugged, as if discounting the interest of this to anyone but herself.

Dr H offered an image that surfaced and crystallised in his awareness: 'It's like you've had to deal, very much on your own, with two broken hearts; the one that killed Harry and the one that you're left alive with, that hurts when you're most alone in the middle of the night.'

'I don't know which I am; full of pain, hurting because I'm still alive when he's gone, or whether I'm just dead somehow, like Harry on the inside, although on the outside I'm just the same . . . can you understand that?'

'Yes, the broken heart that gave up, and the one that has to carry on painfully — it's like you have them both inside of you . . . it takes a long time for that kind of pain and emptiness to go away; to have your heart touched or warmed, so that you know you're alive, and you know you want to be alive. There are times when we have to die a bit first... to come alive again'.

'I think I've known that, at times, anyway, but it feels so much better just hearing you say it. It makes it more real somehow . . . like I know where I am and what I'm going through'.

Mrs G looked at the doctor sadly, but with less desolation than before; as if her heart was enlivened just a little already. The two of them sat together quietly for half a minute in a silence that was consummate and autumnal, as if they both needed a little time to digest, each in the company of the other, what they had produced together.

Mrs G, slowly straightening herself from the doctor's desk that she had been leaning against, gathered her coat and bag together, saying thoughtfully: 'I think I'll be alright, but it's hard. It's good to know you're here. Shall I come and see you next week, doctor?'

'Yes, I think you need to, and I shall want to know how you are', replied Dr H, aware of a glowing sensation in his chest. Perhaps his heart, too, so often numbed by business and his didactic functions, was beginning to warm.

Mrs G did return regularly for some months, but on a very different basis from before. Her chest pains became far less alarming for her and eventually disappeared without any further medical initiative from Dr H. She seemed to seek him out as a companion, helping her through a difficult passage; she knew that he could not take away her dis-ease, but he could help understand it, bear it and perhaps resolve it.

The doctor understood that his 'heart to heart' with his patient had eased the aching in her heart in a metaphorical and emotional sense; had this been reflected at a cellular level too? Dr H wondered. Was she now perfusing her heart when before she was, literally physically, blocking it off? In any case, the doctor mused, their encounter seemed to have penetrated beyond the reach of his medication.

The process and outcome of this last situation are clearly very different from the other two. Dr H did not here attempt to quickly subsume his patient's account of her experience to his own prior concepts, but allowed himself a period of uncertainty, where various notions and possibilities were invented in the moment and could be offered to Mrs G to sample, 'play with', explore, develop or discard as she wished. In doing this, the doctor paid equal attention to all the fragments of percept, affect and concept arising in both him and his patient; his own 'heaviness of heart' when she walked in the room was seen not as a contaminating influence to the medical interview, but as a potentially valuable emanation or expression which could be explored to find some kind of shared meaning. Likewise her involuntary physical reactions to his asking about her troublesome thoughts: when she turned her moistening eyes to the ceiling and bit her lip, Dr H had a new if tentative understanding of her – 'In her mind's eye she continually sees Harry; the sadness she experiences is beyond her capacity to tell the living. She searches for him with her eyes but bites her lip to stop herself speaking of this', Dr H had thought to himself, but also realized it was a subjective hypothesis to be offered to her to see if she would make sense of it. Mrs G. not only made sense of Dr H's metaphor of the 'broken heart', she elaborated on it, thus helping to create between the two of them a new and unique system of understanding, with its own symbols, metaphors and use of language. The physical movement of each toward the other physically, enacted what was happening at the psychological level; there was a convergence, even fusion, of their two worlds, so that the doctor's technical observations (P), his ideas about grief, body language, heart disease, ego-defence mechanisms and so forth (C), and the feelings arising in him (A), could be combined with the patient's disturbed bodily experiences and visual fantasies of her dead husband (P), her feelings of sadness and fear (A), and the notions she had about her physical disturbance and the life-passage she found herself in (C). The understanding that is constructed is new and unique and could only have arisen afresh in this situation; it could not have been organized or prescribed as a 'treatment'.

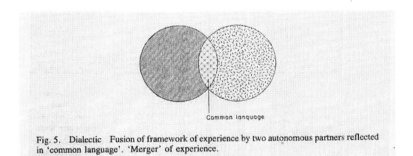

Common language

Fig. 5. Dialectic Fusion of framework of experience by two autonomous partners reflected in 'common language'. 'Merger' of experience.

## Common language

Figure 5 illustrates this process of 'dialectic', where a 'common language' is created in the area of fusion of two individual selves and world experiences. This common language is made up of the two individuals, but transcends them both in creating something new. In many ways it is equivalent to sexual union where fusion and interpenetration leads to new life which is made up of, but transcends, the two participants. Using the economic metaphor again, dialectic is akin to a 'merger'. It is similar, too, to the psychoanalyst

Winnicott's[1] notions of 'playing' and 'intimacy' where these are considered as the creation and elaboration of a 'transitional zone' — a fertile area of interchange and improvisation between the self and the other. The fact that this dialectical approach involves a certain mutuality or intimacy, implies certain conditions, restrictions and prerequisites; it is only possible and only of value, for example, where both partners are prepared to abandon their own frame of reference and integrate it into something as yet unknown. It also implies a giving up of the `control dimension' of the relationship, so that neither controls the other with regard to defining reality, using language, structuring the interchange, or prescribing what should be done. Clearly the didactic approach occupies the opposite pole from dialectic in these considerations.

This intimacy, necessary for, and generated by, dialectic is crucial to certain phases and aspects of healing. In situation 3, Mrs G had the sense of both understanding and being understood in a way that involved her own creativity and participation in the construction of the common language she achieved with her doctor. This being so, she felt empowered, dignified and compassionately accompanied in the experience, and enhanced in her capacity to clarify and express more. It is a fundamental psychodynamic principle that conflicts and dilemmas that remain unexpressed, unclear and unshared with others become amplified inside us and likely to become manifest in symptomatic difficulties. The act of understanding and entrusting our difficulties with another is often the first step in mastery and resolution. An important distinction should be made here between didactic and dialectic forms of insight and understanding. If Dr H had prematurely said to her: `Part of your problem is that you have a masked depression. Your chest pain is due to you not letting go of Harry', he may have been correct and have been saying something similar, in content, to what he and Mrs G had arrived at in situation 3. However, this didactic insight would have been inflicted on her, and would be far less likely to be helpful; the essential processes of trust, rapport, mutuality and common language are missing, and Mrs G becomes, as she was in situation 2 with Dr J, the passive recipient of the doctor's organizing concepts.

## The art of integrating science

Perhaps, though, Mrs G needed to pass through a phase where she abdicated any knowledge of, or responsibility for, her symptoms and be cared for and defined by an authority figure, as she was by Dr J In such a situation she may not have yet had the internal resources, or known Dr H well enough, to have entrusted him with the faltering first steps involved in self-exploration and intimate disclosure. In short, she may have needed 'treatment' by Dr J's organizing scientific concepts – didacticism – as a necessary phase or 'regression' where she felt protected, unchallenged and unalone. Only later, with the passage of time and the development of dialogue with Dr H, could she go on to take some responsibility for, and see some meaning in, her symptoms. The shared development by which this happened – dialectic – passed from a 'treatment' to a 'therapy' situation, where the doctor was more responsive to, but less responsible for, Mrs G. The framework of understanding, and the language used to achieve this, changed from the doctor's scientific ideology to an 'existential' mode, jointly formulated.

Figure 6 illustrates the shifts involved in the three different kinds of encounter and the processes by which they occur.

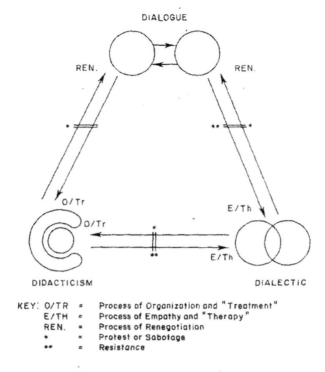

KEY: O/TR  =  Process of Organization and "Treatment"
    E/TH  =  Process of Empathy and "Therapy"
    REN.  =  Process of Renegotiation
    *  =  Protest or Sabotage
    **  =  Resistance

Fig. 6. The interpersonal dynamics of encounter.

Scientific medicine, as traditionally conceived and practised, involves a transmutation by the doctor of the dialogue he has with the patient, so that the patient submits to the treatment and abdicates responsibility for his distress. If either partner does not wish to continue this, or the treatment does not work, then, if the two wish to go on together, there must be a renegotiation through dialogue. If both are willing, able and motivated to find a more personal understanding and language for the problem, then there is a shift to a dialectic via the development of empathy. The naming of this change as 'therapy' (as opposed to 'treatment') implies the increased responsibility and activity of the patient. This can be abandoned by either renegotiation to dialogue, or reversion back to the treatment situation.

Where one of the partners wishes to change the form of the encounter unilaterally, without some readiness on the part of the other, then certain defensive or sabotaging strategies will be used by the one pressurized to change. For example, the doctor who makes a premature shift into didacticism by diagnosing, say, premenstrual tension, is unlikely to get the patient to take the medication as prescribed. Another common example of this is the patient labelled 'schizophrenic' who will not adhere to drug regimes. The psychiatrist might say – didactically – that the patient's noncompliance is part of his 'schizophrenic illness', but it may instead reflect the psychiatrist's personality and training whereby he is resistant to, or incapable of, meeting his patient in a dialogue or dialectic.

While 'protest' and 'sabotage' occur at largely conscious levels, 'resistance' operates unconsciously to defend a person against the authenticity, closeness and self-responsibility that ensue in any shift toward the intimacy of dialectic. Psycho-analytically, this term has traditionally been applied (didactically!) to patients, but it often works the other way round. Most hazardously in psychiatry, there is frequently a rapid moulding of a patient's communications so that they will fit into the doctor's diagnostic and treatment schemes; those that cannot be so tailored are either simply not heard or seen, or dismissed as lacking in 'clinical significance'. The fact that the doctor's didactic pronouncements and plans are often not effective may not lead him to renegotiating a dialogue, or attempting to construct a common language with his patient. In his own, and his profession's form of resistance, he may fall back even further into his didactic position by, for example, elaborating theories of 'psychopathology' of the patient's condition – an attitude and endeavour which may be institutionalized and applauded by his colleagues but, paradoxically, lead to increasing alienation from his patients. Such a doctor's investment in maintaining a didactic position is often based on a fear of the reverse; that he himself becomes the one that is dependent, turbulent, powerless or vulnerable.

Didacticism, at least while it operates, seems to confer immunity against such perils; the illusions, mechanisms and trappings of this have been dealt with in a previous article.[2] Even if the doctor is not resistant to shifting away from his didactic position, many of his patients will be. The investment in another person for certainty, the power of transformation, warding off dangers of the unknown in ourselves and the world around us may be an illusion, but a comforting one. Authoritarian relationships and institutions often provide, too, a certain security and familiarity. Freedom and autonomy are often too much of a challenge and a burden.[3] Thus, a doctor's attempt to provoke an unwilling patient to move away from their passive and defined role in the didactic arrangement will be met by some kind of sabotage or resistance. I remember a woman doctor who had been 'treating', in an impotent and ritualistic form, a man for an endless stream of minor functional disorders, the favourite of which were 'sick headaches', for 15 years. He appeared, to the doctor, a stable, dull man whose lack of curiosity about the nature or meaning of his symptoms seemed part of his general passivity. One morning he came yet again, perhaps for the hundredth time, complaining in his stereotyped way of his inexorable complaints, asking:

'Isn't there something else you can give me doctor?'

'I wonder if there's something you ought to be giving yourself?', replied the doctor, for the first time attempting to break the pattern, she thought rather succinctly and profoundly.

He looked askance at her. 'Have you been on one of your new courses, doctor?', came the caustic retort, sly and rhetorical. She got the message, and he left with another prescription.

In this situation the patient clearly wished his doctor to assume a didactic role and 'treat' a 'disease'; he resisted any attempt she might make to destructure their familiar roles, so that he might become more self-governing, self-responsible or self-aware by exploring the basis of his dis-ease. He wanted to be a patient. It can be seen here how the doctor wished to redefine the problem existentially, while the patient wished to continue with an organic or deterministic approach to his problem. Here lies a central ideological distinction between the dialectic and didactic approach. Didacticism tends to scientific determinism and the notion of mechanical disease, which can only be cured by the expert. Dialectic is an activity arising from an existential outlook, with an emphasis on pursuing personal responsibility and creating personal meaning. Psychotherapy, an area whose psychological and social politics is quite as difficult as conventional medicine, has practitioners whose method is often dominated by one of these modes. The orthodox psychoanalyst, for example, works on the assumption that the patient's 'psychopathology' depends on unconscious processes that only a trained psychoanalyst can understand and treat; Freud himself talked of patients 'submitting' to analysis. Existential psychotherapists, in contrast, emphasize mutuality, authenticity, intimacy and the attainment of common language as being therapeutic; there is here no prescribed treatment or organizing technical language.

Clearly, in medicine, psychiatry, psychotherapy and all other forms of healing, we need to be able to shift with great dexterity between all three approaches with those that came to us. The skills of negotiating in dialogue, taking responsibility didactically, declining responsibility but allowing a new responsiveness in dialectic, are all cornerstones in the rich pattern of human intercourse that make up the healing arts. As in most other forms of intercourse, the problems arise when we are out of touch with one another's internal worlds, or wanting to interact in the external world in different ways. For the healer rigorously trained in the didactic sciences, it often requires a significant change and development of personality to foster equal skill in the artistic exercise of dialectic. The perennial and rather simplistic question: 'Is Medicine an Art or a Science?' can be reformulated more precisely and meaningfully by asking instead: 'How can we, with art and empathy, apply our medical science, and what is the science of applying this art and empathy?'.

It is hoped that this description of the three types of encounter provides some basis for an answer.

Ω

### References

1. Winnicot, D.W. *Playing and Reality.* London, Tavistock Pubs., 1971.
2. Zigmond, D. 'Physician Heal Thyself: The Paradox of Wounded Healer'. *British Journal of Holistic Medicine,* December 1984. Vol 1: 63-71.
3. Fromm, E. *Escape from Freedom.* New York, Holt, Rinehort and Winston, 1941.

Publ. in *Holistic Medicine,* Vol 2, 69-81 (1987)

# The Psychoecology
# of Gladys Parlett

*'Peace dies when the framework is ripped apart. When there is no longer a place that is yours in the world. When you know no longer where your friend is to be found.'*

Saint-Exupery, *Flight to Arras* (1942)

Proud, elderly and sprightly, Mrs Gladys Parlett does not betray her inner burdens and chasms openly. Slightly tinted, sharply coiffed hair surrounds an alert, kindly, discreetly rouged face. Freshly pressed and quietly co-ordinated clothes accompany a manner that seems merely consonant and pleasant to the unwatchful. Those more canny might become aware of more disquieting signs; her tinted spectacles both frame and conceal restless and sorrowfully glistening eyes, white knuckles keep a grip on her handbag with primitive tenacity, her ankles lock together as if to prevent impulsive and involuntary movement.

Until her beloved George's death, Dr L.'s dealings with her had been infrequent, simple and matter-of-fact. To the doctor they had been undemanding, courteous and easy people, and his pragmatic contact with them reflected a cordial and uncluttered alacrity. Her bereavement, though, soon heralded an unprecedented change. She came to him frequently and with numerous and protean complaints; a previously dormant stratum of self now erupting with a lava of fermenting and inexorable dis-ease. Dr L., a busy practitioner, but not illiterate in the task of reading what is not directly conveyed, at first responded with familiar precedent, sympathetically and symptomatically. Her collage of headaches, giddiness, respiratory infections, arthritic pains and nausea received the kind of specific remedies that keep Dr L. in respectable, if undistinguished, company.

Recognizing that he was dealing with a woman, for all her years, unused to verbalizing her pain and conflict, he was patient and delicate in making deeper contact. She needed, he thought, much encouragement and support in clarifying and validating her underlying turbulence and sense of injury. He supposed, or hoped, that exposure and apposition, to himself, of her internal wound might guide her capacity for restoration. Exploring discreetly beneath her sense of physical peril and instability he suggested she take him into her gallery of memories; cherished sepia-like episodes and life-fragments, some idealized, many bitter-sweet, receding back to a post-Edwardian childhood.

Gladys, a middle child amongst many in a poor Methodist docker's family, perceived her world then as loving but harsh. She had few doubts regarding her place and role amongst others, but the conditions demanded of her for such kinship were strict and uncompromising. She grew shyly and demurely into a womanhood of loyal but limited bonds. She met George, a young docker, also in his early twenties, at a local wedding. He was then, and remained for nearly 50 years, with few deviations, a sensitive and steadfast companion. More socially confident than she, he provided through their long interdependence, both a bridge to, and a buttress against, the outside world's demands, vicissitudes and opportunities. By nature a retiring and retroflective person, she had, nevertheless, for several decades, a milieu in which she had an unquestioned, largely unconscious, sense of purpose and attachment.

## No inconvenience to others

What is conveyed to the doctor now, though, are memories and vestigial fragments of Gladys's previous ecology. Her two sons, currently married, middle-aged and with their own families, have enacted with great success the aspirations of their prudent, once poor and conscientious parents: propelling themselves upward and outward in a society increasingly occupationally and socially mobile, they now occupy homes and work-roles beyond any experience or familiarity of their parents. Pursuing better employment opportunities, both sons have settled far from the declining and ghost-like community of the old docks. They are dutiful and attentive sons, reliable in maintaining contact by telephone, and driving the many miles from the salubrious suburbs to visit her. Sometimes from concern, sometimes through guilt, they wonder whether their stoic but hurting mother should live with one of them, but this possibility is fraught with practical difficulties — neither can offer a home capacious enough to provide Gladys with her own bedroom without depriving one of their children of theirs; an arrangement they perceive as erosive to their own family's ecology. Gladys, in any case, overtly and overly proud and self-sufficient, has pre-emptively parried, in many utterances, any arrangement where she feels she may be, as she puts it, 'a burden' or 'inconvenience' to others.

In Gladys's childhood it had been quite different, she remembers, for her own grandmother, Milly. That old lady, like Gladys, had lost her husband 15 years before her own death. But there were important differences. Milly remained very much at the centre of a large family which, through hardship, poverty and social inertia, had little opportunity for mobility, change and, therefore, disintegration. The old lady, the senior matriarch, living in cold, crowded conditions in the family home amongst three generations, was the repository of female know-how, oral family history and tradition, and, often with mollification, sometimes with contention, of counsel, judgement and verdict. Increasingly disabled with arthritis and lingering pulmonary consumption, Milly nevertheless lived out a frail yet powerful widowhood of central importance to those around her until her eighty-eighth year. Consulted for her experience of the tangible tasks of recipes or the management of childhood ailments, or the more intangible problems of how to find happiness, or at least peace, amongst others, Milly had little reason to think of herself as her granddaughter does; 'a burden' or 'inconvenience' to others.

## Somaticized distress

Dr L, in his surgery and home-visits, spends much of his time attempting to decode, if possible detoxify, the somaticized distress of his many elderly patients. It was not always so. A young man when he first entered practice, intellectually crisp and eager to apply, directly and succinctly, the concise medical notions and tools he had imbibed assiduously in his hospital training, he found himself responding with a polite, brisk veneer which masked an intense irritation when he encountered those, like Gladys Parlett, who somehow defied his efficient and medically rigorous ministrations. Like a sheep dog he would, with energy and vigilance, attempt to round them into his pen of medical diagnoses and managements only to find, repeatedly, that his 'good work' was to no avail. Many of them, with apparent obstinacy or perversity, didn't follow his instructions, developed side-effects to his prescriptions, wouldn't give up the medley of their complaints and symptoms. 'If it weren't for these damn patients, I could be a good doctor', retorted a wry and weary older partner when the young Dr L sought commiseration and advice for his increasingly chronic sense of frustration and impotence. 'Frankly, when I see them coming through the door, the question I ask myself is "How can I get them out as soon as possible?"', was his senior colleague's acid and nihilistic counsel.

It was some years before Dr L could understand and make creative use of these feelings of redundancy and defeat, to realize that this somehow mirrored his patients' experiences of decline, abandonment and nullification. He had, first, to face his own losses, witness his parents become elderly, and sniff his own mortality and transience. Dr L's private struggles and dilemmas in this arena have slowly transformed his way of understanding and responding to these refractory and disequilibrated people. He sees now that this public role as a family doctor has a symbolic significance for them, far more subtle and demanding than the problem-solving, technically-based functions in which he had previously immured himself. From a world rotating and changing increasingly rapidly around a technological axis, those at the periphery, particularly the elderly, unplaced and unable to contribute, are thrown off by a kind of social centrifugal force to become society's 'loose-bodies', disconnected and disinherited.

Gladys's grandmother, Milly, was part of the Stream of Life until her own death. Gladys, in contrast, must face her involution and ending, unaccompanied by the evidence of fresh life, the tending of which is one of the few things to make approaching death meaningful and bearable. Human contact and nourishment, having a social role in which we find meaning and which is valued by others, are the social prerequisites for inner and outer peace.

Gladys, and so many of Dr L's elderly 'regular attenders', have little such social role, contact and nutrient to sustain them. Their dis-ease, for them often ineffable and intense, finds inchoate articulation in their bodies. Sometimes, with encouragement from Dr L, there can be a translation into words. At other times this seems pointless and unnecessary, and a tacit understanding grows implicitly. Dr L has come to recognize the symbolic, perhaps unconscious, investment that is made in him and his surgery-environment. The waiting area is often a kind of village square where the elderly and isolated are, for a while, part of the milling of a local community; familiar faces encountered, fragments of gossip exchanged, babies paraded, admired and envied, older children reprimanded and humoured. The doctor's room becomes a sanctum or retreat where secrets, pains and private burdens may be, if only briefly, unloaded, alluded to and shared.

Dr L's physical presence, reassuring in its familiarity and constancy, has great importance for those whose personal landmarks have gone, receded or become rare and ritualistic. For those seldom touched, the physical examination becomes imbued with potent ingredients of care and recognition, something that eluded his earlier judgement when such activities were determined more rigidly by 'clinical indications'. Any medicines he may prescribe, too, have meaning and functions he would have overlooked before he came to understand the anguish that can he born of aloneness. The bottle of medicine or tube of cream becomes a kind of talisman or reminder of the doctor's continuing existence when he is absent.

## A waiting room for death

Gladys Parlett's anguish and sense of desolation have been intense and profound and, at times, beyond the reach or influence of Dr L's empathic interest or rationalized medications. One week she sat, almost immobile and mask-like, and talked obliquely, with a darkly-veiled foreboding, of ending her life. Managing for the first time to persuade her to see a psychiatrist, he arranged an appointment for her to see a consultant known to him as an approachable, sympathetic and psychologically skilled practitioner. This initiative was curtly and bureaucratically rebuffed. A phone call from the outpatient secretary indicated that all patients of her age had to be seen in the Psychogeriatric Unit; no exceptions could be made. Dr L balked, complied and acted accordingly.

The psychogeriatric young registrar pronounced the old lady 'significantly clinically depressed' while also surveying her isolation and 'vulnerable, insecure personality that has led to her notable lack of confidence and tendency to depressive illness since the loss of her husband . . .' A change of antidepressant medication and attendance at a Geriatric Day Centre 'for support and socialization' were recommended.

Much to Dr L's disappointment, but little to his surprise, Gladys developed intolerable 'side-effects' to both the chemical and social prescriptions and discontinued both. It was difficult to assess the possible physiological basis to her reaction to the drug, but her intense dislike of the old people's Day Centre was more easily understood: 'It's like a waiting room for death' she said with a stark, ruthless economy that arrested Dr L's breath for several seconds. 'They're very nice there, very kind, but I don't want to sit around with all those old people that I don't know, being "jollied along" . . . I know you don't have much time, doctor, but I'd rather come and talk to you, it's more natural, more like real life . . . I've known you and Sheila [the receptionist] for years, so it's like family, if you know what I mean. I hope you don't think I'm being difficult.'

Many might have done; Dr L did not, though the task of surrogate kinship, he reflected, was paradoxical in its ordinariness and complexity.

### Separation from life's flow

For a profession currently festooning itself with variations on the themes of 'holism' and 'community care', people like Gladys Parlett confront us with daunting and growing challenges. By well-rehearsed rote we are liable to ascribe her distress to some type of psychiatric phenomenology or psycho-pathology, thus deflecting from a perspective which sees her disintegration as an individualized microcosm of a dislocation and decay happening increasingly in our socially fragmented times. Gladys's symptoms can, perhaps, be most clearly understood in terms of her growing and profound alienation from those around her. She is deprived of social function, substrate and network.

Milly, through a long, often cruel and tragic life, never lost a sense of belonging and purpose amongst others. Gladys, by contrast, in a life increasingly free of the kind of violent vicissitudes, thraldom and injustices her grandmother was subject to, enters her last stretch without this essential *raison d'être*. Her life now lacks an 'existential holism'. Her anguish flows from not being part of the Whole. Dr L, whose waiting-room bustles with human traffic, whose familiarity brings continuity, whose words and touch imply knowledge and interest in her private world, provides a sadly sparse but cherished sense of contact and inclusion. Despite its assigned function, the Geriatric Day Centre was perceived by Gladys as being a form of caring which separated her from the rest of humankind.

There is a certain irony and paradox in treating Gladys Parlett within the special designation of 'psychogeriatrics'. Certainly, her intense misery and despair warranted more time, attention and facilities than Dr L could muster but, as she made trenchantly clear, she could not tolerate this in a form which underlined her separation from life's flow. With the solid but spurious logic of our times, we assume that a growing problem must be given special and separate facilities, practitioners and premises. But if Gladys is to be reinstated into any Family of Man it makes little sense to attempt this in a manner which purports to create a 'community' comprised solely of the aged. The meaningful and healthy ecology of the aged cannot evolve from isolation. It must include the young.

Among the intriguing and tragic perversities of the human condition is the fact that the most enduring and certain of our bonds arise in the midst of hardship, adversity and common struggle. There were few lonely and alienated people in the last World War. When we are not engaged in the struggle to survive we are occupied by the task of creating personal and social meaning. The burdens of (relative) peace, prosperity and proliferation of choice may be often unacknowledged, but are inescapable. In an age where it has become the desired norm to define and pursue our own *modus vivendi*, where technology both generates and catalyses social diffusion and mobility, it is difficult to keep crucial events of our life-cycle within a familiar and ecological human matrix. The hospitalization of birth, decline, grief and death are all, to some degree, indices of our failure to live 'holistically' with one another.

As our real community dwindles, and neighbours become strangers, family becomes (albeit loyally) nostalgic visitors, the church is vandalized and empty, and the corner-shop closes down, we create fictional or symbolic substitutes. Perhaps television's *Eastenders* and *Crossroads* and the doctors' new ideologies of *Therapeutic Communities* and *Community Care* are akin in their efforts to provide 'societal prostheses', devices that provide, by artifice or illusion, a sense of community when the natural community is perishing. Gladys's shrill protest about the Day Centre, a kind of phantom-limb pain, alerted Dr L to her defiance of the alien and the unnatural. Holism, he has come to recognize, extends tantalizingly and without limit beyond the simple and tidy notions he had assembled and displayed, Lego-like, in order to become a doctor.

Publ. in *Holistic Medicine*, Vol. 3, 9-14 (1988)

# The Front Door of Psychotherapy

## Aspects from
## General Medical Practice

*He who knows others is learned*
*He who knows himself is wise.*

Lao Tse (6th century BC), *The Character of Tao*

*It is far more important that one's life should be perceived than it be transformed; for no sooner has it been perceived than it transforms itself of its own accord.*

Maurice Maeterlinck (1896) *The Deeper Life, The Treasure of the Humble*

Healing and growth, through the exploration and expression of the hidden inner-world, is certainly as old as the written word, and probably as ancient as the earliest forms of communication of abstract thought. The last few decades have seen a rapid and diverse organization of such quests, in the form of 'psychotherapy' in its many guises. What these variegated and sometimes discordant schools have in common is the point of departure: the person seeking psychotherapy is already consciously committed (albeit ambivalently!) to the task of expanding their realms of self-awareness and self-responsibility. All such people may be said to commence from the 'lobby' of psychotherapy.

The General Medical Practitioner, however, is faced with very different, though related and equally challenging, psychological and existential tasks. Those who come to him for help are often unaware, or denying, of how their physical or mental dis-ease may derive from their on-going conflicts and dilemmas, and thus see any affliction or help as coming from outside their personal sphere of influence, awareness and responsibility.

The doctor's opportunities and challenges thus occur at the 'front door' of psychotherapy and it is always uncertain whether or not the patient will wish to enter. The doctor's role of 'doorman' here is a complex and interesting one, demanding much in the way of tact, timing and imagination, all of them skills particular to the setting. Unlike the professional psychotherapist, he has often had a long, punctuated and varied contact with the patient, often at crucial life-events, and this can offer him a vantage point and informal, though powerful, rapport that is unique.[1] The following descriptive and narrative case-histories or scenarios illustrate not only the problems of dealing with 'psychosomatic' syndromes which may be construed as the doctor's special territory, but more generally with the 'elements' of psychotherapy which underlie every genus of verbal healing.

## Case No. 1:
## Clarification or exorcism? Very simple psychotherapy

Mrs R seemed edgy and truculent when she entered Dr S's consulting room. Amanda, her four-year-old child, looking frightened and bemused, was thrust sharply towards Dr S. as an accusatory portent, an Item of Evidence for the Prosecution. Amanda stood with pale and compliant immobility as her mother quickly and purposefully unbuttoned her daughter's blouse, to reveal a small annular lesion on her chest, which the doctor immediately recognized as Tinea. He sighed privately with relief; he had expected something far worse.

'It's only Ringworm, Mrs R. Nothing to worry about. I'll give you some cream to apply, and it will clear up very quickly.' Dr S averred with bright and brisk reassurance.

Both his conviviality and authority were unexpectedly assailed:

'That's exactly what you said last year, but it's back again', retorted the flushed and angry mother, disconsolate and her eyes beginning to brim with hapless tears.

Dr S sighed again, now less privately and with the exasperation of a busy man obstructed. Biting back a mounting petulance, he struggled to retain a courteous image of helpfulness.

'Look, Mrs R., Amanda's skin has got a small Ringworm infection, that's all. It will soon clear up, even if she has had it before. But I don't understand your anxiety about all this – there seems to be something else that's bothering you that I don't know about...'replied the conciliatory doctor, now feeling as bemused as the silent and compliant small girl between them. It seemed to him that the mother had her own private, and as yet indecipherable, agenda, and he needed her to share this with him.

'It's all very well for you to say that, doctor, but what am I to think when she's full of worms...?' exclaimed the preoccupied mother.

'Worms!! Ah! I see ...' exhaled the doctor, a sense of benign command returning with a fresh and growing comprehension of this uneasy and cramped impasse.

'Yes, doctor. She can't go on like, this with worms inside of her. ... it can't be good for her...' continued the pressured Mrs R., hoping that enough leverage against the doctor would somehow rid her daughter of this largely invisible pestilence.

The doctor was now quick to understand and salvage the dialogue that had so nearly foundered from the mother's misconception, arising from the colloquial misnomer of this superficial yeast infection, Tinea corporis. Mrs R., witnessing her doctor's fresh comprehension, was now receptive to his explanation and reassurance. She softened and listened, the colour returned to Amanda's cheeks and Dr S stopped his impatient sighing. Their departure was one of tacit affection, peppered with jokes and reciprocated apologies. The doctor later that morning shared his story over coffee, an offering of comic relief, with his fatigued and embattled partner. It could, he realized, have turned out very differently.

What Dr S had here achieved with Mrs R. cannot be called 'psychotherapy' in its more formal sense, and yet the successful outcome of this short, highly-charged and rapidly shifting interchange depended on principles of communication and response which are cornerstones of psychotherapy at all levels of intensity and complexity.

The doctor had first to listen and observe afresh – the mother's shrill and remonstrative manner clearly conveyed much beyond the small, harmless lesion presented, and he had thus to consider that the meaning of the 'Ringworm' had very different connotations to himself and to his two frightened patients. It was only by allowing a hiatus in the usual structure of his interview, that Mrs R.'s fantasy or misconception of worm-infestation, her 'internal reality', could be crystallized, communicated and understood. Only then could both patient and doctor arrive at a new understanding of one another.[2]

Had Dr S needed to be in control at every stage of the interview, and forged ahead uncompromisingly with his initial frame of reference and didactic reassurance ('Nothing to worry about Mrs R., just use the cream ...') all three participants in this transaction would have left with further difficulty in store: Dr S would have gone home with a headache from frustrated ingratitude, Mrs R. and Amanda a symbiotic complex of anxious and unattended dread, coupled to an increasing mistrust of their conscientious but harassed doctor.

The medical prescription, the fungicidal cream, would be an adequate antidote to the physical lesion, but it was the development of understanding in the relationship that healed the growing emotional lesion. Mrs R.'s gruesome misconception – of 'Amanda being full of worms' – seemed to the doctor fortuitous, and due to misconstruction from the oddly termed 'Ringworm'. His task of exorcizing this damaging notion was thus much simpler and swifter than the psychodynamically generated complexes that challenge the skills of the psycho-therapist or analyst. Had Mrs R.'s fantasy of worms arisen instead from deeper, perhaps unconscious compounds of guilt, nameless dread, and inchoate destructiveness – the elemental stuff of psychoanalysis – she would not have departed as easily and lightly as she did, and would surely return with other tense and tangled communications.

## Case No. 2:
## Inner and outer listening: emotional literacy

A large and plethoric man, Mr B. looked briefly and searchingly toward Dr C, smiled nervously, moved away, and then shifted his doleful, heavy frame back toward the doctor.

Dr C, realizing his patient's first utterances would be difficult and important, put down his pen and sat back quietly.

'Doctor, I think I'm an alcoholic ... well I know I'm an alcoholic, I suppose. I know you can't do anything about that, so I'm probably wasting your time ... I just thought there might be something...'

Several routine questions offered to retrieve the fading Mr B. revealed to Dr C the severity and pattern of retreat into the haven of alcoholic oblivion in this unhappy and anxious man. But it was Mr B.'s underlying unhappiness itself, rather than a medically precise definition of his alcoholic abuse, that the doctor gently probed towards:

'Most people who have your kind of difficulty are attempting to get away from a feeling, or a situation, that is difficult or painful for them to manage or put into words, and I have the sense that's so with you, Mr B.', proffered the doctor, in a tone inviting but, he hoped, unintrusive.

'Yes, that's true. I do most of my drinking when I'm upset and all churned up. I think I can't stand all this aggravation, I want "Out", and then start drinking', elaborated an alert and engaged Mr B.

Dr C usually found himself pessimistic and patronizingly 'tolerant' with alcoholics, who, in his experience, seemed to have more guile in dissembling their problem, than he had talent or commitment to intervene in any way that might be hopeful or helpful. But Mr B. was a disarming and refreshing contrast in his candour, and the transparency of his underlying difficulties.

'I have a sense of you as being easy-going and genial on the outside, but hiding your hurts, grievances and resentments inside, where no one can see them ... so that there's a big gap between how people see you and what's really going on inside of you, and that gap makes for a lot of loneliness and fear ...', Dr C suggested, attempting to integrate his own experience of Mr B. with what Mr B. was saying about himself.

'Yes, that's just how it is ... there's this whole other side of me, like a small kid that's really angry and unhappy, and doesn't know what to do...'

'And drinks as a way out?' the doctor suggested before hearing more specifically of Mr B.'s lifelong difficulty in facing conflict and 'aggravation'.

The only child of an unhappy and tense union between a timorous, phobic mother and domineering, bullying father, he had learned early to survive by obedience, almost to the point of invisibility. But such early survival strategies, now fixed and long outmoded, had long ago rendered Mr B. mute in the face of challenge, passive in his needs, and emotionally inarticulate in his closest relationships. It did not surprise the doctor to learn that Mrs B. reacted to her husband's stalwart but hurt silences by bullying provocation, in an exasperated effort to create some sense of contact and definition with her sullen and inscrutable partner. The fact that her attacks led only to his further retreat into the morass, accelerated by his drinking, did not lead her to abandon her pattern, but amplify it.

In this first, and a later, longer interview the doctor gently guided this perplexed and hitherto inarticulate man in his efforts to make sense and connections, amidst the cycles of impotent resentment and retaliatory and palliative drinking. Thus encouraged, Mr B. took up the doctor's suggestion of seeking further counselling.

'I'm not drinking at all now, doctor', reported a direct and proud Mr B., and when the doctor asked him how he saw these first important steps of mastery, the reply was of great interest and edification to Dr C.

'When I first came to see you I thought you'd have little time for me, tell me to stop, that it was my problem and I was damaging myself – that sort of thing. That's what I expected, and I knew it wouldn't help. But you did something quite different: you really listened to me, and thought carefully about what I said. That hadn't happened to me before, and it's very important because it's started me listening to, and thinking about myself. With my counsellor now I'm beginning to see all sorts of things that I'd spent years running away from. I'm really pleased I came when I did.'

Dr C was pleased, too; it is not often that a patient comes to him in such a state of readiness to express and explore the underworld of conflicts and dilemmas, that are essential for radical and healing changes in the attitudes to oneself and relationships to others. The doctor had read much psychiatric literature concerning the efficacy or viability of psychotherapy in different clinical syndromes, suggesting that it is the clinical diagnosis which will determine the outcome of such endeavours. Such 'scientific' formulations never appealed much to his more humanistic temperament, and as the years have gone by he has been more impressed by determinants that can be more ordinarily expressed.

The capacity for candour, courage, curiosity and contact – both with what is within oneself and the other person – have seemed more accurate indicators of a healing dialogue. With many of his patients suffering from 'minor' neurotic complaints, he has never, despite his best efforts, been able to find a way through to these health-generating qualities: his words and attentions seem to bounce back at him. Others with more 'major' psychiatric stigmata, which numerous learned and specialist tracts would deem unsuitable or unlikely recipients of verbal healing, have surprised and inspired him with their readiness to enter the cauldron of challenge and change.

In these many journeys and encounters he has come to a new understanding of the word 'encourage' – as a young practitioner his encouragement consisted of convivial utterances designed to 'make the patient feel better', or at least appear grateful, if only for short periods. Fostering and nurturing the courage that inspires all health and growth, a more literal and substantial 'encouragement', had taken years of his own inner struggles and searchings to develop: encouragement must arise from a position of resonance, not rhetoric. We heal from our own healed wounds. [3, 4]

In parallel with Dr C's growth of understanding of encouragement has been his perception of 'emotional literacy' as a core element in health, growth and psychotherapy.[5] To remain 'in balance' with ourselves and others we need to be clear about our feelings; to name them, to read them, to articulate them. Without this emotional literacy there can be no solid sense or affirmation of the Self, from which any meaningful negotiation or mutuality with others becomes possible.

Mr B. was suffering from such illiteracy; raised in a family where needs and feelings were persistently distorted and discounted, he grew into a man effectively mute and affectively stunted. His alcoholic balm, intended to ease the pain of alienation from himself and others, only deepened the chasm. Many patients, it seems to Dr C, consult him because of such patterns of the inchoate and ineffable. With Mr B. it was his behaviour that led him to seek his doctor's counsel, but more often it is the patient's body that signals and expresses such disease and disequilibrium. The doctor's task is then clear, but often difficult, in helping his patient in the reclamation and deciphering of their disowned and neglected Self.

The long abandoned term of 'Alienist' for what we now call the Psychiatrist – a title connoting the re-engagement of those afflicted by alienation from themselves and others – seemed to encapsulate much of what Dr C must achieve in any healing endeavour with his patients. The doctor, though, is mindful of how demanding this is of the practitioner: as his use of 'encouragement' reflected the painful growth of his own courage, so his efforts at fostering 'emotional literacy' in his estranged patients could only parallel his own capacity for emotional clarity and articulation. To hear others we must listen to ourselves.

## Case No. 3:
## Feelings as wounder, feelings as healer

Dr T was only outwardly acquainted with Bill, an angular wiry man in his mid-fifties with an air of contained and circumspect vulnerability, and when he came with a recent exacerbation of his duodenal ulcer, the doctor wondered what had rekindled this invisible and self-generated wound. Prefacing his tense, though not unpleasant, communications with self-discounting apologies for bothering the doctor, Bill appeared to regard his hurts and needs as being unworthy of others' attention and care. A Council gardener in a small and meticulously tended local park, this well-regulated and compliant man always attended an evening surgery after his day's work, attired in his regulation green overalls.

From previous contact, Dr T had been witness to his limited but loyal life: his father dying in wartime combat, an only child, he had lived with his mother in their small late-Victorian flat until her death five years previously. Her demise had been slow and demanding, and he nursed her throughout this long and gruelling decline with fierce but quiet dedication, parrying any suggestion of her 'going away' to hospital. She died at home, a task painfully and painstakingly completed. When, some months later, Bill had requested an embrocation to soothe an overworked muscle in his thigh, a casualty of his silent and earnest training for the Marathon, Dr T mused on how, symbolically, his stoic self-sacrificing relationship with his beloved mother had been soon replaced. The doctor, while dealing with the matter of Bill's strained muscle, recalled with poignancy the title of an old black and white film: 'The Loneliness of the Long Distance Runner', but Bill's manner then had seemed dour and uncompromisingly matter-of-fact. The doctor did not share his image.

On this occasion, though, Bill seemed softer, and the doctor felt less prohibited from approaching his personal World, and when Dr T carefully asked him if there was anything in his recent life that had opened up his old internal wound, Bill's jaw trembled, his sinewy, tight-body sagged and he wept the copious, ancient tears of a man released from a long imprisonment.

'It was Frank going like that ...' he sobbed, attempting to stem the tears with a peremptory and remonstrating hand. 'He was my best mate. There was nothing the matter with him, but he just went... just went.'

From Bill's spontaneously articulated fragments of narration, and from his own delicately interposed questions, Dr T was able to assemble something of the significance of this much beloved and irreplaceable companion. Frank, another single man of similar age, had worked alongside Bill for a decade in the small and intimate park that had become a kind of child for these two childless men. Frank, apparently healthy and sanguine, had collapsed and died, at the verge of a flower bed, suddenly and without portent.

Bill was able to command back his tears and create a brave, red-eyed hiatus as he shared with the doctor something of his cherished friend and the painful void his sudden departure had left. As Dr T understood, more than ever before, the fragile and lonely courage lying behind the rather impassive exterior, Bill convulsed with another involuntary wave of recent and archaic grief. Dr T sat touched, attentive and silent, feeling like a mother cradling an anguished infant.

'I'm sorry, doctor to be like this… it's stupid, a grown man like me crying like a baby…', a finger and thumb pressed tightly and censoriously to his eyes, a vain attempt to enforce his usual containment.

'Not at all', Dr T uttered softly. 'I'm sad with you that you have this pain and grief, but very pleased you're able to share it with me; that's not at all "stupid". There are times for all of us when we need to cry and be cared for by others. I've long had a sense of you as being both courageous, but very hard on yourself in this way; that you won't allow yourself these very natural and human needs. I'll give you some tablets which will help cure your ulcer but, you know, what you've started here with me, sharing and expressing your feelings, may be the best medicine you can give yourself. I know it's hard and strange for you, but it's something I'm more than willing to help you with if you wish. It can be a great comfort, to have a safe place to talk about things that are kept hidden in other relationships in your life. I don't want to intrude, but I'm here to listen if you want me.'

'Yes, I do see what you're saying … and thank you, doctor. It's good to know you're here'. Bill replied, his voice more sonorous; a quiet, economic and characteristic coda.

Dr T remembered from his earlier training, reading long and complex treatises on which, among the innumerable physical ills to which the flesh is prey, were thought to be 'psychosomatic', and what the diseased part was symbolically, unconsciously, but precisely expressing and enacting.[6] Dr T's view has evolved into something rather more ordinary and less scholarly, for it has seemed to him that any illness can signify the discordance, the 'unfinished business',[7] the mere unhappiness of its host, and that the important question is not 'Is this illness "psychosomatic"?' but 'How may this person's inner and relationship life contribute to their illness, and (how) can I usefully and tactfully intervene?'[8] Aware, too, of the growing research on how immune and repair systems in the body reflect unexpressed and unresolved feeling,[9] Dr T has now a far wider perspective of how the expression of hidden and trapped feeling is so often crucial to recovery and the maintenance of health: Bill's expulsion of painful and palliating tears, a 'natural' therapy, are quite as important as the synthetic compound the doctor gave him to quell the acid production in his stomach. Such is 'Holistic Medicine'.

But there is more to this 'in vivo' psychotherapy than mere catharsis; for Bill may learn, through his experience with Dr T, that he can share powerful feelings with others, that both can survive it, and that from these a new growth and modus vivendi becomes possible. Whether or not he takes these tasks into the more deliberate territory of 'in vitro' counselling or psychotherapy, he has encountered, in its humblest form, what the psychoanalyst Michael Balint terms 'a New Beginning'.[10] While the doctor's interest, skill and 'encouragement' are clearly important in these first steps of encountering such challenges, it is ultimately Bill's own capacities of courage, curiosity and candour that will decide how far through this 'Front Door of Psychotherapy' he decides to travel and explore.

## Case No. 4:
## Being there

It was an exceptional and dramatic illness that Alice had suffered when vacationing with her husband and two teenaged sons in a West Country resort. A detailed hospital letter, replete with technical details, chronicled how she had, from apparently good health, almost died from a rapidly spreading perineal infection which, within twenty-four hours, had spread to her blood-stream, rendering her comatose and moribund, to be plucked from death's door by the vigilant dedication and expertise of the Intensive Care Unit. A horror and a miracle, Dr D had thought as his eyes scanned the scores of investigations that had guided the medical salvation of Alice, but which left

Dr D perplexed and ignorant as to why Alice had been so savagely felled in the first place.

She had rarely seen Dr D, and when she entered his room looking pinched, tired and grey, his attention was focused almost solely on the physical ramifications and sequelae of her nearly fatal complaint. An examination revealed a small residual abscess, and with a manner both apologetic and authoritative, the doctor referred her promptly to a surgeon to drain what he hoped would be the last outpost of this grim and mysterious foe. His hopes were premature or ill-informed, for she soon developed a bowel complaint with loose, frequent motions and the passage of mucus. The hospital physicians, asked to assess this problem, investigated her story and internal tissues with zealous and impressive thoroughness, fearing that her relentless and severe constellation of complaints might be due to some concealed fault in her immune system. Perhaps to their disappointment, but to Alice's relief, they found nothing.

When she came to tell Dr D of her 'progress'(!) and her most recent hospital odyssey, the doctor listened with courtesy and concealed despondency, before embarking on a lame but well-intentioned ritual of 'performing' a physical examination: he could not hope to unravel this Gordian knot, but at least he could be seen to be conscientious in his efforts. With a consoling but clueless hand on her abdomen he said:

'Events have moved so quickly and unpredictably that I haven't had a chance to get to know anything about you, apart from your illness. But I've been wondering if there's anything in your life, worries or frustrations, that you think might have brought all this on.'

Alice's abdomen tensed as her breath stopped momentarily, and Dr D did not expect the succinctness of the reply:

'I think you've got something there, doctor. You know, I just can't settle into this second marriage...'

Realizing the pregnancy of Alice's confidence was likely to be both fragile and crucial to understanding her menacing afflictions, Dr D acknowledged the importance of her statement, but desisted from asking anything more explicit from her, instead inviting her for a longer appointment where she could, if she wished, unfold and reveal her personal world.

Until ten years previously Alice had regarded herself as happily married to Tom. Their sexual relationship had always seemed a celebration of this; vibrant, full-blooded, enlivening and tender. Tom's confession had come with horrific suddenness: with shame but conviction, he told of an affair he was having with Alice's cousin, a woman much loved and valued by Alice. In a conflagration of shock, hatred and grief, this apparently loving and companionable relationship became a bitter and empty ruin. Alice, shamed, resentful, and uncomprehending, became circumspect and prickly, directing what bruised love she felt safe to entrust, toward her two sons.

This turbulent and bleak period of her life was eased somewhat by a kindly and attentive, though somewhat phlegmatic, neighbour, Cyril. Cyril too, had recently suffered a painful and central loss through his wife's death from breast cancer. Now a childless widower in his middle years with no family around him, his loneliness was soothed and expunged by his growing acts of concern and protectiveness towards Alice, a widow of sorts, an injured soul-mate. The two became bonded by mutual commiseration. Her two sons, hungering for paternal presence and interest, accepted Cyril's good humoured and stable involvement with an almost incredulous joy and gratitude: they had expected to remain fatherless. Alice's siblings and, now elderly, parents, at first warily protective of Alice, grew steadily in their warmth, admiration and respect for this unassuming and devoted man. It all seemed like a miracle of restoration when Cyril proposed marriage, and Alice, to the joy of all those around her, accepted.

But Alice's secret and inner world rumbled, faintly at first, with a doubt she could not communicate. While her gratitude and affection for Cyril warmed her heart, her flesh remained dispassionate to his touch. Tom had been a vital and charismatic lover, who had rarely failed to arouse and satisfy her deep visceral hungers, and to her dismay Cyril's body had seemed waxy and lifeless; at this primal level she could find no love for him.

'At first I thought I could grow to love him in that way, that it would come if I was patient. He's been so good to me and the children – the boys adore him. And I kept thinking: "It's not much to do in return. I should be able to offer him the sexual love he wants". But I just haven't been able to. At first I'd pretend, though it always hurt, and I tried to hide it. Then it got worse; I felt repelled and sick and terribly guilty for marrying him when I didn't desire him. It's a terrible problem I have, doctor. I can't reject him or leave him now, not after what he's done for me, and what he's been through with his wife dying. I think he'd die of a broken heart…'

'And the terrible infection you developed was like a way of keeping him out, and killing yourself, without you having to tell him anything painful. It's as if your body expressed, and attempted to solve, your whole painful predicament,' Dr D pondered, realizing that such metaphor might seem bizarre or obscurely distasteful to many of his colleagues.

'Yes, that's just how I've felt. The doctors at the hospital seemed amazed at my condition, but all the way through it didn't really surprise me. Secretly I thought of it as a way out, and as a kind of punishment … It all made some kind of awful sense,' Alice replied with stoic and dark candour.

Dr D, gratified and deeply moved by his understanding of the deeply tragic nature of Alice's dilemma, found himself feeling disorientated and impotent with his wish to help further. Toward the end of their harrowingly intimate hour together, realizing that the severity and momentum of this woman's problem was quite beyond his usual scope of support and clarification, the doctor suggested that her problem should be shared further with a counsellor.

'No, doctor,' she said with firm conviction. 'I can't tell anyone else, and I know nobody can do anything to change my situation. But you've probably done more than you realize, because it's important that someone, just one person, knows my situation and what I'm going through. It may sound strange, but it will help me manage. Can you understand that?'

Dr D's nod was warm and sorrowful. He did not need to say more.

Alice returned a fortnight later and reported her bowel complaint quiescent. Mindful of Alice's words on the previous occasion he did not enquire about her life, but the mellow and tender tone of the interview indicated that an implicit and important rapport had been created between them: she would return and talk if she needed to.

Dr D's 'psychotherapy' with Alice was not in any way complex or 'clever', the doctor merely provided a safe and attentive place where there was trust, time and containment enough for her to unburden herself in a way that was compassionately accompanied. Dr D, in allowing her to 'pour out' her secret pain and difficulties, had been struck by the way her bowel had no longer needed to fulfil this function symbolically and somatically. Putting her conflicts into words, it seemed, had thus shifted the locus of expression from her body.

There are other ways we can understand the healing encounter of Alice and Dr D In providing a 'Safe Space[11] for Alice to share her most anguished and burdensome secrets, she could, if only in that particular setting, bring together the self that was normally presented to the world and the self that she alone knew. From Freud onwards psychoanalysis has concentrated on the integration of the Conscious and Unconscious Self as the major task of psychological growth and healing. But the example of Alice illustrates a challenge more common in medical practice and counselling: for the integration of the split between her outer, Public Self and her inner, Secret

Self, is in no way 'unconscious', and yet is cardinal to her difficulties.[12]

Dr D's skill here did not lie in subsuming her communications to his own specialist concepts and frame of reference,[2] but rather to create the kind of relationship and dialogue where Alice was 'encouraged' in entrusting and accepting herself. This could only happen if she felt she could trust, and be accepted by, Dr D; and the doctor could create this kind of 'holding environment'[13] only if he could manage a particular kind of unconditional listening and responsiveness.[14] This is more complex than it might seem for, as we have seen with Dr B in Case No 2., such qualities of outer listening to another emerge from the long gestation of listening to oneself. The empathy mustered by Dr D could not arise merely from curiosity and benevolent intentions; the resonance required demanded a deep and hard-earned inner sentience.

Alice's final communications to Dr D at the end of her long interview have an intriguing and instructive message in the endeavour of psychotherapy. In a culture and profession increasingly obsessed with questions of active intervention, terminology and technique, we are, perhaps apt to overlook the healing power of being known, with intimacy and volition, to another.[15] It is often unmitigated aloneness that makes us sick; inclusion and acceptance that heal. It is here that the heart of the Alienist is most tested.

Ω

## References

[1] Balint M. *The doctor, his Patient, and the Illness.* London: Pitman, 1957.

[2] Zigmond D. Three types of encounter in the healing arts: dialogue dialectice and didacticism. *Holistic Medicine,* 1987; 2: 69-81.

[3] Bennet G. *The Wound and the Doctor.* London: Secker and Warburg, 1987.

[4] Zigmond D. Physician heal thyself: the paradox of the wounded healer. *Br J of Holistic Med* 1984; **1.**

[5] Steiner C Emotional literacy. *Transactional Analysis Journal* 1984: 14

[6] See for example,
Alexander F. Fundamental concepts of psychosomatic research: psychogenesis, conversion, specificity. *Psychosom Med* 1943; **5**: 205.

[7] Perls F. *Gestalt therapy verbatim.* Utah: Real People Press, 1969.

[8] Zigmond D. A psychosomatic approach. *Practitioner,* April 1982.
Zigmond D. the psychosomatic mosaic. *Practitioner,* April 1982.

[9] See, for example
Bathrop RW. Depressed lymphocyte function after bereavement. *Lancet* 1977; **1**: 834-6.
Selye H. *The stress of life* New York: McGraw-Hill, 1956.
Friedman SB, Glasgow LA, Ader R. Psychosocial factors modifying host resistance to experimental infections. *Ann New York Acad Sci* 1969; 164: 381-93.

[10] Balint M. The basic fault. London & New York: Tavistock, 1968.

[11] Fry A. Safe space. London: Dent, 1987.

[12] Zigmond D. The elements of psychotherapy. *Practitioner* September 1981.

[13] Winnicott D. *The maturational process and the facilitating environment.* New York: International Universities Press, 1965.

[14] Rogers C On becoming a person New York: Houghton Mifflin, 1961.

[15] Pennebaker JW, Becall SK. Confronting a traumatic event: toward an understanding of inhibition and disease. *Abnormal Psychology* 95 274-81, 1986; 85: 274-81.

Publ. in *Holistic Medicine,* vol. 4, 197-208 (1989)

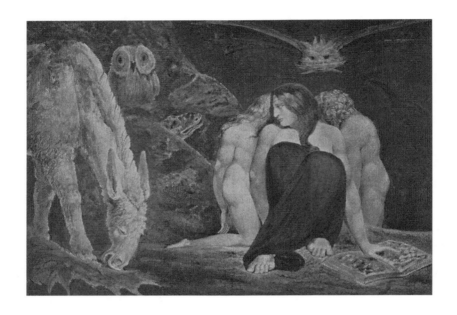

William Blake, *The Night of Eritharma's Joy*, 1795

# Intermezzo

# The Shadow of Venus - Atavism and Sexuality

## How can the primitive shadow side of our sexuality be understood?

We are driven not so much by the need to procreate as by the attempt to master and fixate the past.

*'If venereal delight and the power of propagating the species were permitted only to the virtuous, it would make the world very good.'*

James Boswell, *London Journal*, March 26ᵗʰ 1763

*'Most creatures have a vague belief that a very precarious hazard, a kind of transparent membrane, divides death from love: and that the profound idea of nature demands that the giver of life should die at the moment of giving.'*

Maurice Maeterlinck, *The Life of the Bee*, 1901

Of all human paradoxes, our Sexuality is the cruellest, the richest, the most tragi-comic. For all, it is the Maker of Destiny; but for many (most?), the Scrambler of Design. It is the 'Joker' in the Pack of Intent. Even if we have ourselves escaped archaic and anarchic tides and vortices, we are almost certain to have witnessed other, no-lesser mortals, depart the rational world; Abducted by Aliens. At its best, it spawns the ordinary miracle of new life. It is 'Libido', 'Nachus', the germ of family, the template of growing networks. But as it enters our shadowlands it is transformed, trance-formed, to Destrudo, Mortido: the slayer of integrity, the courtesan of dismembered and dishonoured unions. The fluids that carry the Germs of Life, may also convey the viral Nucleic Acids of Death. The Harbourer of Life beclouds the Harbinger of Death. Perhaps our existential predicaments are, literally, embodied in the anatomical plan: our reservoirs and channels of procreation reside and emerge next to those of elimination. Spring of Life: Waste of Death. Propinquitous adversaries; inseparable neighbours.

Libidinal sex runs to the trumpeted birth, the proud dynasty. But sex is chimeric and fickle: tumescence sometimes transmutes to tragedy with the inexorability of a mighty waterfall. We are publicly and privately fascinated by such sex-in-destrudo. In its noblest and grandest forms we have Biblical Tales, Classical Myths and Opera. For more immediate, salacious gratification, weekend newspapers are cheaper and easier. The Fallen Great always sell news-print. Those less candid savour shrill morality, the more humble know it could be (has been?) them.

Humankind is unique in liberating libido from oestrus. Our sexual activity is only fractionally motivated by our desire for procreation. In other species every 'courtship' gesture is some kind of selection, ranking, monitoring of healthy fertility, and negotiation about defensible space. The sexual act itself is functional and uniformly stereotyped within the species. All is subsumed to procreation. All this can, and does, happen in human encounters, but most sexual acts occur outside the procreational remit: we create a more diverse and unpredictable world where sex, the excitement produced when we are touched at the delicate junction of our inside and outside, can only be understood in terms of experience, not biological function.

This 'experience' is a hind-brain act of creation. With our fore-brain we may attempt to guide, edit, appreciate or moralise —all the ways we have of socialising the 'primitive'; directing the sexual 'current'. But the 'sparks' of sexual excitement are forms of primitive en-trancement and en-thrallment: the gravitational field of our individual and collective past, impelling us to re-enact, regurgitate, revisit, sometimes resolve ancestral homes: our infancy and our biological legacy. These forces, emanating from our individual and species inheritance, act in many ways like planetary gravity. We are mostly unaware of it, until mishap and misjudgement make clear how decisive and irresistible are the influences of planets or stars, which may have long passed out of visibility, and whose distance from us is not comprehensible within our usual frame. In the domain of our sexuality, especially, there are crucial influences whose origin has long vanished: 'Woe betide' is an interestingly constructed phrase to caution those sceptical or casual about submerged tides and currents. The determinants of our sexuality are not part of the usual landscape of conscious and intentional self. Hence the peril and fascination.

What are these primitive realms, these springs of such hypnotic power? A condensed answer is that human sexuality recapitulates both ontogeny and phylogeny. We are driven not so much by the need to assure the future (by fertilisation), as by the attempt to encompass, master and fixate the past. As we shall see, such attempts are only ever transiently successful; but the most fleeting of such satisfactions is still the most reliably alluring and perennial of all human balms and stimulants.

The ontogenic basis of our sexuality is the one that has been recurrently rummaged, especially by psychoanalysts. In brief, we regress to earlier satisfactions or struggles in order either to possess or master them. We become the anguished infant quelled by the stroking hand, the hungry mouth searching for the breast, the newborn gazing at the source of life, or struggling (vainly!) for re-entry through the Arch of Birth. Intertwined, interpenetrated, we relive the fascinated dances of exploration of body parts, the existence of 'other'. The familiar and the alien. Safety and danger. A part and apart.

All this, as in infancy, is lived out through touch, gaze, body heat and fluids, and contact of the most primal and powerful kind: the junction of inside and outside; Endoderm and Ectoderm. Sensation is seared to its earliest and its essence – the Mother of all Experience.

By publicly-avowed convention we regard sex as 'healthy' and 'wholesome' when it derives from the Winnicottian triad of pleasured mother-baby bonds: feeding, nursing and playing. These, with myriad variations and inventions, conjure the 'Joy of Sex', the 'Light Side of the Moon', libido. But the infant is not purely pleasure-seeking, pain-avoidant. Whether by wish, fear or phantasy, the primitive mind tips over into a welter-world of monsters, perils and horrors. The pleasure-triad becomes starkly inverted — a Kleinian cluster of pillage, invasion, spoliation, makes a shadowy, malign reflection. We are in the territory of Crime and Punishment, The Moon's Spectre, Mortido.

This mortidinous dimension of Sex is commoner than 'common-sense' would have us suppose. For the 'public' and simplistic view is that 'healthy' sex is fuelled by solely 'good' intentions and inclinations — kindness, pleasure, safety, mutuality. Most of us know otherwise. These contributions may make sex warm, but not catch fire. Alas, 'normal' sexual excitement often needs an element of danger, challenge, peril, pain. Mostly, fortunately, our forebrain can contain and compromise the hindbrain's hazardous cravings. We settle for the fierce kiss, the sharp ridged sweep of a fingernail, the violent thrust, the understood utterances of erotic abuse, the fantasy never uttered. Here, we can have combustion without conflagration, danger without harm. Flesh and trust are unbroken. An erotico-magnetic field and spark needs this tension and juxtaposition of opposites. Safety and danger, protection and attack, libido and mortido. The balance of opposites is difficult and fragile, especially in long-term relationships. Most commonly, through fatigue, the balance shifts towards safety, leading to a current without sparks and often, sadly, no current at all. Less commonly, the shift will be toward danger, destrudo and death (either literal or metaphorical), which leads to many sparks, but no current. Frequently, in such cases, sex is no balm, but a bait and a weapon, used in symbolic retaliation for ancient hurts and horrors. There is, here, no counterbalancing libido.

Such condensation within our sexuality of early and primitive experiences and struggles often imbues our sexual bonds with infantile intensity and perspective: 'I can't live without you'. It is often impossible to separate primordial bliss from primeval terror: life and death are here explosively close. 'crime passionel' is the commonest (peacetime) murder.

Our hindbrain is the repository not only of the innumerable ghosts of our individual-past, but also the echo-traces of our species-past – our phylogeny. The odyssey of evolution, the aeons passed in life's push from amoeba to flatworm to fish, mudskipper, amphibian, mammal; all exist as remnants in our anatomy and gestation. Miraculously, we condense millions of years of evolution into the nine months in-utero, during the ordinary, extraordinary growth of fertilised ovum to human foetus. 'Ontogeny recapitulates phylogeny.' There are equivalent vestiges in our dreams and sexuality, too. We dream of flight, of sub-aquatic or burrowing existence, of being the bloodied roaring king, or his terror-struck, whinnying quarry. We may dream of our skin shedding, of laying eggs, of pupating into alien forms. These are not the workings of a modern fore-brain engulfing biological data to feed it, fragmented and mutated, into hind-brain's dreams. Such images and notions occur among the earliest myths and art-forms known to us, often from cultures not acquainted with such creatures. The identification with other life-forms seems an 'intuitive' hindbrain act, an awakening of a prehistoric memory trace, a zoomorphic variation of Jung's Collective Unconscious, connecting and echoing life, in all its panoply and history. Such dreams are not merely inventive projections: they are nature's reminder that we are where we have come from.

And so it is with our sexuality; an activity so diverse as to make absurd our endless attempts to contain it within frames of morality, normality or sanity. Even if we do not outwardly transgress, we know that our inner images and wonderings are often generated beyond the frame. We burden and misunderstand ourselves with the assumption that human sexuality should, like other creatures, have a standard and stereotypic form; a 'normality' that can be assessed by the parameters of a biological function. But millennia of evidence indicates that sex is more akin to dream-state than bodily function. In this dream-world, this en-trancement, we may unwillingly and unwittingly find hypnotic echoes and compulsive urges which have no useful role in fertilisation, but in which, by vestiges and relics, the whole of nature finds representation.

Sex is the anchor that we throw over the gun-wale of human-kind to the ocean-bed of the animal. The anchor-points through which we cleave, with such ephemeral obsession, to our animal substratum are, often, so diverse and remote, that our forebrain-self responds with either incredulity or alarm.

A short selection of other species' scenarios gives some illustrations to the notion of our sexual atavism. They range from the benign and sublime, to the malign and hideous. In some we find the parallel is direct and clear, in others indirect and metaphorical. For the sake of brevity, I have bracketed the human equivalent in a cursory, but hopefully comprehensible, form.

- Birds feed their young beak-to-beak. (Sexual mouth kissing comprises many feeding imitations.)
- Mouth-brooder fish fertilise and care for the eggs in the mouth. (Dreams and fantasies of oral impregnation and fertilisation.)
- Snails and slugs are hermaphrodite, enacting both gender roles simultaneously. (We are significantly more hermaphrodite, in secret or private, than our anatomy or social conventions suggest.)
- Cat family males have a barbed penis — this causes intense sudden pain to the female on withdrawal, stimulating ovulation. (Some pain is often aphrodisiacal, either intrinsically, or because of its suggestion of danger.)
- The female praying mantis devours her male mate soon after fertilisation, to serve as nutrient for her motherhood.

(At its most horrific is the post-coital murder, usually perpetrated by males. What is rather more common is an intense, but inchoate, male fear of post-coital engulfment or castration. In my view, these feelings are nowhere near accounted for by psychoanalytic notions of envy, oedipal retaliation etc.)

- In some species of spider, the male will weave a web around the female in order to protect himself from being eaten. Often he will offer her a web-wrapped gift of other food to distract her while he is doing this. (Bondage is often a defence against the danger of coitus, albeit sometimes ritualized. Gifts are often distractions to forestall attack.)

- In many mammals the mother will lick the infant all over for cleanliness and warmth. Common too, is the mother's eating the body waste of the infant, not only for hygiene and the deterring of predators, but also to make an olfactory bond of recognition that may be essential for the infant's survival. (As with mouth-feeding, there are many echoes here in oral sexuality.)

- Barnacles, which cannot move to mate, have developed a unique telescopic penis to enable sex at a distance. (The human equivalents here are numerous and metaphorical, and range from voyeurism to telephone and internet-sex; from prostitution to pornography. The human 'shell' here is emotional, and the 'distance', anonymity.)

Possibly the most universally emotive animal act serving as a metaphor for understanding the experience and metaphysic of human sexuality, is that of the salmon. Such fish swim from their sea habitat, up and against river currents, in order to spawn in the very same place that they were hatched. The journey is gruelling and the mission heroic, for the enfeebled creatures die of exhaustion soon after emission.

There is a poetic equivalence here to our own sexual and life-cycles of excitement and struggle; decay and death. The heightened senses, the thrashing, gasping, rasping struggle of life. The cries and shouts, akin to the holler of labour: the fanfare of imminent birth. Then, explosion-implosion. Transcendence, contraction, mindless, senseless, flaccid, as vulnerable as a new-born; still-born? Quiet and still: barely breathing in the twilight. A sweet-musty odour, a fluttering fall of autumn leaves. Death fleets and vanishes. Beneath the flow, the undertow. Life is fragile and transient: how precious!

It is through sex, through the stellate explosion of our senses into orgasm, that our struggling polarities are miraculously, if transiently, reconciled. Inside and outside, forebrain and hindbrain, human and animal, safety and danger, a part and apart, self and other, microcosm and macrocosm, life and death. Perhaps this last verse can most aptly close this circle of cycles:

*We shall not cease from exploration*
*And the end of all our exploring*
*Will be to arrive where we started*
*And know the place for the first time.*

TS Eliot, 'Little Gidding', *The Four Quartets*.

Ω

Publ. in *Human Potential* Winter 1995 27

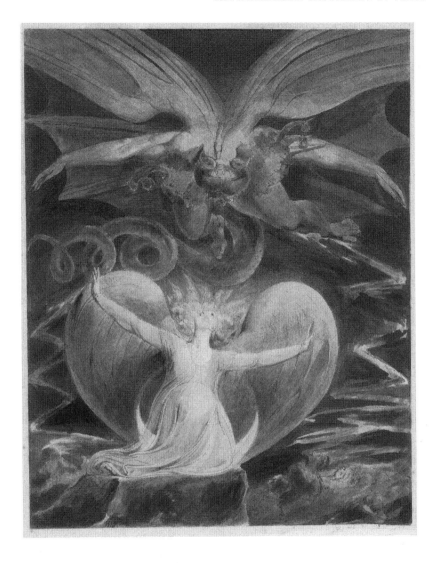

William Blake *The Great Red Dragon and the Woman Clothed with the Sun*
1805 – 10

# Section Two

# What can go wrong?

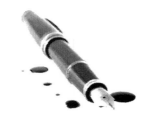

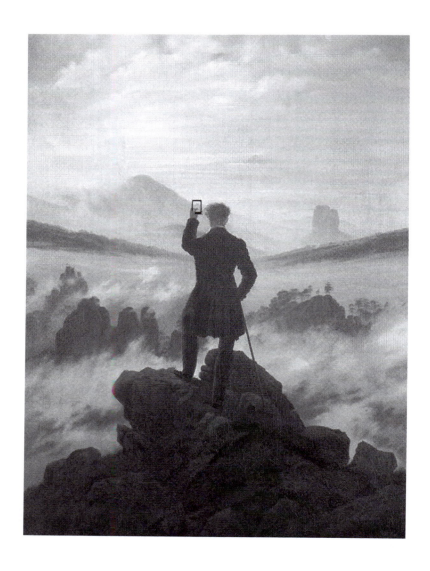

C. D. Friedrich – *The Wanderer above the Mist 1818*
(upgraded 2012)

# Where in the World are You?

## Miraculous cyber;
## insidious dislocation

What do mobile communications, internet sex and modern over-schematised mental health systems have in common?
– a computer mediated disconnection of intended content from embedding human context.
What happens?

## Introduction

Our increasingly easy and instant access to knowledge and products is usually regarded as 'progress', yet, paradoxically, often deprives us of more organic forms of discovery, connection and creativity. This is a growing problem that we are ingeniously disregarding. Mobile phones, internet sex, Sat Navs and computer-systematised mental healthcare are exampled and explored.

*

*'A thing in itself never expresses anything. It is the relation between things that gives meaning to them'*

Hans Hofman, *Search for the Real* (1967)


I miss the call. I recognise the number but cannot identify it: I call back. The voice is reassuring in its immediate familiarity; a softly musical, slightly apologetic lilt, a faint West Country burr. It is a voice I have known for many years; it is so clear that I know she must be calling from somewhere close by. Yet she has recently talked of imminent departure for a late-career gap-year; travelling to long-envisioned, little-known, distant places.

I continue to misconstrue: 'Where in the world are you?' I ask, part genuine enquiry, part misjudged tease about her unstarted travels. 'Oh, I'm in Ashqabat' she says prosaically, as if this should be self-evident. I make some opaque but friendly sound to deflect attention from my geographical ignorance and misfired humour. 'That's in Turkmenistan' she explains without comebackance.

Later I look it up in an atlas: I had no idea of its existence.

*

Still later I am pondering this now ubiquitous greeting from terra firma to mobile: 'Where are you?'. Thirty years ago such an utterance was non-existent: if you called someone on the phone you also knew their location; if you did not know where they were you could not contact them. Such a question would have been nonsensical or ironic metaphor. Contact required locational, and usually personal, knowledge.

Even more has the Internet rapidly dislocated such timeless preconditions for communication. We can now convey precise and instant messages with no identifying features of person or location. The *content* is all: the *context* increasingly unnecessary or lost. As our electronically mediated messages and data become more crystal-clear, their human and vernacular ambience becomes more fog-like. This new world of combined clarity of content and obscurity of context had some early and interesting explorers. Internet sex has managed (for countless many) an astonishing uncoupling from experiences and activities mostly rooted in the primacy of the interpersonal and physically sensate. Internet users could now, with unprecedented ease, replace these with an instant, synthetic composite of the depersonalised and abstracted: a screen glowing with generic alphabetical signs (words) conveyed featurelessly (text) by an unknown person. Even the latter may be wishful thinking: such cyber-erotica could have been generated by computer. Yet even if the transmitter of virtual delights is human, that human form may have little resemblance to the one constructed by the recipient: there is no touch, sound, smell, taste, face, gaze, or even a real name. There is no evolved mutuality or history. We have, instead, highly abstracted, electronically transmitted signals, which the recipient then conjures into a desired fantasy of desire. Such are our substitutes for 'intimacy' when we choose to eliminate context with content.

Such computer-mediated dislocation inevitably darkens with opportunities for malign perversity. We are now a mere few clicks away from masking our spying, intrusions, threats and assaults on others: cyber-bullying and graphic sexually framed humiliations or terrors are the shadow of cyber-erotica.

Under a cloak of anonymity it is easy for us to do our worst: we have democratised *Jack the Ripper*.

*

Such cyber-dysrotica may be one guise of Satan in our digital age and brings to the bystanders a dark wonder of strangers, fear for our children and unsettling frissons of doubt about partners. The most egregious of these will bring us salacious headlines.

The rapid development of such social disjunctions is largely due to digital informatics. There are many other forms that are now so commonplace as to arouse little thought or comment, yet generate new types of oblivion. These oblivia usually incur losses and while the short-term effects of these may seem benign and superficial, the longer-term consequences will turn much less trivial. Here are two apparently disparate examples of evolving dislocation.

### i)  Where am I? Ask the Sat Nav

I am lost in a part of Norfolk unknown to me. There is a complex cluster of non-motorway road junctions with inadequate and discrepant signage that may have recently been changed and does not conform to my map. Close to the junctions is a large petrol station with several drivers filling up. I ask six drivers about the signage and designation of the nearby major roads and they are all amiably and helpfully unhelpful: they do not know.

What is happening? I think this small story is part of a new and growing trend; it would not have happened twenty years ago. Clearly, this is not yet science: my sample is small and there is no control group. I may just have been unlucky in choosing six consecutive non-locals who were all as new to the area as myself. Maybe, but I have other, similar experiences that indicate something more interesting and important is happening: just as we increasingly do not know our neighbours, we are losing personal knowledge of our neighbourhood, our terrain and location. A key to understanding this story is that most (all?) of the drivers had Sat Navs and, I believe, were decognitised by their devices. They habitually tapped in required destinations, thus delegating all navigational decisions: this leaves them 'free' when driving to wander the mind, to chat and to phone. The technology thus unburdens them: they now need little sentience of their journey and surroundings: personal knowledge of whereabouts hence ceases to have any useful function. Whatever needs to be known can be accessed instantly in the vast annals of cyberspace; omniscient and omniprescient – like a secular deity. By constructing this supra-ordinate intelligence we human users are relieved of the burdens of having to plan, notice, remember or make decisions when journeying: our surroundings become irrelevant and we are freer to go on our personally oblivious, computer-sighted way – a procession of antennaed, encapsulated cyber-solipsists.

This computer-mediated oblivion of our geography may be thought inconsequentially expedient and thus benign. I think this is mistaken: such losses may start subtly, but later the price paid is serious. This is currently becoming painfully clear when similar computer-enhanced oblivion loses sight of people.

What then happens?

## ii) Who is he? Ask the computer

Stuart is sitting with me again, trembling and harrowed, in my consulting room. His partner, Jill, has brought him to the surgery with tender but tiring vigilance and now stays with us – he needs many mooring points to stop his drift out into an ocean of perils, unhorizoned and tempestuous.

Stuart is in his mid-forties and after many less catastrophic premonitory symptoms, his mental cohesion and integrity are now breaking down. He has no clear or coherent language for this disintegration: at first he described his frightening experiences in physical terms, then he learned to talk from a basic psychological but impersonal lexicon – of panics, disturbances of mood and emergency escapes by impulsive actions. Healthcarers apply their usual terminology.

Stuart's manner is of a frightened, wary, resentfully hurt child who wants to find someone to trust but fears making that decision. There are good reasons for this, which he has been encouraged to share in numbed or painful fragments. His life was conceived from a careless and doomed union by a young couple, and his father had disappeared forever several months before he was born. His young mother did not want – and then could not cope with – an infant son, but she was blessed with parents who were happy to do both these things.

Stuart had five loving, devoted, stable and happy years with these grandparents before a sudden destructive disruption: his mother found a new partner whom she wished to marry and intended to accelerate the formation of her family group by reclaiming Stuart. The loss of his grandparents was litigious and he saw little of them after the battle-dust settled. Worse was to come: his mother never conceived again and his stepfather's initial tolerance toxified through indifference to contempt and hostility, to eventual violence that ineradicably and intensely frightened and humiliated the boy. Fearful of and for her marriage, Stuart's mother colluded with the stepfather. Stuart's contiguous, through different, mistrust of men and women took root.

Stuart survived these betrayed attachments in his youth by various kinds of numbness, denial, structure and displacement – alcohol, drugs, sexual promiscuity, drunken fights, emigration, army service – but by his middle years his defences are crumbling. His estranged ex-wife and two adult sons are long lost to him and expatriated in the wake of his many years' flailing and dissonant defences; buttresses against his ancient grief, rage and mistrust. But these could bring only partial and fleeting respite – the spectres would surely return. This they did when he attempts to reciprocate Jill's wholesome and unconflicted love: Stuart's bedevilment reconflagrates, but this time he does not attempt to escape.

Instead he breaks down.

If Stuart is to now turn this breakdown into a breakthrough, he will need the kind of caring and understanding stability that he once received from his grandparents. To heal such deep and chronic wounds he will need long contact with, and containment by, a kind of extended 'loving family' in which there are several overlapping and complementary roles. For healing 'love' – a patient, non-possessive, non-controlling, benign, disinterested interest – is most fertile when it can flow between several angles and strata. Jill's love is primal, domestic and personal. What I offer is more boundaried and ritualised by professional role – though heartfelt for us both – and massively symbolically significant for Stuart: I become the benign and committed father who does not leave. But the strains on me in doing this are great: I, too, need a supportive and therapeutic extended 'family'. I will need my psychiatric colleagues to widen the net and share the strain.

But the NHS psychiatric services that I ask to help me help Stuart do not now have the kind of consciousness or organisation to step into this kind of role – one guided by powerful metaphorical realities of stable family surrogacy and loving therapeutics. Instead they offer a carouselled medley of long, formulaic interrogatory assessments, risk-management protocols, behavioural modification programmes, Treatment Plans and (transient) Care Coordinators to attempt cohesion and comprehension. These latter flail and fail: Stuart often sees someone different each time he attends, and when he does so they ask him similar and repetitive questions without, apparently, any growth of personal or mutual understanding. This is negatively reflected in Stuart's recall: he cannot remember their names, job designations or much of what was said. 'They look at the computer a lot and seem to be mainly interested in whether I'm taking my tablets and whether I intend doing something pointless or horrible. They keep on asking the same questions like some kind of Official Inspector … No, I don't think they're really interested in me, only what I might do …'

The depersonalised fragmentation of care worsens with time, as Stuart's possible attachments never develop naturally, instead they are recurrently displaced by administrative formulae, timetables and plans. Over several months he is passed between many different teams, which he cannot remember, but I do.* All of these encounters of *Therapeuticus Interruptus* add to his core sense of futile and despondent unwantedness and the inscrutable, random, uncaring, unreliability of others and their power.

Stuart understandably loses faith in them, but not (yet) in me. I make several phone calls over these months in an attempt to retrieve and repair the situation. I speak to Team Managers, Care Coordinators, Duty Desks, various types and grades of Psychiatrists and – eventually – the Clinical Director of these services. The pattern becomes familiar: the responsible practitioner may have been briefed about Stuart, but rarely know much more about him. But I am told this is not significant: 'all relevant mental healthcare workers can locate him on our shared (computer) System'. No, they cannot have a more detailed discussion with me, but my concerns will be noted for the next Team Meeting. They politely deflect my suggestion for more personal continuity of care: 'Stuart's Patient Journey is carefully considered and planned by each Multi-disciplinary Team. In all this we follow our NHS Trust protocol as an assurance. There is thus no need for any one practitioner to have the more particular knowledge or longer-term commitment or relationship you speak of. Our System will tell us what we need to know.'

Despite Stuart's lack of meaningful engagement with these professionally sequestered colleagues I still want him to attend. They may not offer what either he or I need, but at least they are around to provide a modicum, or symbolic presence, of caring: I do not want to be left to struggle as a 'single father'. Neither do I want him to collect a fresh label of 'uncooperative patient': his ancient label of 'illegitimate' is already more than he can bear.

*

I am thinking of similarities between Internet sex without personal intercourse, the Sat Nav directed drivers who can designate their destination but never know their journey, and the Mental Healthcare workers who know how to access Stuart's healthcare data but are not concerned to know Stuart. All assume a supra-ordinate system that short-circuits the need for personal connection, responsibility or sentience – all elements of *relationships*. The cyber-knowledge of the Sat Nav impoverishes our *relationship* with our traversed geography. The cyber-knowledge of the Healthcare Computer too easily replaces our *relationship* with people whose lives we accompany at critical times. The healthcarers I spoke to talked of Stuart – often, I thought, to their complete self-satisfaction – as if they had successfully Sat Naved him on his Patient Journey, and no further discussion was necessary. Such cyber-parenting may reassure the institutional healthcarers, but is experienced quite differently elsewhere. Now I must largely cope alone as a 'single father', without an extended therapeutic family. For Stuart it is far worse: his ancient history of family instability, unpredictable strangers and recurrent powerless subordinations to others' decisions is re-experienced painfully by him, but never discussed with them. Their relationship is mostly with their System; Stuart may be granted some of this, if he conforms.

*

Holism – our humanly flawed attempt to see wholes – can never be perfectable or completeable and is thus an eternally precious but doomed project. It is an aspiration, an inspiration, a philosophy and an ethos: we travel, but never finally arrive. It is the antithesis of expedience, device or procedure – although we must make compromises with these. Amidst this, holism is untidy and risky: we must employ imagination to make unobvious connections with the apparently diverse – activities that cannot be measured, managed, packaged or proved. Holism thus needs, at least, our tolerance of – at best, our creative play with – ambiguity, uncertainty and unproveability. Paradoxically, it is when we risk and venture these that we develop our most meaningful understandings of one another. Just as the Sat Nav's crisp, authoritative certainty may blind us to our geographical journey, an over-systemised, computerised healthcare system may unsight us to the hidden humanity of our fellow journeyers.

*'The quest for certainty blocks the search for meaning. Uncertainty is the very condition to impel Man to unfold his powers.'*

Erich Fromm, *Man for Himself* (1947)

---

*In one year Stuart was seen by the following Psychiatry and Psychology Teams: Hospital Liaison Psychiatry (three hospitals); Community Mental Health: Assessment and Brief Therapy; Mood Anxiety and Personality; Increased Access to Psychological Treatment Services; Emergency Psychiatry; Home Treatment; Hospital Inpatient; Early Discharge; Assertive Outreach.

The putative integration of fragments is called a 'Patient Journey'.

The administrative fragments themselves are propagated, defined, reified and justified by an increasing volume of tautological (often) academia, derivative algorithms, and think-tanked services-redesign documents.

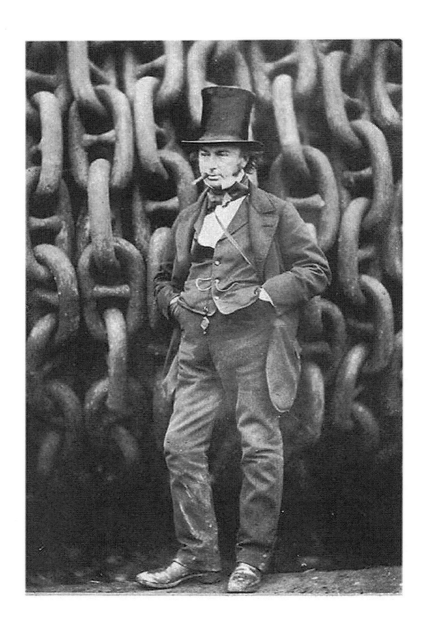

Isambard Kingdom Brunel (1806 – 59)

# Edward
# shot in his own interest

## Technototalitarianism and
## the fragility of the therapeutic dance

As long as I can remember I have been a searcher and a sceptic. This often uncomfortable predicament has led to my tendency to perspectives that are relativistic and kaleidoscopic. For a man so afflicted, my NHS practitioner roles have been contrastingly stable and durable. Nearly 30 years in the same general practice and hospital posts have offered me a remarkable long-term vantage point for the destiny of individuals, families and the tides and style of organisations and working ideologies. Through all this, my intense interest in the complexity and power of human contact and attachment has remained vital.

Charlie Chaplin *Modern Times* 1936

*Even in slight things, the experience of the new is rarely without some stirring of foreboding.*

Eric Hoffer, *The Ordeal of Change* (1964)

*Change is scientific, progress is ethical; change is indubitable whereas progress is a matter of controversy.*

Bertrand Russell, *Unpopular Essays* (1950)

It is well past midday. For nearly four hours I have variously survived a chimeric procession of human contacts that push and crowd a Monday morning GP surgery. I am turning light-headed, retreating with compassion-fatigue, and losing my sharper abilities for convergent thinking. When Edward enters I know I will have to recover my receding faculties, if we are both to feel well-disposed to one another.

Edward is a complex man, and has long evoked much frustrated confusion in those who attend him. His large physical frame has carried his 82 years mostly with great reliability and robustness but, I sense, without much expression or pleasure. His physical complaints of mild hip arthritis and angina have been well suppressed by usual current treatments. Not so his 'illness behaviour'. Edward's frequent attendances, over many years, despite his lack of serious illness, had first perplexed, later irritated and finally enervated his previous doctor, Dr T, a man long admired for his good-humoured restraint and diplomatic wisdom. With Edward, Dr T tired from an attrition of his higher powers; his colleagues sighed with relief when he declared an uncharacteristic abandonment of this 'heartsink patient'. They had secretly and individually feared far worse. Edward, removed from Dr T's list, was assigned to mine; a blind and involuntary coupling.

Six years later, I have identified and commiserated with Dr T, his travails and honourable self-discharge. Edward has been a 'difficult' man, often experienced as contrary and contradictory, ambiguous and ambivalent: his neediness mistrustful, his responses to attention often spiky and diminishing. Beneath this surface of confused signals and contacts, I have imagined a life of thwarted yearning, of previous struggles, and now, turbulent submission. Edward does not want his private life probed, but he does, somehow, want it understood. He recurrently declined invitations to enter the more directly investigative and interventive domains of psychiatry and counselling. Early on in our encounters I framed these suggestions, I smugly thought, with much skill and artistry. His retort was tart: *'I'm no more crazy or disturbed than you, doctor'*.

I had insight enough not to contest him. Explicit enquiry remained subtly parried. My interest in explanatory history, or explicit portraiture, would not be met. I was slow to learn that well-travelled approaches of medicine, psychiatry and psychology could not help me to help, or even contain, most of this man's complaints. I was in the world of the shaman and the cryptographer.

In the analogy of journeying, I was now confined to the use of narrow winding tracks in poor visibility over uneven, often steeply inclined, surfaces. The steady, even, well-lit, straight, broad roads of 'conventional' medical practice were elsewhere. Off the major thoroughfares, hazards are more numerous and various. To stay on such paths requires vigilant anticipation and attention. With Edward I learned to offer him not just the usual, pre-packaged questions, explanations and reassurance, but also bespoke medical ritual and respectful play. Lingering over a manual (not electronic) measurement of his pulse and blood pressure was usually unhelpful medically, but offered a form of structured, caring touch and contact that was tolerable and safe for this lonely and armoured man. 1 learned, too, of an acerbic and anarchic wit beneath his previously gruff, combative presentations: our banter developed an accompanying, unspoken affection. I was rewarded for taking The Road Less

Travelled. He agreed to come every two months for 'routine review', and stopped his more frequent opportunistic, antagonistic attendances. Receptionists reported a baffling patience and politeness. I cautiously enjoyed my brief but regular appearances in a marathon role as secular priest. Edward became less querulously hypochondriacal, his presence in the room was lighter, his gaze softer, he left the room willingly and without a trail of unfinished, unspoken business. He stopped being a heartsink patient. I thought often of the innumerable ways that we humans devise for engineering contact, but ensuring structure and optimal distance between us. Intimacy threatens more dangers than most of us wish to acknowledge.

*

When Edward enters, I am marshalling the end of my working energies. Not only must I redirect myself to our uneven, tortuous track, but I am running out of fuel. I remind myself of the probable importance of this visit for Edward, and conjure sufficient attention to satisfy us both. As Edward seats himself, there is a brief, silent peace between us. This is punctured by the imperative trilling of the telephone. Yet another distraction: I am aggravated. The practice manager's voice sounds courteously singsong but curt and peremptory: the fresh vigour of new authority, a commissar of the New Contract.

*'Doctor, don't forget to weigh and measure Mr C, and put the data on the computer. You didn't do it last time, and the nurse can't do them all. I don't want us to lose points because you haven't entered the data.'*

As she rings off I experience a flush of impotent, irritated resentment. Instantly, and without design, I amplify and caricature my instructions; a contagion of uncoordinated authority. I speak to Edward with unprecedented suddenness;

firmly, clipped and without compromise: 'Stand up, take your shoes off and stand over there, with your back to the wall'.

Edward, startled by abrupt change, involuntarily winces, stops his breath and jerks back in his seat, as if struck by a sharp stone. With silent obedience he stands, shoeless, where instructed in front of the measuring rule. He looks frightened and gulps.

*'What are you going to do?'* he asks, stiff with wariness.

*'Oh'*, I answer with distracted new-cheeriness, *'we just want to measure you, information for the computer ... what did you think?'*

Edward sags, sighs, and breathes freely with relief. *'I thought you were going to shoot me'* he replies, a starkness that shocks me, before dissolving into nervous laughter that embraces us both with the recognised menace of the absurd.

Fortunately, my relationship with Edward has survived this (partly) comedic convergence of mistiming and misperceptions. I never established how much Edward's notion of his 'execution' was transient fantasy, and how much it was darkly surreal humour, mocking our relationship and my job. Aside from such idiosyncratic factors, more general and important themes can be perceived. As with many executionees, Edward was haplessly caught in a cross-current of two very different approaches, occurring at a time of rapid change and reorganisation. The first represents my efforts in the *art* of medicine: consultations that are private, individually crafted and attuned, often using data which is personal, transient and unquantifiable. This approach is at the heart of empathy, creative (more than 'satisfactory') dialogue and healing. Its language may be rich and varied, but correspondingly inexact or ambiguous. The second represented the practice manager's endeavours to impose a publicly formulated *science* to my consultation. The activity here is standardised, quantifiable, mass-produced; heedless of unprogrammed individual variables, and conveyed by language which is neutral, exact and deliberately restricted in vocabulary. Such lies at the centre of 'hard' research, treatment procedures and public health measures. Between individuals it can garner very particular knowledge, but it is unlikely, unaided, to lead to a growth of emotional or experiential understanding.

The tale has other valuable, metaphorical pointers. The practice manager's executive intrusion into, and redirection of, my multi-layered and fragile dialogue with Edward is a microcosm of many dilemmas posed to contemporary healthcare planning and provision. That systematic data-collection, measurement and 'evidence-based practice' should be a cornerstone of safe and effective practice is now axiomatic. But a cornerstone, crucial as it is to a building's integrity and stability, can only function purposefully if securely attached to walls running in different directions, which are themselves attached to other cornerstones. A cornerstone not thus related has little useful function.

Asking for Edward's height was a redundant cornerstone of activity, but one which involved team effort. At 82 years, his height can only change by amputation or involutional shrinkage. Otherwise it is a stable bit of data, of no use or interest diagnostically or therapeutically. The systems, which automatically and rhetorically demand such data, and the mind-sets and social-structures that develop in response to these, are of greater significance.

*

Sheila is the locality-manager for general practitioners in my area. More than a decade ago she had several years of various nursing experiences, and has since equipped herself for her executive role with further training in organisational management, and a wardrobe of demure, but sharp, dark suits. She is a pleasant, intelligent, open-faced woman, focused and efficient in her work. I imagine she is ambitious for promotion and will soon succeed. Currently, a large part of her job is to ensure conformity to the burgeoning requirements of the 'New Contract'. She comes to meet with my manager (Kate) and I, to 'encourage' such compliance.

Our meeting is brisk and mutually respectful, the agenda completed rapidly. This yields an unprepared and unstructured hiatus of time. I want to describe my recent story of Edward's 'execution', partly for light relief and partly because, beneath this small-scale surreal drama, larger themes and forces have aroused my curiosity and unease. The light relief comes with a gust of shared laughter.

We are laughing, I think, at the improbable and the absurd. We are laughing, also, for some respite from our own burdens, fears and spectres. The fear of harm-through-care is especially dark and universal. So, too, is the awareness of our tinsel-like autonomy, evident when we perform acts, knowing them to be futile, even harmful, because a 'higher authority' demands and monitors compliance. The example of the mandatory measurement of Edward is small but instructive. He is an intelligent, alert 82-year-old with a vigilant awareness of his bodily processes, and the kind of care he is receiving. Measuring and weighing Edward makes no sense to either him or me. It is the group's submission to the diktat of a distant planner. In themselves, these activities are neutral and unlikely to harm, but enacted in an industrialised or authoritarian manner, any procedure risks eclipsing or extinguishing more personal reflection or communication. It is hard, then, to combine mass-production with mutuality; corporate compliance with fertile dialogue.

The seismic effectiveness of applied science and mass production in the last century is matched closely by the reciprocal decline of individual craft and non-performance art. Generally, occupational activity is said to make 'progress' when individual dexterity, judgement or intuition are replaced by mechanised or electronic precision and speed. In medical practice there are areas of diagnosis and treatment where such 'progress' is hardly to be questioned: the intensive care unit, the lithotripter, the MRI scanner, are clear examples. These cumulative medical triumphs are the evolved legacy of Newton and Brunel; a medical model of applied and empirical science; biological engineering. Here 'diagnosis' is made objectively, by observation and measurement from the outside. Similarly, 'treatment' is mediated by a manipulation of 'external agents': chemicals, lasers, radiation, scalpels, stents, sutures and so on. This kind of medical model assumes engineering principles, and operates from outside the person's subjective experiences; such experiences may be dealt with courteously, but are usually thought of as distractions from the 'real work'. As with other forms of engineering, it is readily conveyed by authority, instruction, management, hierarchy, flow-charts, pie-charts and algorithms. It has its roots in scientific determinism, and has been ineluctably successful in our 'control' of many serious and demonstrable physical illnesses.

But there have always been a large (the larger?) proportion of people who seek help, but are not so afflicted. These sufferers of dis-ease, dis-equilibrium or dysfunctionality often cannot be understood or relieved by such objectively conducted bioengineering. If we are to have any success in these areas, we must somehow address the *inner* psychic and experiential world of the other; not just their fears, conflicts, fantasies and dreams, but also their positive, self-generated resources for immunity, growth and repair. Such (re)generative capacities operate at both psychological and physical levels, and are sensitive to many influences. The importance of these factors is not matched by their poor accessibility to biometric sciences. Even psychoneuroimmunology, a sophisticated sounding mouthful, often manages little more than attempts to define, in pathophysiological terms, micro-mechanisms for larger pictures, such as 'people who feel hopeless are more likely to get ill, from both trivial and serious illnesses'. It remains the *art* of attunement that helps the hopeless person feel that there can be positive possibility in contact, and to wish for a wider empowerment in their fate. It is the *art* of conveying faith, hope and charity\* that can catalyse the other to heal and grow. This is a world more of induction that conduction: an inter-subjective realm of energy fields, transponders and eco-systems. Here a person's illness or difficulty may be understood and influenced by attention (not always directly) to their personal inner-world and relationships.

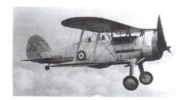

In this dimension of medical practice, the art of the consultation itself may become a powerful source of understanding and change. Like any art, it cannot always be applied, and thus cannot be mass-produced. Often it evolves by dancing in the dark; a coded bond, an improvised choreography – such activities are akin to living organisms that are delicately environment-specific. Attempts publicly to illuminate, transplant or formulate are likely, inadvertently, to distort or destroy. As in the world of agri-business, the industrialisation of living processes in medical practice can offer high yields, but there are serious dangers. We have to take care not to mutate adversely, not to poison in the process of our crop's provision and protection, not to obliterate bio-diversity in our engineering of monocultures. This latter consideration is not merely important for our aesthetics and souls; casual destruction of other life forms – 'collateral damage' – may have an amplified echo through surrounding eco-systems. Hedgerows and trees are not just sources of beauty and wonder; they also prevent soil erosion, thus enabling our crops. Politicians, health economists and service planners necessarily make decisions for thousands or millions of individuals; their task-view is like that of the owner of an intensely-farmed vast prairie. The individual practitioner's view is much smaller, his understanding more intimate. On this scale the hedgerows can be preserved and tended; human idiosyncrasy is here both familiar mystery and essential currency.

A final squeeze on this metaphor; the practice-manager was like a 'beater', harrying creatures concealed and protected in the hedgerows out onto the open plains for dispatch. Edward's stark fantasy, 'I thought you were going to shoot me', may refer to the vulnerability of both his own life, and the few relationships that he believes sustain him.

*

My friend, Charlotte, gazes glumly to the bottom of her glass. The last drops of a mellow, fine claret. In her early 50s, she is an attractive, accomplished example of contemporary professional womanhood: bright, candid, warm, funny, compassionate, resourceful and strong. She is surprised, she says, to hear herself talk of giving up her job as a general practitioner and trainer. For years it had been a love of her life; the investment high, the rewards deep. She had not imagined changes that would so deplete her motivation, her hope.

*'My last two trainees were very unrewarding. They were personable and intelligent, but really only interested in IT, devising ways of getting more data onto the computer, more 'points' for the practice ... that sort of thing. In spite of their intelligence, they have been dull in their curiosity They're not interested in the more subtle aspects of communication, the quirky humanity of our lives generally, our work in particular. At first, I thought "it's just the individual". With the second trainee, and talking to colleagues, I can see it's a trend or, worse, The Future...'*

I offered her simultaneously more misery and commiseration: a sampling of my own experiences and concerns. She became encouraged by our joint gloom

*'In nearly 30 years, I've never felt more deskilled. Despite my years of professional and life experience, the interest and imagination I want to bring to the work, I feel my judgement and choice are increasingly squeezed out by a kind of slavery to procedural lists and computer-templates. I feel controlled and diminished in a way that's unfamiliar for me... I now talk about my surgery as "the ants' nest...".'*

\*

Sheila seems a willing recipient of my lunchtime panorama. I describe the two metaphors of Edward's shooting and Charlotte's ants' nest. They usefully capture a zeitgeist, an emerging world of paradoxes where the 'ordinary citizen' is increasingly restricted and controlled by the same technology that is designed for his benefit: a high-tech cuckoo in the nest. A new totalitarianism.

Not framed by grand and dangerous ideologies, nor delivered by evil demagogues as had so shattered and terrified the earlier twentieth century, this current totalitarianism is administered by such apparently benign beings as Sheila, Kate and myself – conscientious officers in a democratic state. On reflection, all participants agree that the weighing and measuring of a healthy 82-year-old man makes no sense to any of us, but diverts us from things that do. It is the computer program that increasingly decides what we should do, and how we are performing. The individual's judgement or wish – however well-intended, designed or considered – is simply irrelevant to the computer's executive demands and monitoring. This is *technototalitarianism*; electronically coordinated mass-management.

The enthusiasts and advocates of this regime are likely to talk, realistically, of increased efficiency through compliance, clarity and precision. What they do not talk about are the unwanted side effects. At their most mild, these are manifest as superfluous and redundant activity and data; this is akin to the current over-packaging of groceries, creating waste and clutter. The more serious side-effects are those common to many command-and-control systems; they tend to run counter to flexibility and creativity. For the IT-saturated practitioner, this can easily lead to a production-lined and humanly impoverished degradation of contact skills, where individual faces are not remembered, important stories not listened to, voices not heard – the institutionalised and narrow-gazed behaviour of healthcare factory workers. Such command-and-control mindsets are inimical to the types of encounter likely to induce autonomous growth and healing. These inductions are fragile processes that require communications often more resonant than explicit, more artful than automatic.

Imaginative receptivity here is crucial and cannot be pre-programmed. In the realms of general medical practice and psychiatry in particular, consultations generated in this way lie at the heart of ancient forms of how we may best understand and help others. Many difficulties currently arise through this genus of activities being dys-compatible with mass-production, statistical research and electronic-management technologies. For all this, they require our special protection, rather than extinction through neglect and destruction of natural habitat. Treatment can be readily mass-produced; healing rarely so. Ensuring co-existence of these approaches requires much corresponding imaginative receptivity from our planners and managers.

\*

It is time for us to stop. Sheila must return to debrief with her own managers; reporting on her management of me, our 'progress'. She frowns, and then purses her lips as she gathers and packs the vast scattering of data-dense papers that guided the earlier part of our meeting. She gazes at the heavy pile, symbolically I think, before turning to me, a smile intelligent with sentience and sympathy.

*'You know, doctor, if you want to prosper, let alone survive, in this new era, you've just got to get on with it, like the rest of us, and not ask so many questions: you'll slow yourself down for the important work...'*

This tease-in-the-tail is her offering of consoling irony, not hierarchical sarcasm. She sighs with both fatigue and, I imagine, undisclosed complicity. Her voice is less resolute now.

*'I think your notions are really interesting ... I just wish we had the culture and time to really think and talk about these things.'*

'Ah! Small mercies!', I mock-exalt, a small eddy of optimism, a coda: *'we glimpse democratic technototalitarianism'*.

'What?!' she says, but her frayed response is more exhausted exclamation than enquiry.

We are both, for now, too tired and busy to attempt an answer.

*

*He who is being carried does not realize how far the town is.*

Nigerian Proverb

Ω

---

'Faith, Hope and Charity were the names given to three obsolete Gloster Gladiator biplanes which defended Malta in June 1940 against a vastly more modern and numerous Axis bomber force. Against overwhelming odds Faith, Hope and Charity on several days harried, parried and dispersed the attackers, with great courage, skill and guile. This created a seemingly miraculous hiatus, which ensured the survival, and then recovery, of the autonomous Maltese population. The wider implications of this were fascinating and enormous. Possible healthcare analogies here are legion.

Publ. in *Journal of Holistic Healthcare* Vol.2 Issue 4 Nov. 2005

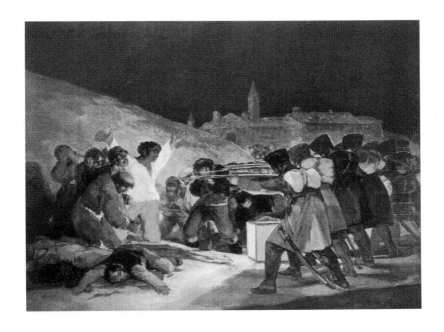

Francisco de Goya *The Third of May,* 1808

This patient reputedly did not survive.

# Planning, Reform and the Need for Live Human Sacrifices

## Hegemony and Homogeny as Symbols of Progress

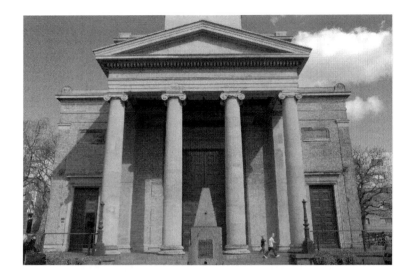

St James Church, Bermondsey, London
Home to an NHS GP surgery for nearly 30 years.

Zealous or rigid attempts to get others to standardise or 'modernise' are often shrugged off as a kind of Zombie-Curse of large organisations. But what are the hidden psychological and social currents that so burden and reduce us? How does it start? Who is responsible?

**Biographical Note**

I have spent most of my four decades in the NHS as a single-handed GP and part-time psychiatrist. I was always interested in the subtle shifts and balances required between opposites, to make our better understandings and interventions. Central to these is the general truth of the species ('science') *v.* the particular variation of the individual ('art'). As electronic technology makes mass management of communications and information more efficient, I fear the loss of creative diversity to increasingly standardized, anonymised procedures, professionals and premises. I fear the loss of art in medicine and heart in practice.

# Prologue

Inescapably, the world becomes more populous, and our lives longer and more complex. Governments' responses tend to increase goals and targets, directives and legislation. Official policy turns easily to officious practice. There, any holistic considerations are disregarded in favour of visible submission to itemized edicts.

In healthcare this can, paradoxically, be discouraging, even destructive of best practice. Such requires conditions of flexibility, discrimination and personal investment. Institutions, by their nature, require homogeny and hegemony. Inevitable tensions arise between the institutional and the interpersonal whenever there are large-scale and complex human variables. Dextrous and imaginative care is needed to navigate and balance between these. A current narrative of an anomalous NHS practice, and a brief sampling of other, darker times, serve as metaphors to explore these themes. The descriptions, events and encounters are authentic. Usual devices disguise the characters only.

*'Our sense of power is more vivid when we break a man's spirit than when we win his heart'*

Eric Hoffer (1954), *The Passionate State of Mind*

*'The wise become as the unwise in the enchanted chamber of Power whose lamps make every face of the same colour'*

Walter Savage Landor (1824-58), *Imaginary Conversations*

When I sought sanctuary, twenty years ago, in a large, fadedly-handsome and age-weary 1830 church I was equally amused and bemused by my fate. The previous lease for my General Medical Practice had been terminated in rapid and unforeseen circumstances. Amidst my anxious and fevered searchings I found this cavernous, deserted, forlorn space. Despite the superficial decrepitude of neglect, I immediately sensed an august serenity, a rare comforting quiet in this ancient recess. As an agnostic Jew, I chuckled at my location and fortune. I was in my fortieth year.

Those early omens foretold a fertile and appreciative relationship between occupants and space. At the start of these two decades I resettled my practice and celebrated my feelings for my occupational new home with a profusion of delights for the eye and comforts for the body: impressionist and expressionist period prints, hand crafted and painted objects, plants, substantial and comfortable furniture, warm and luminous background colours. All recorded and amplified a long and loving investment: the satisfactions of the patient gardener.

This eccentric locus and mode of institutional healthcare has provoked a steady stream of spontaneous comment. Most often people would speak, with surprised warmth and bright-eyed delight, of the informal, inviting ambience, its oasis-like incongruities. Very rarely I was encountered by surly, malcontent modernism: 'What are you doing in an old building like this? Can't the NHS afford anything better? ...' These brief, cold gusts were rare, but they chilled me: I somehow knew they were harbingers of a vigorous new culture, sharply focused and uncompromisingly business-like. From the fragile peace of my oasis I glimpsed the approaching dust-clouds of new orders and reform.

*

The NHS surveyor's report felt like a thud of both inevitability and threat. Amongst the many alleged deficiencies or aberrations of 'current acceptable standards' stood an obelisk of 'lack of provision for the disabled, especially access and WC facilities.' There is no counter-balancing comment on the unusually aesthetic or comfortable environment and its great popularity among staff and patients (including the disabled), which are much in evidence. To the uninitiated, the report conveys a picture of neglect, negligence, hazard, drear of the premises and certain abject discomfort (and worse) of its occupants. This is not a place for safe or viable contemporary medical practice. This is the view of an expert on premises with a narrow, executively prescribed brief, who does not speak to its inhabitants.

*

What of the inhabitants of this alleged nest for potential malfunction: myself, my many staff, my two-thousand patients. The human eco-system of perpetrators, victims, both?

The unheeded evidence is decisively and dramatically opposed.

In summary: Results from my patient-experience questionnaires have been consistently and exceptionally good, and among the best on record. Most of my various staff (nurses, assistant doctors, receptionists, administrators etc) stay for many years, leave on good terms and have little sickness leave. I, myself, continue blessed with good health and have never taken sickness leave or had a substantial complaint made in twenty years. There has never been a significant accident. Disabled patients have cheerfully accepted help with access (when needed), and our explanations and apologies regarding any difficulties (when needed). 'It's worth it,' they have said, 'I prefer to come here ...'

Holistically, this eco-system is working well in its anachronistic home.

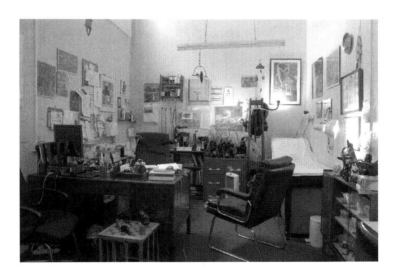

*

If 'bad' premises are defined as those likely to lead to a 'bad' effect on its occupants (surely the most meaningful definition), how can we best understand a 'bad' premises (as defined by an expert surveyor) hosting remarkably 'good' results (as defined more holistically by medical and personal feedback)? When expected correlation breaks down (as in my practice) which set of data and concepts should be discarded, and which retained and valued?

*

It occurs to me that much of this management difficulty arises from a confusion between 'correlation' (a 'sometimes' relationship, which allows exception of many kinds) and 'equation' (an 'always' relationship, often causal, that allows no exceptions). At its best such confusion may lead to clumsy, indiscriminate decision making. At its worst it is a major source of the most frightening and destructive human acts. There is a spectrum from dogmatic over-inclusiveness, to fanaticism and elimination of the most horrific kind.

Correlation mind-sets may lead to aspiration and guidance. Equation mind-sets tend to intractable ideology and mandate.

*

I do not need persuading that disabled people and their needs (among numerous groups) have been poorly understood and represented. I see clearly how improving awareness, dialogue and facilities can help them with their predicaments.

I point out to my managers that I am a relatively small inner-city practice in an area where patients have many practices to choose from. The disabled patients I have are all intelligent, informed adults who understand my predicament (lovely old building, very difficult to radically transform etc) and are well able to make their own choice. They choose to stay.

I also point out that with the cumulative growth of newer premises designed with full disabled facilities, that the problem is bound to disappear. Older practitioners and their premises will be naturally retired, to be replaced by more contemporaneous designs. With guidance and careful projected planning, the provision for the needs of this group (and others) will grow solidly and surely. There is no need for ideologically postured coercion, or destruction.

What, then, is the need for an urgent cull of the obsolescent?

*

In my frustrated dystopia I seek the counsel of two NHS managers.

The first, Sam, a genial man, stooped-before-andropause, with a passive, damply-anxious hand-shake. He listens initially, I sense, with gratuitous fascination. Soon, he shrugs, a mixture of apology and embarrassed dismissal. He looks away. 'Look,' he says, 'I probably agree with you, but that's got nothing to do with it … I don't make the rules … I'm just doing my job …' As his voice fades away, my mind involuntarily reels back some forty years to a black and white television image of a bespectacled, unremarkable looking man in a glass armoured box in a court-room. Quiet, unassuming, clerically mannered and plausibly rational. Adolf Eichmann on trial. I shock myself and shudder invisibly, grateful that my life is of this generation. I ponder how close is imaginative intuition to paranoia.

The second, Paula, shakes my hand with a dry, sure, decisive grasp. Her sympathy has a canny edge. I sense she has a well-ordered and well-filled stock of elegantly pre-packed answers. She offers me one: 'Yes, I understand, your points are very valid … Unfortunately, our hands are tied by current legislation. We cannot allow any exceptions, as we have no power or right to exercise discrimination in these matters.'

This declaration is concise, courteous and consummate: an impeccable wrapping of political correctness. I flounder with clumsy perplexity. Surely this cannot be true: ordinary policeman arbitrate about whom to confront with (say) speeding or illicit drug use. This happens thousands of times daily. And when were the laws on blasphemy last applied consistently? A lather of protest foams from my mouth.

She quietly listens to my foaming, looking down at a pen which she revolves between her fingers. A gold-plated rollerball; smooth hegemony. She then looks up at me, radiating a consoling, winsome smile; patient, experienced, forbearing. I understand I am misunderstanding something fundamental.

'Yes' she says euphoniously, 'but how is any of that going to help you? Authorities won't make that explicit. They talk only of official policy: "x is the law: offenders are liable to prosecution" ... Don't you see?'

I do, but I don't want to. My foam is difficult to swallow.

*

When Jed is addressing the media his voice has a tough, compact alacrity. Now, at his kitchen table at the end of a long Westminster political day, he sounds wearily ironic.

He had earlier been humoured though harangued by my semi-parodic analogies of contemporary politically fuelled NHS reforms with 1930's Soviet Five Year Plans. We share a fascinated scholarship of the follies, horrors and genius of the 20th Century.

'I'm a happy Kulak', I lampoon-protested. 'I'm productive and settled on my small allotment... I definitely don't want to be forced onto a Collective Farm ... I don't even want to be shot'.

Jed knows that my jesting both expresses and conceals much fear, anger, and anticipatory grief about my uncertain fate. Our shared laughter dies and the mood darkens. He rises and shuffles slowly to a favourite old armchair, a trusted friend to contain and support his strong but work-enervated frame. He well understands my relationship with the old church. He unbuttons the top of his shirt, a further loosening of the bonds and demands of public service.

'We politicians, planners and change-merchants often make almost impossible tasks even more difficult ... One of the things that happens is we lose the bigger picture, and with that much else goes; flexibility, creativity ... our imaginative humanity. But difficult change often needs a lot of effort and resolve. So, we change-merchants, and our buyers, both need evidence of 'progress', to keep going (and keep our jobs). This easily leads to the kind of deception and self-deception that, decades later, startle us with grandiose ideology and then the eventual grotesque cruelty ... The Communist Commissars developed such a strong belief in the Collectivization Programme that they would go to any lengths to ensure recruitment and conformity. The human cost, and even the clear evidence of tragically large production losses, became utterly eclipsed by the enormous ideological bulk of "The Plan" ...'

'What's often most frightening is how sincere, vocational and visionary the agents of change can believe themselves to be. People often think of Nazi SS Officers or Stalin's Communist Commissars as being sadistic opportunists. The truth is more shockingly ordinary and paradoxical: they often truly believed they were making the world a better place. 'Doing what needed to be done.' Many were sincere ideologues who needed 'evidence' of their success.'

I consider my own current drama: massively small and benign, in comparison. I think about the predicaments and modus operandae of my NHS Managers whose reputations, jobs, mortgages, maybe even self-esteem may depend upon offering up (to their managers) visible tokens and totems of change. To leave me be, in my benign and atavistic place, would be symbolic of their inertia and inactivity as agents of change. Allowing natural evolution through retirement might feel and appear like managerial impotence. A live human sacrifice will propitiate.

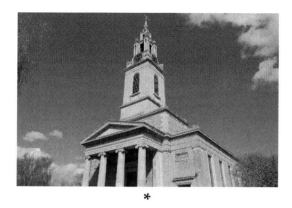

\*

'How do we maintain vision, momentum, resolve *and* caution, flexibility, openness all at the same time?' A rhetorical question, Jed knows. He groans, a tiring acknowledgement of his insoluble dilemmas, the conundrae of power.

'On reflection, I don't think I'll bother any more … I'll just sit here, where I have peace and quiet … ', he pats the arm of his old chair, his comforter and container. He darts me a witty mischievous smile, a mock-surrender to my self-interested, insistent doubts and questions.

We sit in a restorative silence. Jed, I think, needs some respite from clamour and challenge. I want time to assimilate this bigger picture to my own small story, so important to me.

As my mind recedes from its 20th century panorama and returns to my current preoccupations, I think again of how fortunate I am to be living where and when I am.

In my fortieth year I chuckled insouciantly at my fortune. In my sixties I am less mirthful, but more mindful. The consolations of ageing are hard-won and subtle.

\*

*'Conformity is the ape of harmony'*
Ralph Waldo Emerson, 1840, Journals

Ω

Publ. in *Journal of Holistic Healthcare* Vol. 9 Issue 3 2012

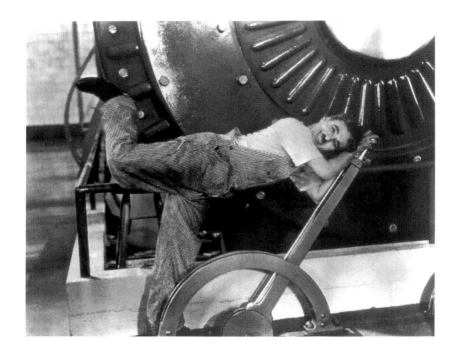

Charlie Chaplin – *Modern Times* 1936

# Modern Times

(True) Parables
from the frontline of the NHS

## Introduction and summary

The massive expansion of the NHS has led to a burgeoning of organisational and procedural changes deriving from mass-production industries and corporate capitalism. This 'industrialisation' of Health-Care is likely to confer clearest and greatest benefit when dealing with well-defined bodily complaints, 'physical pathology'. When dealing with the evanescence and complexity of human unhappiness or mere dis-equilibrium, 'functional pathology', considerably more difficulties are encountered and generated.

Such disorders as those of behaviour, appetite, mood or impulse ('BAMI') introduce innumerable human variables, and from all participants involved. Measurement, standardisation and technical language all become highly problematic, if not contentious. Ensuing operational difficulties are inevitable. For those interested in ethics and epistemology, important questions arise. This presents a vast and ambiguous area, particularly in General Medical Practice and Psychiatry. Inadvertent damage may result from indiscriminate and automatic use of mass-production protocols. The cost, in both human and economic terms, is probably enormous, but receives little attention.

In all human life inevitable compromises have to be made: between structure and flexibility, control and creativity, Group conformity and individual integrity. Such dilemmas have a universal span from the lives of individuals to the largest groups.

From the basis of current NHS events, these and related themes are illustrated. The narrative and dialogues are authentic. Only peripheral descriptive detail is changed to guard anonymity. Although the personal nature of the recording may be uncommon, the dilemmas they describe are not.

## 1.  Imagination

*You can't depend on your judgement*
*when your imagination is out of focus*

Mark Twain, *Notebook* (1935)

'This one's going to be trouble …'

Sophie approaches my desk with officious pleasure, a privileged messenger of bad news. As senior receptionist she opens and pre-digests much of my post, both to prime and protect me. Or so she supposes.

'You've been assigned this man, Stefan M, because he was extremely rude, and threatened violence against Dr K … Dr K had no option but to remove him from his list … Dr K's surgery had to call the police … I hope you won't keep him longer than you have to …'

I sense in Sophie not just concern, but a hidden, elliptical gratification, an anticipation of righteous vindication. Her expression carries gravitas skewed by a faint twist of a smile.

*

Stefan M's self-introduction to me, the next morning, disturbs me with the unexpected. His proffered handshake is warm and firm; receptive but not at all overpowering. Watching him walk across the room, I am reminded of an ageing, wounded male lion – previously a powerful predator but now incrementally vulnerable and unable to hunt. He meets my gaze with subtle and kaleidoscopic complexity: pride, hurt, defiance, pleading, enquiry. His intelligence is sharp, sprung, mobile.

The answers to my opening salvo of routine medical questions further alerts me to the breadth, depth and weight of this man's troubles. Among my notes I write:

Medical: Age 38. Heart attack last year. Lassitude and weakness since. Says he can't work because of this (never previously 'off sick'). Smokes 40/day for 15 yrs. Sister died aged 39, two years ago, amidst political asylum litigation (in Scandinavia). Psych/social: From previous African conflict zone. He and (now deceased) sister fled to different European countries as racial minority persecution mounted in danger and savagery. Both he and sister fought hard for political asylum, in different countries. He succeeded. His sister's case became impacted as a 'cause célèbre', when she died suddenly. Plight of his remaining, once-hunted family members unknown: presumed dead. Since in UK (10 yrs) worked 16 hrs/day as advocate/spokesman for his much-mauled national group. Deeply disturbed by sister's death, but worked harder and smoked more to obscure grief. Collapse of relationship with girlfriend after heart attack: says sexual potency problems (1st time) then. ?Blocked grief etc. ?Medication effect ?Smoking/vascular. Enquiries re: depression: explicitly denies this. (Tightens his jaw and hands and says: "What good would that do ... who could care for me now?" His eyes moisten, but he rapidly dabs them. He looks away – ?hoping I will, too.) Imp: ?Masked Depression ++.

I ponder this psychiatric term, now little used: an explanation, a description, a hypothesis spawning its own questions about the masker and the maskee, the relationship of the 'ghost' to the 'machine'.

Stefan M's cumulative life-traumas seem enormous, matched almost by his formidable courage, resolve and wilful integrity. Almost, but not quite. It is the 'not quite', I suspect, that has led to his incapacitation. Fighting against such mountainous adversity for so long, he has attempted an indefatigability of the superhuman. Only his body can stop him.

*

Only later, when Stefan has mapped me as a Safe-Haven, do I enquire about how his (mis)communications with Dr K had become so conflagratory.

'He told me that, from the information he had received from the cardiologist, there was no reason for me to stay off work … he asked me psychiatric-type questions, which I felt patronised by … When I tried to discuss this with him, he turned away from me toward the computer where he was consulting investigations and some kind of recommendations. I said I just can't work with this weakness I have. He said that, from the information he had, he couldn't help me further. While still looking at the computer he asked me to leave.'

I asked Stefan if Dr K had known much, or anything, of his story.

'No, he didn't ask much, and I didn't think he was the sort of person I could talk to … He seemed much more interested in what was on the computer. After he had glanced at me, I don't think he could remember what I looked like …'

\*

Soon after, I attend a local medical meeting, a congregation that owes its longevity more, I suspect, to the reliably good curry served there (a silently appreciated bribe by International Pharmaceuticals), than to important shared concerns and commitments.

Dr K and I are long familiar cohorts. He is a 'busy GP' with a large practice and a bluff, no-nonsense, impatient amiability to help his long-term survival. Our affinity is stable and considerate, but not deep. In greeting he shakes my hand, a limp detached ritual as he looks away, toward the banqueted table, his gaze dully observant.

'Bad luck! I hear you've been assigned that very rude and troublesome man Stefan M, ' he mocks, with the relief of the released.

Soon after, amidst the steaming fragrances of massed curries, I try, with lightness and diplomacy, to interest Dr K in how our own common aggravations may easily blind us to the exceptional tragedy of others. He glances at me briefly with a slight twitch of a shrug, while spooning another large self-serving of Chicken Dansak:

'You like all the difficult ones,' his jest seems half-tribute, half-consolation, 'I just think some people are impossible'.

## 2. Belonging

*Every exit is an entry somewhere else*

Tom Stoppard (1967) *Rosencrantz and Guildenstern are dead*

Karen greets me by her bed, B23, with the social facility of a TV chat-show hostess. Her hair is dark, wavy and lustrous; a generous and sensuous frame to a soft, cherubic face. In counterpoint, sharply mascaraed eyes warn me of other agendas, of danger. Given the seriousness of her overdose a day previously, this now silk-gowned young woman seems disarmingly urbane and insouciantly welcoming.

Behind the curtained screen Karen and I are now invisible to the gaze and traffic of the ward. This seems to free Karen to hesitantly disclose a little-known self, more usually obscured by her competent, voluptuous masks or painful shards of self-harm.

The brief, typed referral form had forewarned me of the latter: '3rd serious overdose, with alcohol binge, in recent months. Recent stresses: break-up with boyfriend and alleged rape (different relationships). Denies mental illness and wants to leave ...'

The story Karen tells me is as perplexingly discrepant as her calm social persona and her juxtaposed, profoundly hazardous behaviour. Within the envelope of her salubrious suburban home, her publicly polished, professionally respected parents were locked in decades of a grimly hypnotic power struggle. Their two children became both weapons and casualties. Common emotional violence would erupt, often through a haze of alcohol, in periodic convulsions of physical violence. In her early teens, under cloaks of darkness and alcoholic amnesia, her father culminated the domestic damage in a sexually intrusive visit to her bedroom. Karen, with admirable but precocious resolve, left her parents and never returned.

*

This first time I meet Karen she is entering the Eye of the Storm that will determine her mortal existence. In the months that follow, her life is like a narrow path skirting the edge of an abyss. Several times she lunges, with angry despair, both softened and fuelled by alcohol, to her own self-annihilation. The serial projects of foiling her self-killing are administered by teams of physicians and psychiatrists at various other inner city hospitals: the Blue-Light Ambulance disgorges this dangerous cargo with blind haste. Precedent is neither known nor important. The practitioners immediately charged with saving her life are similarly blinded by emergency: there is no place here for nuance or finer historical reference. Medication and the Mental Health Act will contain: if not, 'Severe Borderline Personality Disorder' will explain. Karen becomes both lost and lime-lit by the doctors' (self?) defensive conferral of 'dangerous mental illness'. She may be transiently contained, but she is not understood.

This follows a pattern where the (usually) young and inexperienced practitioners, fearing for both Karen's life and their own professional career, act with zealous and crisp efficiency. In order to forestall disaster, Karen becomes crippled by pre-emptive strikes: Sectioned, medicated, monitored, 'specialed'. Karen is managed: dialogue is discarded.

Karen remembers the earlier exchanges she had with me and re-contacts my small department, a different venue and culture from the busy, bustling, prescriptive Community Mental Health Team now in charge. In this small, relatively quiet hospital department, there is great stability and accessibility for Karen. Over several years she keeps deliberate and regular contact with me via my long-serving secretary, Dorothy, a woman of unpretentious warmth and robust but respectful intelligence. Her considerable range and length of life experience may discretely illuminate, but will not dazzle. Dorothy and I are both gently silvering with age, a source of wistful banter between us.

*

The consultant in charge of the populous but constantly changing Community Mental Health Team, Dr Q, thinks more management is called for. He writes: 'We need to rationalise and unify this woman's care. It is clearly not in the interests of the patient or the Service for her care to be fragmented. For this reason, I have asked the patient to continue her attendance to this department and arrange cessation of her sessions with you...'

I telephone Dr Q in an attempt to widen our understanding of this alluringly haunted young woman. He is more interested in speaking as Commanding Officer: Karen's care would now be systematically planned, coordinated and monitored by his Multidisciplinary Team at HQ. With well-manicured authority he instructs me about the incipient New Order. Dialogue is skilfully bypassed. I am aware of holding my breath; I feel I, too, am being processed.

Karen's compliance to such prescription is fragile: she meets with the many mental health professionals assigned to her, but is progressively confused and wearied by their complex and rigid protocols, their unpredictable impermanence. She describes it later: 'They were all different, of course ... A few I thought I could really trust and talk to, but twice they suddenly disappeared – gone for another job or training, or something. It hurts and I don't feel safe ... my barriers go up again ...' Karen's offerings there turn shell-like: she yields only what she must.

She seeks connection and asylum where she feels less diminished and defined: she is discretely resolute in her regular contact with myself, and thus Dorothy. I have some unease about colluding with her unusual dissent. Dorothy and I are now as Foster Parents to this grown woman, with the added illicitness of an extra-marital affair. I convolute my mind with a cabal of dark interpretations: Freudian Triangles, Deposed Fathers, vengefully reprised children. I do not exonerate myself from these constructions: I can locate enough of my residual developmental sediment to secure my place. I have training and imagination enough to ascribe a variety of such roles to each of us. It is all plausible. It is, professionally, the safest thing to do.

I take the riskier course: I follow Karen's thoughtful dissent, sensing that she has an instinct now to create new and positive patterns. I remember a harsh and pithy judgement of a non-medical friend: 'The problem with most psychiatry is that, at best, it can stop some "bad" things happening ... but it doesn't usually help people heal and grow ...'. I had ruefully agreed, hoping I might be an exception, at least sometimes.

*

The months that follow bring a seemingly impossible mix of alarming headlines and growing peace. The first headlines shock with a precipitous, ill-judged but highly-charged affair. She embarks on this with an impecunious, unrooted, political Balkan refugee. Unwary, he enters a Lioness's Den of erotic attachment. With dismayed foreboding, I see her demeanour transform from a soft mist of adoration and total trust, to a terrifying furnace of raging accusation, incandescent disillusion, Total War. I see him briefly at this time: he is emotionally stunned, lost and inchoate – signs of Emotional Blast Concussion.

Amidst these emotional explosions she announces her pregnancy, her first. This news invokes waves of alarmed consternation across professional networks. How will this demonstrably unstable woman deal with the inexorable changes and responsibilities? Professional anxiety and vigilance increases. 'Risk-Management' becomes the gravitational nucleus round which their many activities orbit.

\*

Karen then confounds and disarms us with her peace: a rapid crystallisation of structure and stability in her life. Faster than we are able to comprehend, she ceases her many ways of imperilling, alarming or punishing herself. Increasingly her emotional intelligence turns from hurt wariness to a capacity for reflective receptivity.

'I'm a mother now … I have to make sure I don't pass on my mess to the next generation,' she says, patting a ripely-pregnant belly. The sagacity here is fresh and self-realised: the integrity of such self-regeneration rapidly renders obsolete the hundreds of pages of specialist, 'expert' communications in her thick folder. In this forest of technically-dense, bureaucratically-moulded prose, it is difficult to discern much of this woman's unique bondage, suffering, struggle and quest for suffrage in her own life. Seeing her now tenderly touching her belly, and uttering such protective and far-foresighted intentions toward her 'accidentally' conceived foetus, I am suddenly and rapidly connected to her in my understanding.

\*

Two years later I am talking with Karen of ordinary but crucial problems: of the difficulty of being a single mother, of being receptive to her toddler-son when fatigued and already multitasking, of finding a pragmatic, appreciative semi-detachment from her son's father, her ex-lover. I have been close to formative events; she is relieved by the common understanding we create without lengthy explanation. Since motherhood, her female demeanour has changed from alluring siren to fecund and earthed mother. Sean, her delightful wide and sparkle-eyed son babbles happily in playful exchange with Dorothy, who welcomes this heart-warming, brief transformation of her office into a crèche.

Karen tells me of growing good contacts she has with other professionals: a Health Visitor, the new Clinical Psychologist, a Community Support Worker. She talks of them with growing trust and faith. Without deliberate design she has assembled around herself a kind of extended family. I reflect on this a while, and lightly contrast her flowering conviviality with our previous shared era, a tangled and dangerous time, when any dependent relationship was likely to carry an explosive charge. For several years, she had managed, time and again, but without any conscious intent, to replay myriad variations of her painful childhood dramas. As we sample these shared historical events, we contrast our different recollections and perspective. We talk of the inevitability of personal relativity, and the importance of creating common language, the most reliable balm for humankind's painful awareness of our individual separateness and mortality.

Equally surprising, to Karen and myself, is the redemption and resumption of her parents' relationship, both with Karen and one another. After many painful years without contact, her mother and father are back in her life, but dramatically transformed. They visit and welcome as calm, kindly, ageing parents and doting grandparents. Karen learns of the paradoxes behind the transformation: her parents are living separately, but close. After decades of internecine marital strife, they have found affectionate and loving peace in separation.

I marvel at the mystery of unseen and insensible matrices that guide such parallel events.

\*

'A good 'Clinical Outcome', then?' Keith gently teases me with mock managerial formality and falsely dry tone. Another veteran practitioner, he, too, struggles to maintain his élan vital amidst the increasing constriction of institutional rules, diktats and deadlines; the rhetorical boa of planners and politicians.

'Seriously, though, what do you think most helped Karen's transformation?'

*

I ask Karen.

She looks down for a few seconds. I imagine she is rapidly respooling the last five years. Her answer is scattered, but thoughtful:

'You gave me time and space, faith and guidance …' She hesitates, checking for my understanding. I believe I do, but I prompt her elaboration.

'Well, you've always been here for me, and for a very long time … You helped me find my voice and rediscover a self I'd been running away from … If you ever offered me guidance or suggestions, I've always thought it's from a real and growing knowledge of me, not some theory, or book or plan about The Mentally Ill … I'm not mentally ill, I was very disturbed: it's very different…'

This notion is expressed with a brief burn of sardonic anger. This yields to a smile of recognition between us. I raise an eyebrow; my curiosity about her distinction.

'What I mean is … Yes, I was like a person blinded with fear and confusion, and like a dumb person in not being able to talk about it. But I was never deaf: through talking with me, you guided me back to my voice and my vision. Then I could get my life back and start to make it really my own. Can a seriously mentally ill person do that?'

Her question is genuine. I delight in her simultaneous ingenuousness and sophistication. I wish often that my colleagues would ask such trenchant but unaffected questions. I inhibit my urge to now explore this question, a favourite haunt of mine. She goes on, to talk of Dorothy and our small department.

'Dorothy has been great ... always helpful and interested, but never bossy. A lot of the psychiatrists have wanted to control me, without understanding very much at all. Some have talked to me as if they know everything already. I felt very diminished: "shrunk to fit" their professional theories and procedures.

'Coming up these stairs to be greeted by Dorothy's friendly manner, sitting in this cared-for space, surrounded by growing plants and homely, colourful prints, has somehow given me the same kind of messages that I've talked about with you: that I can heal and grow ...'

She becomes quietly thoughtful, and I enquire about why she thought she had received these vital messages so rarely.

'Well, a lot of doctors don't seem to think like that, but even if they do I've got to have a good relationship with them for it to mean anything ... It's like talking about love.'

This last utterance was a short circuit I had not expected. The shock enlivens and awakens me. In unmanaged and unengineered contact, human electricity can flow in unexpected ways.

*

Keith talks of the death of a neighbour. She had lived many years in the large multi-occupancy house next door. He has only just heard of her death, three months after the event. He is disturbed by his remoteness from someone so close. We discuss the broader theme of how new technologies lead us to live such lives: where we communicate electronically-mediated words and images instantaneously to the other side of the world, but are insentient of our surrounding environment, oblivious of our neighbours.

My mind returns to an event Karen described three years ago, shortly after one of her turbulent stays in Dr Q's unit. She had resisted a brain imaging scan, feeling both repelled and afraid of the formidable machinery. The young doctor, she said, was curt, prescriptive and didactic: it was 'imperative to exclude significant pathology' (such was most unlikely, and thus hardly 'imperative'). Karen submitted to the scan, but never trusted them with much of her story.

This brief tale can be readily dismissed by more common or cursory analyses: the doctor was inexperienced, busy, unimaginative; or Karen is oppositional, oversensitive, paranoid. Much more interesting is this account as a microcosm, cultural metaphor, Zeitgeist. We are constructing a world of sharp new paradoxes and polarities. We have grown used to, expect, rapid and precise information and images: we are impatient and intolerant of the indistinct, the ambiguous, the slow. We pour massive resources into machinery to provide us with such unprecedently detailed and accurate images, but hardly notice that our own subjective image-making, our imagination, is atrophying. Karen is more easily electromagnetically scanned than imaginatively heard. Keith e-mails unknown people with effortless regularity across continents, unaware of his long-term neighbour's slow death, fifteen yards away. We increasingly delegate our tasks and responsibilities to inventions which save us time and effort but, with cruel inversity, we observe our lives as incrementally more rushed and less savoured. The mostly inexplicable, but thriving, new syndrome of children with Hyperactivity/Attention Deficit Disorder may serve as a pathological index of our accelerating, kinetic and rootless lives. To belong, we have also to be-long; we have to stay, be still and receptive.

Long enough to relate and to bond.

$$\Omega$$

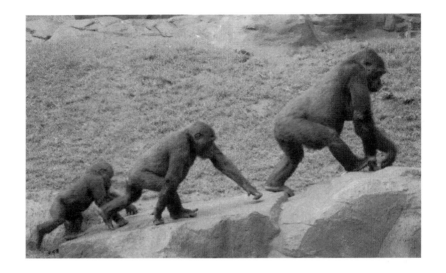

# No Country for Old Men

## The Rise of Managerialism and the New Cultural Vacuum

*'Knowledge is proud that he has learned so much; Wisdom is humble that he knows no more.'*
William Cowper, *The Task* (1785)

My early apprenticeship in psychiatry, from the early 1970s, was blessed and guided by two older men, my supervising consultants. These fatherly mentors were models for compassionate and creative professional dialogue: head, heart and soul interwoven seamlessly into their many-faceted communications. Although young and otherwise restless, I valued the cultures and communities they 'fathered' and wished to prolong their influence on me. Between them, I stayed five years. Now, more than thirty years later, I evoke these mentors and memories with warmth, admiration and gratitude: sweet–sad clouds that guide me still.

Dr G was a South African Jewish man whose family had fled Nazi Germany. As a young adult he became increasingly troubled by his comfortably privileged status in the Apartheid State. The two types of authoritarianism confronted him with resemblances, if not equivalence. To live more amicably with his conscience, he shipped his young, burgeoning career and family to England: he would train as a psychiatrist here, in the Mother of Democracies.

Fifteen years later I joined him, to begin my own training. This apprenticeship was in a large, grandiose late-victorian asylum, more recently poor and provincial mental hospital. He had a soft green-eyed gaze; observant, enquiring, encompassing. A sharp intelligence was swathed in a softly reticent, self-deprecating courtesy and deft, gentle irony. The beginnings of a stooped posture reminded me of his many stoically carried burdens and his ancestral losses. On many occasions we sat together to make some kind of 'assessment' of an individual's bruised and faltering struggle with, and against, their biological predicates and their existential tasks. He would listen with empathic detachment; his attention sometimes free-floating, sometimes sharply converged. Drawing together our ensuing discussion he would often say: 'I suppose we could call that …'. His cautiously and ambivalently hued language was no accident: he well understood the inadequacy of our tools of language or science, in their assigned tasks of defining or changing complex human predicaments. When the psychiatric language seemed to offer some pragmatic guidance or clarity, he was transiently and conditionally grateful. We would talk of how easily an over-extension of our quasi-medical vocabulary would turn help into hegemony; compassionate containment into prescriptive control. We considered the seductive dangers of aggrandising our partial metaphors into didactic conclusions. I remember an especially fruitful dialogue, over coffee, exploring how the 'Lord of Language' becomes 'The Definer'. I thrived in the inviting and reflective space he created to initiate such discussion. In my youth and optimism, I did not anticipate how rare such sanctuaries would become.

\*

The next mentor I sought out worked in the very different setting of a large, (then) prestigious teaching hospital. Dr R had, I thought, similar qualities to Dr G, but in a High-Anglican form. Spawned from an old and respected 'medical family' in the Home Counties, his salubrious, educated background progressed with a kind of blessed and urbane inevitability, through Oxbridge to his medical training. World War II interrupted such euphony with discords of terrible violence. As a young army doctor he tended the battle-shattered and trauma-deranged in North Africa. Earlier, at a distance, he had inferred the Black-Hole of human destructiveness, growing up in the legacy of the previous war. Now he witnessed it directly. Thirty years later he talked to me of this awakening: how a tidal wave of experiences impressed on him, as no theory could, the complex, fragile interconnectedness of all: mind and body, friend and foe, libido and mortido. Garnering whatever could help men restore and heal, he began his life-task and scholarship; to offer a sensitive but pragmatic service of 'Psychological Medicine'.

By the time I joined him, his department embodied the sophisticated pluralism of his experiences and intent. Although a busy service, covering a large General Hospital, there developed through and around such tasks an informal University of ideas. Alongside psychiatrists, I was engaged and guided by open-minded psychoanalysts and refreshingly rethinking medical anthropologists. Fertile experimentation enlisted other groups: GPs exploring the unexplicit psychological subtext of their work, medical students taking on patients for psychodynamic psychotherapy (the results were remarkably good, and probably not just for the patients). Without any higher edict, plan or mandate, we were all studying the Psychology of Affliction. Remembered now, from a current perspective, it seems almost impossible that this fecund community of learning and healing blossomed independently of any centrally directed NHS management or plan.

Dr R was tall and imposing, though he chose not to impose. His considerable intelligence and knowledge were quietly flanked by a kindly wisdom. I remember us listening to a many-chaptered, harrowing account of a woman's long and complex difficulties; how the medical and psychiatric organisations and mind-sets had habitually missed the personal meaning of her struggle. He looked up from the voluminous case-notes, weighing heavily on his lap. His blue eyes glinted both gentle humour and sorrowful recognition. 'It may be the best this kind of psychiatry can do', he had said. This was no condescending judgement, rather a stoic lament for how our complexity so often eludes our determined attempts to encace and understand ourselves.

*

In that decade, rapid technological advance proceeded amidst swirling philosophical challenge. From the structured, scholarly enquiries of Medical Anthropology and Sociology, to the more poetic and maverick challenges of Szasz, Laing and Illich, the stolidly revered worlds of medicine and psychiatry were being deconstructed. Fundamental questions regarding the relationship of subjective to objective knowledge, and of these to language, power and agency – all of these became matters for public and professional debate. As in all genuine philosophy, it was the process of enquiry and dialogue that was enriching, not the (impossible) end of providing definitive answers. I did not, then, appreciate how robustly dialogic those times were. Remarkably, I cannot remember talking with Dr G or Dr R much, or even, explicitly, about the challenging scholars or the rebellious luminaries, but they had somehow distilled their spirit for private consumption. These 'Two Wise Men' had developed a kind of potent humility, a demonstration of how wholesome (self) doubt could be harnessed to great therapeutic leverage. Philosophical curiosity need not be the reserved preserve of the leisured, or the academic.

*

More than three decades have passed. I am now older than either Dr G or Dr R when I apprenticed for them. My work in Medical and Psychiatric Practice is as near the end now, as it was in its beginnings, then. Despite, and because of, the passage of so many years and so many different experiences and influences, I value their values and modae operandae even more. But though my faith is solid, my optimism is not.

*

'Manage or be managed!' an executive young NHS consultant, Dr T, had exclaimed sharply to me in recent years when I lamented the loss of familiar forms of colleagial and cooperative dialogue. I was not sure if her remark was meant with any humour or irony, but I reflected later on how pithily it captured our changing world. Simultaneously it conveyed description, prescription, prophecy and ethos. This utterance came from a world far from my early influences of the Hippocratic Oath, or the gentle sagacious guidance of any Dr G or Dr R, or the better kinds of confederate socialism that had nourished and encouraged the NHS in its earlier years. This now is a world of corporate industrialism, large competing organisations, and the then inevitable hustling, hassling, spinning styles of authoritarian management.

\*

More recently still, for the first time in many years, I am involved in disputed negotiation with, and between, mistrustfully aligned NHS Trusts. The problematic area is one which used to be called 'Psychosomatic Medicine': substantial chronic physical disease, fuelled and exacerbated by the sufferer's ongoing life-problems and conflicts. Such an association has to be discerned, not only by the experienced and imaginative practitioner, but increasingly by the (self) afflicted patient. It is an operational arena of interfaces, often paradoxical: Psyche–Soma, Subjective–Objective, Art–Science, Determinism–Choice, Procedure–Innovation, Individual consciousness–Generic biology. Unlike procedurally-based areas of medical practice, it relies on 'induction' quite as much as 'instruction', to help in the restoration and growth of resilience and health. *Induction* is the evocation and development of internal, personal resources; *Instruction* is the application of external, impersonal resources and notions. Generally then, induction is dialogic; instruction is didactic. Induction is (more) receptive; instruction propulsive. Applied with functional synchrony, they are two essential components of holistic care: like the pulsing heat; receptive in diastole, propulsive in systole.

Problems arise. The 'systolic', instructive, propulsive aspects of medical practice can be (relatively) easily measured, managed and standardised. The 'diastolic', inductive, receptive components cannot. Politicians, health-economists and planners, managers and clinical directors are likely to see the way to greater effectiveness and economy through increasing standardisation, mass-production, instructive management. The burgeoning plethora of audits, goals, targets, 'treatment packages', NICE guidelines, league tables, QUOF points – all are designed to supercharge the 'systole' of propelled, executively-managed care.

What then happens to the 'diastolic' functions of care? Diastole needs time and space for the heart to fill, for systolic thrust to be possible. Likewise, we need the time and space for the art of induction, the inter-subjective dance that makes the objective then possible. As with families, we need freedom-within-structure in order to function well, both individually and collectively.

The structure we can engineer, mass-produce, manage. The freedom we cannot. We must instead assure a respectful space, a skilled conservationism.

\*

I attend this meeting of managers because my long-running 'Psychosomatic' service has been terminated by two mistrustfully allied executive NHS Trusts. This happened by oblivious default, without consultation with those most affected: the patients, referring clinicians or myself. Protests from all were parried by the kinds of skills, 'correct' avoidance and ellipse that large organisations use so frequently as a first line of defence. The new trusts, and their employees, are now part of a corporate quasi-industrial world. This confers a new, but continuing, Darwinian struggle for survival of the fittest, with all the evolutionary feints, deceptions and traps – the behaviours of threat and fear. There necessarily follow changes to our mental life; our priorities, then our values: our individual thought-process, then our collective culture.

The psychosomatic work I do may have been valued by patients and clinicians for many years, but it has not been executively planned and is thus not a contractual obligation of any trust. Occupying a territory of interfaces, it does not feature in the thrall of official goals or targets, or the threat of complaints or litigation. For the survival of the trusts, it confers no evolutionary advantage. Ipso facto, there is no problem and no need.

*

As I listen to the guarded forays, assertions and retorts of these corporate managers and managing clinicians, I am struck by their acquired sureness of style and resolve of language. In this new world of competitive commissioning, expressions of doubt, ambiguity or respectful hesitation are likely to be seen as hazardous indecision, implied submission. To survive, an aura of potency, resolve and business must be maintained. These Commissioning Officers, who are now paid to commodify and trade in areas of outstanding natural complexity (human suffering), become powerfully and subtly changed by this new kind of market economy. Trusts' negotiations and spokespersons must now appear, like senior politicians or multinational corporate bosses; authoritative, confident, decisive. The product marketed must appear definite, clear and assured. 'Confidence', as with the banks, becomes less an internal state of real assets, more of a hypnotic strategy, illusion, even deceit.

## The economy determines the language.

'Providers' now spawn 'treatment packages'. Fascinatingly kaleidoscopic forms of difficulty and distress are speedily designated to 'mental illnesses' or 'disorders', and hence streamed to the 'appropriate intervention'. There is no language (or time) here for the ambiguous, the nascent, the naturally evolving; the semiotics of symptoms, the creative possibilities of uncertainty. The language is systolic.

\*

And then the language determines the thinking.

The monoculture language, intended to expedite the functions of system and symptom management, does not merely provide utilitarian thoroughfare. Like tarmac roads, such prevailing or exclusive language destroys other forms of intellectual life or thought. An unmitigated use of psychiatric or organisational language will, for example, lead to reification; an unwittingly obstructive consequence of language. Mental illness becomes a 'thing', akin to a Cataract or Inguinal Hernia. Sometimes this is unrivalled in effectiveness as a guiding metaphor, a procedural template. At other times, other kinds of language and understanding will yield more: the symptom as lever, language, sacrifice, catalyst or code; the sufferer as messenger or conduit; 'illness' as encoded social or personal construct or contract. The development, and discriminating use, of a wide repertoire of such 'modae cognitiae', constitutes the bedrock of any 'Art' we may bring to our medicine or psychiatry. The heart of this art must have diastole and systole in constantly changing, but functional synchrony. When this does not occur, the interpersonal or clinical disturbance represents a kind of dysrythmia.

\*

**And then the thinking determines the (inter) action.**

'There's only one way to manage this kind of psychotic patient...' avers Dr T in a way that seemed to impute to any attempt at discussion, qualities of incompetence, ignorance or insolence. In fact, both the patient and situation were rich with possibilities of understanding and encounter. The man's psychotic difficulties turned out to be a minor part of what responded to a more holistic and personal approach. But Dr T's utterance reflects far more than her particular nature, or her response to this scenario. It exemplifies the problems of excessive government, management and executive control in matters that are also personal, protean and delicate. The highly structured, proactive 'bullish' vocabulary and style is endemic amongst corporate captains. It now risks becoming epidemic in areas of complex human care, where it can do real harm.

\*

In my many youthful years of apprenticeship to Dr G and Dr R, I never heard such sharply prescriptive or didactically summary communications. These recollections are not only about departed individuals, their sterling and subtle qualities and my long-enduring admiration. They are also about changed times and cultures, and about the loss of values that could flourish in organisations that were more collaborative, colleagial and cooperative; when doctors were more vocational and less careerist; when managers did more to facilitate and less to control.

How would Dr G and Dr R have fared in this current world, to which Dr T is so much better adapted? To my consternation, my imagination deserts me.

\*

*'A wise man hears one word, and understands two'.*

Yiddish proverb

Ω

Publ. by *Public Policy Research* 16:2 2009

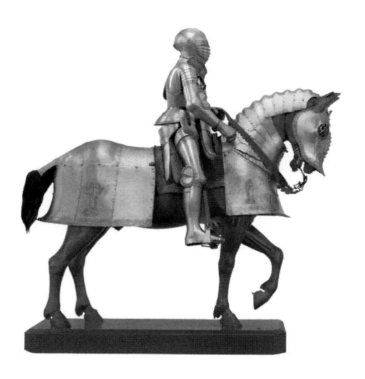

Armoured knight early 14ᵗʰ Century
NHS mental healthcare manager early 21rst Century?

# Psychiatry
# Love's Labour's Lost

## The pursuit of The Plan
## and the eclipse of the personal

Attempts to gain greater safety and efficiency in Psychiatric services have led to a redesign which mimics the increasing streaming and fragmentation of Medical Services. The results are, very often, dislocating, depersonalising and demotivating for both staff and patients alike. Human and economic costs are considerable. This article explores by narrative and analysis.

## Introduction

It is a little over thirty years since I gave up my full-time job in Psychiatry. I reduced this work to part-time, became a single-handed Principal General Practitioner and ran a small, private psychotherapy practice. Amidst this busy multivalent work, I turned oblivious and vague from the confusing mosaic of organisational plots and plans gathering around me.

The metamorphosis within the NHS would be much different to what I had indifferently supposed. More recently I have awoken to the nature and consequences of changes that incubated and hatched in this last decade, my period of circumspection.

The psychiatric service now settling is a much more complex compound of numerous, specialised, boundaried teams. These mostly operate with strict intake criteria and sharply delineated, short-term goals. Algorithmically, such a managed medley may look elegantly precise and machine-like. Such is the likely and wishful perception of managers, policymakers and (increasingly) practitioners.

This sharply contrasts with the experiences I hear elsewhere. Frequently I receive patients bewildered and adrift. They attempt to describe a plethora of different teams and formulaic, interrogatory styles of interview. I strive to counter their fatigue and dispiritedness. These often ensue from the recurrent breaking of short-term therapeutic bonds. The engineered neatness of diagnoses and clinical plans does not often correspond to the natural untidiness and inconsistencies of people's lives and distress. Or their complex and changing needs for reparative contact. Older practitioners, too, talk of their frustration; of being deskilled and disempowered in their fragile endeavours to respond with care that is personally attuned, and with an open view to the longer-term. It is not just patients who may be 'shrunk-to-fit'. These tribulations derive, paradoxically, from designs and styles of management attempting to address 'efficiency' - a Higher Good, a necessary Utilitarianism.

This collage of recollections and notions, from both General Practice and Psychiatry, serves both to illustrate and explain some major, current healthcare conundrae. The Law of Unintended Consequences is evidenced from diverse viewpoints.

Increasing hegemony and rigidity within and between institutions, at the expense of interpersonal attention and sensitivity, is a central and recurring theme. Inevitable, though inadvertent, losses to our understanding of individuals, and thus our therapeutic effectiveness, are difficult to measure directly. Indirect evidence is plentiful. It signals exponential losses to the kinds of therapeutic benefits that need quality and continuity of human contact as a bedrock. The new services are thus very much more expensive,[1] but, in crucial ways, less effective.

In the following accounts, events and dialogue are authentic. Usual devices of disguise protect anonymity.

*

*I would rather ride on an ass that carries me,*
 *than a horse that throws me.*

George Herbert, *Jacula Prudendum*, 1651

The telephonised voice is unfamiliar. It is bright, young and crisp, with the assurance and pre-set utterances of a corporate officer, officially and well briefed. Amanda tells me she is the Duty Manager for the Community Mental Health Team:

"We have had our Referrals Meeting. We have considered your letter and do not think that your patient, Tessa, meets our intake criteria. We noted that her attendance here previously was poor, and we didn't think she benefited from our Service ..."

*

Three weeks earlier Tessa comes to see me, her GP of twenty years. Now in her late 30s, Tessa enters with a reticent demeanour of bruised trust and flickering hope. I have long known these to lap a larger internal land-mass of bleak fatalism and despair. She offers me a very brief direct look and a hint of a smile of greeting: I imagine she cannot risk more.

More than a decade ago I attended the multiple and fresh wounds in, and from, Tessa's family. The fewer were stark and shocking: a young brother's violent suicide, in prison; an older brother's serious residual brain damage, from drugs. Tessa, thereafter, was his Carer. The many were more 'ordinary', but cumulatively destructive: chaotic and emotionally illiterate parents, compounding their (family's) problems with alcoholic oblivion. Then the consequent physical damage. Then came disability and, ineluctably, their dependence on Tessa. As a droning bass-note: the symptoms and trap of endless, ugly, economic poverty.

Knowing something of this background and story I understand the meaningful evolution of her psychiatric Stem Cells: her swamp-like poor self-esteem, insecure attachments and default position of helpless depression. Simultaneously, I have long admired the battered and malnourished hulk of her will to survive and connect. These are the germinators of her health: I encourage them in myriad ways. Over many years I have offered her, piecemeal and compressed, refuge, reflection, and asylum. Often we have needed expedient, intermittent bolstering from others, from Psychiatrists, Social Services, Day Centres and Counsellors. Like the Asthma and Diabetes she has 'inherited', her Mental Distress is not decisively curable, though it (she) is responsive, ameliorable and containable. Mostly I guide and I palliate. Often, I help her perceive and act in ways that do not make difficult situations worse. I may sometimes help her succeed. Far too late to make major reversals of Fate, I offer valued morsels of parenting that were tragically lacking in her biological family: safety and reliability. Then space and sensitivity, for respectful, imaginative dialogue; sometimes, even, wisps of play. All have been necessary, but rarely sufficient. To alleviate some of the insufficiency, I welcomed synergy from like-minded colleagues.

*

One such was Dr M, a senior psychiatrist at the local (teaching) hospital. A little short of twenty years ago I am meeting Dr M every few months. Our conversations generate mutual interest, guidance and clarification. We share care for many puzzling, distressing or enervating patients. Our roles, locations and periods of contact are different, sometimes disparate. It is the exchange of these that may enlighten work that is so often uncertain and uncompleteable. Sometimes it will not: then there is support and affiliation from a trusted colleague; a humble balm for long-term professional goodwill and morale.

The cordiality and informality of our meetings is framed by a light lunch or early evening meal. There are no recorded agendae, bullet-points, power-points, or action-plans. This is learning by mutual enquiry; Education at its most feral and refined.

Over many years I had several such alliances with Senior Psychiatrists from this hospital. Although the style varied with the individual, the pattern of commonality endured: we were fortified by a pragmatic rapport of uncertainties. Such extemporised dialogue made us a little more able to perceive and address the chimeric complexity of people's lives.

*

I remember a conversation with Dr M about Tessa, early one summer evening. As usual, we each brought our samplings of newly garnered notions and reports. Again, his perceptive compassion and imagination freshened my own efforts, sometimes lost and stumbling. Thus enriched through our fallibilities, we grew an implicit bond of gentle, ironic affection.

Tessa, too, benefited from this unplanned but now deliberate and fertile overlap of 'multi-agency care'. I thought of the secure and happy child who senses good contact and connection between her parents, but does not necessarily know (or care) what they are talking about. Tessa partially articulated this, shortly after her brother killed himself:

"Mum and Dad can't offer one another, or me, or anyone any comfort … Thank goodness you and Dr M talk together and are here…"

Later that evening Dr M told me of mooted plans to reorganise Psychiatric Services. He was not directly involved, but had heard:

"They [the planners/authorities] think that the hospital-based services are too large, impersonal and distant (both geographically and psychologically) from the populations they serve – the frightening, forbidding 'Castle on the Hill', above us and surrounded by mist, that sort of thing.

"Their idea is to have smaller, but more community-based, centres instead. These will be 'friendlier'; they will certainly be geographically closer to most patients. Also, they will be excellently placed to build up personal working relationships with GPs and their Counsellors, Health Visitors, Social Workers, District Nurses … even Work-placement Officers and FE Colleges … What do you think?"

It all sounded good to me. My hesitations were trivial, brief and personal: I rather liked the system as it was, and my relationships within it. Also, I'd never really been interested in that kind of Grand Planning … I soon stopped my timorous muttering. I assured him I would look forward, with alacrity.

*

Twenty years later I am struggling to learn the language and etiquette of this 'community-based' system. The current consultant, Dr Q, has been in post five years, but has had only essential and remote contact with myself and the few other GPs similarly interested and motivated. I once attempted to speak with him, about an obscured and worrying patient-situation: I hoped for the kind of dialogue I had, fruitfully and repeatedly, many years ago, with Dr M and his contemporaries. Dr Q's response was stiff in formality and cautious to the point of inertia. He quickly demonstrated (to himself) that there was little to discuss. As he spoke, I remembered old monochrome newsreels of the 1950s: the veteran Soviet Foreign Minister, Gromyko, and his stern monosyllabic camouflages, neutralising western journalists' eager questions. This opaque gravitas seemed both comic and threatening.

The threat is felt because the (Non) Spokesperson may foreshadow an enigmatic and concealed multitude, not a mere (and maybe) curmudgeonly individual. Silence can be interpersonal darkness, in highly vulnerable territory.

*

Other Practitioners are having similar problems. Like Dr K, a Local Medical Committee member. She is a warm-hearted, sharp-witted woman with a reputation for intelligent but humorous persistence. In an unscheduled encounter we briefly discuss my doldrums with local psychiatric services.

Her initial receptivity soon dissolves with gestures of thwarted aggravation. "It's hopeless," she summarises with testy terseness, "they're so boundaried and seem accountable only to their own management ... I can't get any real dialogue from them, just organisational ripostes ... I've given up ..."

I think of Dr M's metaphor of the previous psychiatrists working in The Castle on the Hill, and how we have somehow, at great expense, replaced it with local armed garrisons of foreign soldiers, who speak only their own language. I share these evolutionary images with Dr K. We laugh heartily at this vignette of The Law of Unintended Consequences, but it is the manic, displacing laughter of doomed respite.

As our laughter falls away, I am aware of a sadness; a grieving, a realisation that valued activities and contacts are gone. Relinquished for those that seem (to me) to lead to such misalignment and derogated contact. Is the problem, mostly, that in my fortieth year of practice I am too rigid to mould to the cusp of change? Or is this more a cultural grief, for the passing of a colleagueial culture that was more responsive in its informality, pluralist and 'organic' in its growth. Replaced by a managed culture of sharply boundaried and structured multidisciplinary teams, themselves issuing and receiving 'information' and 'action plans'; where any 'development' is engineered and sanctioned by official diktat and now, increasingly, 'market forces'?

*

I try to get Amanda beyond her templated telephone 'management' of Tessa and I. I am becoming impatient. I feel obstructed by an armoured inflexibility. These colleagues seem immured and impermeable. Most worrying, they seem unstoppably confident in making remote, procedural decisions about a complexly troubled person who they have never met.

Clearly, there is little precedent, capacity or inclination to engage with me: an observant, thoughtful practitioner (I like to think) who has known the patient twenty years. I need to inject (my) reality into this surreal impasse. I can do this by talking collegueially with Dr Q. I ask to speak to him.

"Dr Q is very busy in meetings, all day … In any case, as I told you, the decision was taken as a Team."

Her crisp voice now seems edged with reprimand. I am being managed. I imagine the bright, brittle shell of a mollusc, a protective exo-skeleton. An 'executive persona'.

*

Thirty-five years ago I worked with Carl in a large victorian mental hospital. As young, trainee psychiatrists we enjoyed a friendly network of peers and older mentoring consultants. The ancient institution's heavy, forbidding architecture was, paradoxically, home to a warmly personalised 'village' within the NHS. In my two years there, friendly colleagueial relationships extended far beyond my closer professional 'family' (psychiatrists, psychologists, PSWs); I developed affable and effective alliances with art therapists, rehabilitation officers, the laboratory manager, even the hospital telephone switchboard operator. All these were known by name, face, voice, styles of banter. Reminiscing, Carl and I remember them with surprising precision. Beyond our individual memories, this says a great deal about that old institution and its connection to people.

Carl and I were mostly blessed by similar personal continuity and attention in our clinical apprenticeships. We both were guided by Consultants who (often) had known their patients for many years. This knowledge was likely to be quite as much 'in vivo' as 'in vitro'. Individuals were 'known' not just by questioning in the consulting room. Often they had been seen, over many years, in their homes, with parents, partners, children, friends, neighbours, even the (then) 'family' doctor. Our mentoring consultants thus taught us a kind of 'Field Psychiatry'. Here was a long time-span, and a wide matrix of human connections and understandings. By example as much as theoretical formulation, we learned to be imaginative about the unspoken, respectful of the complexity of attachments (including our own). We were gently shown creative discipline amidst inevitable uncertainties. Likewise, a pragmatic scepticism of the incompleteness of our consensual psychiatric language and tools. We discussed how many individual exceptions there are to our theoretical generalisations. "The more you see of somebody, the more of somebody you see" was an anchoring, guiding principle.

For many years, after he became senior, Carl continued this trajectory; he managed and delivered a service that got to know well its many kinds of sufferers, often over several years. For those whose problems were longstanding and variable, he was unhampered in his experienced choice of approach. In calm times, he would offer accessible, gentle interest. When trouble brewed, he could fast-track to a more interventive and urgent out-patient appointment. When serious trouble impacted, he would admit the patient, to be cared for by the staff he knew well; another part of his therapeutic family. Amidst the stresses and tensions inevitable in psychiatry, he grew a quiet love for the satisfactions of his role as a kind of pater familias and patient gardener. During these two decades, I did not hear him speak of 'Holistic Practice', but recognised the radiation of these values.

*

In recent times, Carl and I are talking of our individual and common travails. At this august stage of a diligent and creative career, he is disheartened and despondent. Not from his marathon contact with the anguished, but with the ever-tightening structures and strictures of management.

"I'm now just stuck in an Out-Patient Clinic, which is run by managers ... I can't, myself, make an appointment for a patient I've known for years: it has to be referred by the GP (who, increasingly, may not know the patient) and then be assessed for 'suitability' by the team (ditto) ... If my well-known patient may need admission, I have to send them to another team they don't know, because I no longer have beds ... and if it's decided they don't need admission there's yet another team (who probably don't know the patient ...) to look after them at home ... So, we have the Community Mental Health Team, The Emergency Psychiatric Clinic, The Home Treatment Team, The

In-Patient Unit, The Early Discharge Unit, The Assertive Outreach Team … that's not all, and there's more on the way: shall I tell you?"

I raise my hands limply in surrender: my comprehension is coagulating.

He continues in angry jest:

"Well, if you don't understand it, or can't remember it all, what do you think it's like for patients who are dizzy with *their* distress, chaos or instability? Very often the most basic and important thing we can do for people is to provide a familiar and stable source of understanding, comfort and recognition; an accessible and humane form of asylum. I've tried to warn and remonstrate about how this complex multi-team approach leads to personal disconnection. It's not just frequently distressing; it's cumbersome, inefficient, and thus much more expensive. An aggressively defensive manager recently said to me: 'Our job, and your job, Doctor, is to make sure there is continuity within and between teams. It's the team, not the person. That way the Patient Journey is integrated …' *'Integrated Patient Journey'*: what a professionally self-referring shibboleth! I hope it makes the managers and planners feel calmer and better, because that's not the experience I usually hear from patients. With them, much of my work is about trying to soothe administratively torn connections. Imbue a sense of personal, durable and sensitive contact … that's not easy when, at the same time, I am attempting to explain and apologise for a system that is (for them) recurrently unfamiliar, and thus (for them) incomprehensible and undependable.

"Yes, we talk of 'Agreed Care Plans' but these are usually *our* schematic actions, to which the craven patient will usually concur (or pretend to). Those who explicitly will not, are likely to evoke our subsidiary, often tendentious, diagnoses: the patient is 'non-compliant', 'chaotic', 'uncooperative' and so forth. I find these 'Care Plans' are much more prescriptive and authoritarian than the more informal, conversational ways you and I used for decades. It's only the clothing, the spun language, that illusion the democratic. More smooth deceits of Political Correctness!..."

Carl seems a little self-surprised by the size of this bolus of professional frustration, and the force, though ease, with which he has expelled it. Knowing my kindred experiences, we are, both, more emboldened than embarrassed.

How has a practitioner of Carl's calibre, experience, and personal qualities become so restricted, deskilled and impoverished in his work? I want to know the hidden organisational history.

"Carl. You've been the Senior Consultant at your hospital, the Clinical Director of your Trust, Regional Postgrad Tutor, Fellow of your Royal College ..." I pin the medals to his chest, and then ask: "Who are the people who designed such a system? How did they decide on this? Who did they ask? When? You must know these things ..."

My clustered questions are insistent, but softly spoken.

Carl looks disarmed and discomfited by them: shards of freshly realised but compromised ignorance.

"Ah!" I exhale, now canny in recognition. I imagine a stage-curtain descending. The Triumph of Bureaucracy-become-Culture: The Dictatorship of Everyone by No One.

"It's fiendishly clever", I say with affected, boyish lightness. "I mean, how can anyone ever undo it ...?"

*

We decide we cannot discern the persons behind the plans, those behind the unplanned drift into depersonalised care. Our attention turns now to more generic influences: culture, economics, new technologies, the media ... We rummage in this attic-full of tangled puppet strings, previously unheeded. Carl and I, veteran cohorts, rejuvenate our fading energies with regenerated language and questions.

"If you're writing about this new, skewed rigidification of Psychiatry, you really should include these undiscussed influences", Carl says.

"But there are so many, and they're so subtle ... the article will be far too long ..." I falter, daunted.

"Well, condense it and offer it as an Appendix. You can always write it up more fully, later," proffers Carl, saturated, succinct and prescriptive.

I agree. Herewith.

## Appendix:

Current and recent influences displacing Person-Centred, Holistic Healthcare, especially in Psychiatry and General Practice. Some brief notes.

### 1. Industrialisation/Mass Production

Now determining influence in most human activities and their objects. May be the most important and difficult to counter. Leads to standardisation and pre-packaging. Loss of individual input: craft, attention and interest. 'Factory sizes' only: no bespoke. Difficult to prevent anomie. Best only when human variables are minimal, e.g. Cataract extraction, Vaccination, Acute and severe physical illness. Least good with complex, changeable processes and atypia. (As 2 +3)

### 2. A(na)tomisation

Medical Model = MM= best when dealing with localised physical macropathology. (Much less effective in other areas.) Psychiatric services now very dominated by MM. Anato-atomisation = AA = Multiplying and confining specialisations according to smaller body areas. e.g. General Orthopaedics ----- Hip/ Knee/ Shoulder etc. GI - Upper GI/ Hepatobiliary/ Colorectal etc.

AA and MM lead to limiting analogy of 'Mental Disorders' being generic 'states', rather than individual 'processes'.

AA and MM are structural and mechanistic models. Thus v. compatible with Industrialisation/ Mass Production/ Management Hegemony/ Goals and Targets (see later).

Recent massive attempts to mimic AA in Psychiatry, by mixing patient behaviour with organisational expedience, e.g. CMHT, Dual Diagnosis, Assertiveness Outreach, Eating Disorders, Alcohol Dependence, Emergency Psychiatric, Home Treatment, Early Discharge ... Medieval Theological Problem = How many Angels can sit on a single pin-head? Current NHS problem = How many Clinics can medicalise human anguish and be paid for by one PCT?

Such designed complexification generates its own problems. Akin to fitting a 117-speed gearbox to a vehicle: gears will tend to miss or jam, power is lost in propelling the larger bulk of machinery, which is much more expensive to produce …

### 3. Computers and IT

Based on binary code: 0 or 1. Difficult medium for creative uncertainty. Algorithmic processes/choices coded as clear and definite. Incompatible with ambiguity, multiple meanings etc. Likely to lead to reification: Mental illness seen as a 'thing' rather than an organising concept for complex, evanescent processes: leads to Knowledge as a 'commodity' rather than 'activity'; a 'product', not a 'creation'.

### 4. We know how to work things, but not how things work

Objects of our use increasingly maintenance-free, disposable, sealed-for-life. A growing conundrum and syndrome in our Hi-Tech world. Few users now understand the innards of their car or computer. Leads to widespread mastery-without-understanding mindset. e.g. psychiatrist who follows 'correct' (decreed) 'Treatment Pathways', but has little understanding of/interest in the unique experience and 'innards' of each patient. Management without personal understanding.

### 5. NHS Commissioning: Territoriality and Commodification

Commissioning conceived (presumably) to tighten and sharpen working awareness and performance. Does it? Model derived from corporate competitive commerce. Many unintended side-effects: Practitioners frequently more boundaried = affiliation to Trusts' short-term, measurable, G & T (Goals and Targets) rather than patients' longer-term, less measurable, health and welfare. Increasing resources spent on window-dressing, PR/'Spin', legal process. Officious practice = adhering to 'Letter of the Law', not cleaving to values underlying it. Rules devoid of jurisprudence. G & T very compatible with MM + AA (above). Fosters competitive, territorial behaviour, rather than cooperative, colleagueial alliances.

### 6. Governmental Modelling: Less Conscious influences

a) Since 1997 the previous (New Labour) government has had more lawyers in Cabinet than any previous. Hence accelerated tendency to rules, regulations, prescribed procedures in most difficult human problem areas, especially Health and Social Care, Education. Intelligent and creative flexibility initially displaced, eventually proscribed.

b) In recent years a very influential senior Minister of Health[2] has been a Laparoscopic Surgeon. His expertise re: illness and treatments is via well-defined (mostly successful) procedures to very confined body areas. (Where MM and AA are most effective.) His perspective on planning and funding derives from these. Problem = if too dominant, leads to impoverishment of more holistic approaches. Especially important re: syndromes that are chronic, incurable, fluctuating or non-localisable = much (most?) of Elderly, Primary, Psychiatric Care. Much more than MM/AA required with these.

### 7. The Climbié-Clunis Factor:[3] The ratcheting of Defensive Practice

In our media-dense world, we now mass-produce and sustain interest in the most extreme enactments of 'madness' and 'badness', as never before. These sporadic horrors are rare, through perennial. New (and understandable) government initiatives to assert 'authority': systems for early identification and sequestration of perpetrators. 'Never again.' Resulting mass micromanagement is doubtfully effective. May be less effective, due to secondary inflexibility. Services dominated by 'worse case scenario' become anxiously and narrowly focused: like phobic patient with rigid and controlled relationships. Another analogy: the over-armoured medieval knight who cannot walk, mount his steed, or respond dextrously to attack, when it comes. Lesson: too much caution creates new hazards.

Practitioners strangulated by procedure lose capacity for reception, perception and reflection.

## 8. Not only but also: unintended multiplications and extrapolations

AA will tend to fragment holistic care and its long-enough healing attachments. Increasingly, ever more numerous and boundaried teams then have to be staffed and trained for. Trainees (who may provide most consultations) are then necessarily rotated more frequently between these many teams. Q: How will doctors learn about the power and subtlety of caring attachments? Are we already losing arts and crafts in these? How can the emotionally vulnerable connect, trust and heal by submitting to a carousel of professional 'strangers', united largely by the managerial designation of a team?

This discontinuity recently and coincidentally amplified by EC Working Hours legislation. 'Rationing' of working-time necessitates even more complex rotas and teams.

## Epilogue: Distant Voices – Paradoxical Times

Intentions and consequences can be very different. In the early 1930s few realised how long and dense would be the shadow cast by the sinewy and virile youth of Totalitarianism. Giovani Gentile ghost writes for Mussolini, with Olympian righteousness, *The Doctrine of Fascism*:

"Anti-individualistic, the fascist conception of life stresses the importance of the State and accepts the individual only in so far as his interests coincide with those of the State, which stands for the conscience and the universal will of Man as a historic entity. It is opposed to classical liberalism which arose as a reaction to absolutism and exhausted its historical function when the State became the expression of the conscience and the will of the People ..."

About 75 years later in the National Health Service of our liberal democracy, Dr Steven Ford, a medical practitioner, writes to *The Independent* newspaper:[3]

'The thrust in the health field is towards the establishment of legions of meekly compliant, cloned health-droids with narrow spectra of competencies, tightly yoked by legally enforceable contracts, protocols and guidelines. The fate of patients in the new regime is to be parcelled into managerially tidy job-lots and auctioned off to the lowest bidder. Managerial and commercial skills are more highly valued and rewarded than clinical ones ...'

Few have claimed to design this new legacy, but many, already, are clearer about its effects. Whoever redesigns this redesign will have much to draw from.

\*

*A mariner must have his eye on the rocks and sands, as well as on the North Star.*

Thomas Fuller MD, *Gnomoligia* (1732)

## References and footnotes

1.   NHS expenditure shows an accelerated increase in the last two decades, far beyond any inflation. Statistics published in Hansard show this to be nearly 300% in the period 1995-2007 (c. 220% when inflation-adjusted). GDP fractional expenditure shows a similar trend in this period, from c. 6% to 8%. Some of this increase is due to factors inevitable, widespread and desirable, e.g. more people getting relief or cure from more conditions, greater longevity, more sophisticated and effective investigations, interventions and medications.

Psychiatric services share most of these. Where the new design of such services is exceptional is in its generation of complexity, with all the more and less obvious additional costs.

2.   Lord Ara Darzi

3.   Victoria Climbié was a child murdered by her aunt and partner in 2000. Christopher Clunis, known to be disturbed and labelled 'Paranoid Schizophrenia', murdered a stranger 'randomly' in 1992.

Both cases led to castigation of relevant professions (Social and Psychiatric Services respectively). Followed by demand for more management, supervision, documented procedures. 'Never again.' Major historical influences in current overgrowth of 'defensive practice'.

4. *The Independent*, Letters, 13/12/08

At the time of writing Tessa has been lost to contact. This followed my rejected referral. The connection seems significant, and I fear the gravity of the consequences. More positively, after many initiatives I have arranged a meeting with my CMHT.

$$\Omega$$

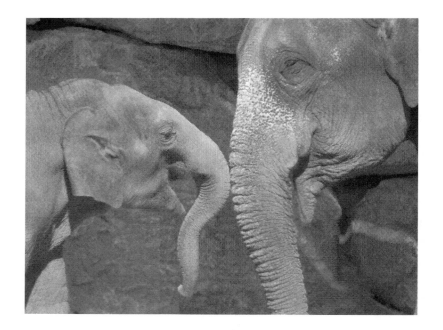

# Why would Anyone Use an Unproven Therapy?

## Treasures in the Mist:
## Another personal view

*Not everything that can be counted counts. Not all that counts can be counted.*

Albert Einstein, 1879-1955

*Religion is regarded by the common people as true, by the wise as false, and by the rulers as useful.*

Seneca the Younger, ca 4BC-65AD

Professor Edzard Ernst's 'Personal View'[1] is a short, robustly sensible piece. He leads us briskly along a much used path, pointing out how straying into surrounding, unscientific territory subjects us to the lures of fantasy, corruption and personal influence. The tarmacked path is smooth, firm, safe and even; the wilderness is unmapped, hazardous, disorienting. It is stalked by predatory creatures. Why would anyone choose to traverse this Wilder Ness?

I am reminded of many scientific-rationalist thinkers who pour easy scorn on religion: its tenets are absurdly unprovable, its conduct inconsistent, its basest expressions shockingly destructive. Why would anyone pursue irrational belief? But Ernst's rhetorical question is less simple than apparent. It spawns many beyond. Some are explored in this longer reply.

While his critique is importantly true, it is crucially incomplete. In particular, myth and fantasy are often harbingers of our most positive aspiration and inspiration. Belief in the transcendent and the transpersonal can be powerfully transformative, but only for the believer. Far from whimsy, these complex phenomena have been shown to be essential components in studies linking religious faith and health resilience,[2] and multifarious research into placebos.[3] Over several decades, repeated investigation identifies how the emotional state, the belief and faith of the sufferer, and the perceived quality of contact with the Healer, make critical differences in illness experience and outcome.[4]

Such interactional and transpersonal factors may be scientifically discerned generally, though with some difficulty. This cannot be said of the individual transmission and processing of such influences. Here we enter different and difficult territory: the 'art' of medicine and healing. Here are personal perceptions of experience and meaning. These are transmitted mainly intersubjectively, thus generating subtly unique language, metaphors and rituals.[5,6]   Such personal factors can become quite as important as the impersonal science of biomechanism. Dilemmas arise, for it is only the impersonal, the generic, that are readily accessible to the organising code of our quantitative science. With all else we must suffice with other kinds of understanding and evaluation. Biomechanical Medicine has had dramatic successes in the last century. It is also readily understandable, reproducible and testable in ways often impossible with other forms of healing.

But the reach and strength of science is gravitated to the externally measurable: the sharpness of its definition fades as it enters the dappled realms of inner experience and the complexly interpersonal. Absence of (scientific) proof is not proof of absence. We must be wary that this potent and precise, but limited, world of Biomechanical Medicine is not overused, assuming a kind of regal hegemony. Some areas are not its natural territory.

We should be imaginative, therefore, about complexity and thus paradox. It is true that interpersonal healing (in contrast to the Orderly Ness of generic biomechanical treatment) is a Wilder Ness; obscure to scientific mapping. Ineluctably, as Ernst reminds us, more vulnerable to contamination by human folly, deception, greed or grandiosity. But what of its opposite pole? By analogy, arcane and ancient religious texts have led to those most disturbing and cruel perversions of 'righteousness' and superstition. Yet those same texts, very differently selected, have led to millions of undramatic quieting comforts for the anguished, humble acts of inclusion and kindness and (irrational?) faith and hope in our troubled and evanescent lives.

We can think of a genus of basic existential anxieties: primordially the chaotic meaninglessness of life; our mortality, our cosmic insignificance, and our ultimate alone-ness. How well we make positive sense of, or adjustment to, or defences against, these anxieties will have a determining effect on the basic quality of our lives. This is enacted through our relationships, our state of health and our response to illness, when it comes.[7,8]

Core biomedical practice does not address these inner workings. Religion and healing have many approaches, both explicit and inexplicit. The inexplicit are conveyed by metaphor and ritual. Such become the common currencies of healing. Thus, for example, healing 'procedures' involving touch or gaze may symbolically communicate to the sufferer recognition, inclusion and significance; all important requisites to palliation and recovery.[4] The procedure is a kind of language, but it can only be 'spoken' if both participants have congruent belief systems about the affliction.[6]

All this comprises something of the 'art' of healing and medical practice, and why it is so difficult to standardise, measure or mass-produce. Another important way of distinguishing and understanding these activities is to consider the source of resources: external and impersonal, or internal and (inter)personal. Prevailing biomechanical treatment exerts its influence via the former: by externally located agents – be they chemicals, manipulations, instruments, radiations, stents or sutures. Likewise, understanding and explanation are of an objective, generic and impersonal kind. Both are externally 'conducted'.

By contrast the many kinds of healing address and facilitate the individual's innate capacities of immunity, growth and repair: this is an 'induction' of internal resources. It is the product of interpersonal exchanges within a relationship field. Although induction may be individually powerful in-vivo, it is a protean, evaporative process, very dependent on individual attunement. In-vitro attempts to mass-produce or measure are left mostly with empty husks. Experience yields only external epiphenomena to measurement. Inductive healing can gestate only in the Wilder Ness: a conundrum for those health planners and managers who understand.

The film 'The Wizard of Oz' illustrates this fertile but paradoxical subterraneum of healing with charming simplicity. Each major character represents a universal human developmental task; the failure to address these leads to dis-ease or sickness. The Lion must find the courage to be himself (Identity); the Tin Man his heart for others (Love); the Scarecrow his own thoughts (Logos); and Dorothy a place of peace, acceptance and kinship: 'finding my way home' (Belonging). To re-own these they must achieve something that seems impossible to them as individuals: destroy the Wicked Witch of the West – the despair, nihilism and hatred that we can all harbour and inflict. They manage this communally, pursuing a shared belief in a myth: the all powerful Wizard of Oz. It is through faith in this mythical Other that they transcend their habitual (self-)limitation, subtly trance-formed, then transformed.

Dorothy, later, accidentally discovers that The Wizard is an unremarkable man operating a panoply of pyrotechnics to create such hypnotic charisma. Dorothy confronts him:

'You're a very bad man!' shouts Dorothy, through angry tears.

'No, I'm not a bad man. I'm a very good man. Just not a very good wizard ...' comes a faltering, apologetic explanation.

I am reminded of a recently retired bishop telling me that he had lost his faith, but had found verve in becoming a 'born again atheist'. With a further paradoxical garnish, he told me he still liked to attend church services.

'Why?' I asked, perplexed.

'Because it is the prayer that is transformative, whatever the fiction of the myth. Through prayer I find a kind of empowered humility, a sense of myself more clear and connected, though more transient. Through faith in something far beyond myself, I become less defined by my faults, frailties and inevitable mortality. I can now do without God, but not without prayer ...'

'How do you manage that: the one without the other?' I ask, again puzzled.

'Ah, well, you have to be a bishop first!' he replied with teasing wit and ambiguity.

After my amused bemusement had passed, I was left thinking how multilayered and meaningful his reply had been. Or was I imagining his encoded and askance wisdom? Was that a private myth, of mine? In any case, this contact induced in me a burgeoning constellation of new thoughts and connections: I was enlivened, enriched and energised. A small incident, but I reflected on how this offered a microcosmic example of the questions we face with both healing and prayer. How do we even begin to measure, manage or mass-produce such subtle life-exchanges, such treasures in the mist? Do we need a Yellow Brick Road?

*

*We can be absolutely certain only about things we do not understand.*

Eric Hoffer. *The True Believer* (1951)

## References and notes

[1] Ernst E. Why would anyone use an unproven or disproven therapy? A personal view. *Journal of the Royal Society of Medicine* 2009; 102: 452–53

[2] Frank J *Persuasion and Healing*. New York: Schocken, 1972

Frank J *Psychotherapy and the Human Predicament*. New York: Schocken, 1978

Frank, a Professor of Psychiatry at John Hopkins Medical School, was a prodigious academic researcher and writer for several decades. He demonstrated the pathogenic influence of alienation and despondency. As a corollary, and their institutions. He showed, too, how these placebo effects could all be reversed by pessimism, mistrust and negatively-experienced attachments: the 'Nocebo' effect.

Frank's work is equally impressive in its breadth, depth, meticulousness and clarity. The above two books offer the most accessible introduction.

[3] Ibid.

Zigmond D. Mother, Magic or Medicine? The Psychology of the Placebo. *British Journal of Holistic Medicine* 1984; 1:113–9

The paper provides a brief survey of placebo research as well as providing some explanations from developmental and social psychology.

[4] Frank J (1972), op cit; Frank J (1978), op cit

[5] Balint M. *The Doctor, his Patient and the Illness*. London: Pitman, 1957

Balint's informal, qualitative study was of encounters between General Practitioners and their patients. Amidst his clarifications was the importance of the inter-subjective in medical practice, which has become increasingly defined and confined by an objective view and language. He explored the different kinds of diagnostic and therapeutic opportunities that were possible from this interpersonal perspective, as well as the perils that followed its neglect.

Due the difficulty (?impossibility) of standardising, regulating or mass-producing this approach, it has been responded to with bewilderment, indifference or hostility by, first, contemporary health planners and economists and, then, managers and practitioners. In this author's view, the consequent loss of 'emotional literacy' to the cultures of General Practice and Psychiatry, is grievous: therapeutically, economically and experientially.

6) Zigmond D. Three Types of Encounter in the Health Arts: Dialogue, Dialectic and Didactism. *British Journal of Holistic Medicine* 1987; 2:68-81

A short paper considering how practitioners and patients jointly process experience and language in different kinds of transactions. These confer power, agency and responsibility in very contrasting ways. The origins of these and the consequences of misappropriation and misalignment are illustrated and explained.

7) Balint M (1970). *Treatment or Diagnosis. A Study of Repeat Prescriptions in General Practice*. London, Tavistock

Another of Balint's substantial, small scale, quantitative researches, over many years. Explores how many illness behaviours and their medical responses are best understood as ritualistic, encoded communications, which both doctors and patients often resist decoding. As with (6), above, now much neglected, with considerable loss of personal types of understanding.

Quite as important, he showed the therapeutic effect of: feeling re-engaged with peers, having an explanation congruent with native beliefs, a sense of positive personal agency and some evidence of its success. Pre-requisite to these were faith, trust and positive attachment to healers and Another of Balint's substantial, small scale, quantitative researches, over many years. Explores how many illness behaviours and their medical responses are best understood as ritualistic, encoded communications, which both doctors and patients often resist decoding. As with (6), above, now much neglected, with considerable loss of personal types of understanding.

8) This was well illustrated in an NHS project in the late 1980s. An Alternative/Complementary Medicine Clinic was set up for GPs and Hospital Practitioners to refer to. The results, in terms of therapeutic results, and even attendance, were poor. The Alternative Practitioners were equally dismayed and puzzled: they had abundant good evidence of much better results in their private practices.

In this author's view procedures might be the same in the two settings, transactionally they were very dissimilar. In Private Practice both patient and practitioner are likely to assume convergent values, expectations, maybe myths. There is a shared 'language'. In the NHS, where a third party organises the dyad by referral, there is less likelihood of such a 'match', and thus no occult 'common-language'. These exchanges are thus less receptive to the possibilities of 'induction'.

The hypothesis here is that it is the encrypted 'communication' that is therapeutic, not the procedure per se.

[Experience from Author's own practice.]

Ω

Publ. by *Journal of Holistic Healthcare* Vol. 7 Issue 2 Sept. 2010

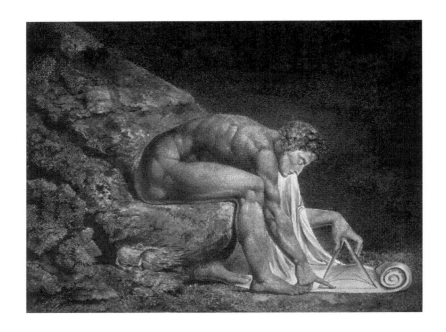

William Blake – *Isaac Newton* 1805

# Idiomorphism
# the Lost Continent

## How diagnosis displaces
## personal understanding

## Introduction and summary

In understanding of the non-human world, our scientific procedures and 'objective' observation and generic clustering serve us well. But human complexity renders such presumptions much less reliable: motivation, protean states of (un)consciousness, encoded behaviours and communications, concealed diversities – all such phantoms are signifiers of the human condition; and all are frequently elusive and impenetrable to our usual scientific endeavours.

Publicly provisioned healthcare is now largely designed and guided by a new cultural convention: 'Evidence Basis'. This is anchored to science whose competence is rooted in the impersonal. While this often works well in dealing with clear physical disease – 'structural pathology' – it becomes adversely inadequate with other kinds of distress. It is these 'functional disturbances' – dis-ease – that comprise the subtlest challenges to healthcare. Our understanding and response to this world of human complexity, paradox and chimera needs very different, though complementary, skills. The illustrating vignettes in this article are authentic and typify what is common in primary care. In psychiatry and psychology it is the subterraneum, though now increasingly, and hazardously, disregarded.

How do we respond?

\*

*'Though all men be made of one metal, yet they be not cast all in one mould'*

John Lyly Euphus, *The Anatomy of Light* (1579)

*'Every man is more than just himself: he also represents the unique, the very special and always significant and remarkable point at which the world's phenomena intersect, only once in this way and never again.'*

Herman Hesse, *Prologue to Demian* (1979)

## A. Idiomorphism – People's stories. Samples from primary care. End: Week 1

### 1. Cathy

Age 63, Cathy has suddenly looked older, since she found her husband, Bob, collapsed and dead in the bathroom. A stalwart and uncomplaining man, his life suddenly ended; a mortality shocking for its lack of warning. The coroner had judged it due to a massive heart attack.

Dr R had had only light and infrequent, though amiable, contact with Bob over many years. Cathy's many encounters with her doctor had been very different. Twelve years ago she had discovered Bob in a secret, flirtatious tryst with a younger woman. Theirs was a long marriage, blighted by infertility; for decades they compensated with affectionate care and companionship. Until this quaking portent of infidelity and abandonment.

Cathy had responded with a primitive and punitive maelstrom of explicit and encoded emotion. Fear, grief, rage, despair all fed into her abject and retributive broth of distress of body and mind. How could either she, or he, be motivated or permitted to go on living in the wake of such betrayal? Earlier Dr R had feared explosive or implosive catastrophe. After six years he felt safer; like a clergyman suggesting, nurturing and guiding buds of forgiveness. Cathy now sustained a warily melancholic marital bond with Bob: 'I love him but I won't tell him, or allow him too close ... he has to sleep on the sofa, doctor'.

Two days after she finds his just-deceased body, warm but unbelievably still on the bathroom floor, she seeks out Dr R. She is ushered in, kindly, by the receptionist as an end-of-surgery 'Emergency'. She is almost mute with shocked intensity, choked and blinded with tears. Dr R knows he cannot hurry – he has to lean far forward to hear her barely expressed voice: ' I thought I heard a "crump" but I wasn't sure ... I waited a minute, then went in and found him ... I think I could have saved him, if I'd gone immediately ... So it's my fault: if it weren't for me, he'd be alive ... I don't think I can live without him ... Does he know that, doctor? ... Do you?'.

\*

## 2. Amir

When Amir first came, he could not talk of his hurts, his shame, his well of sadness, his furnace of fury. Only slowly has Dr R understood the exhausting struggle Amir has to endure and bear alone. Amir is a large-framed, but compliant and placatory man. His story, which Dr R has always believed, was largely made and smashed by others. His arranged marriage in India, to Kalpur, twenty years ago, had been largely fertilised and conceived by their two prominent and dominant families in a small Kashmiri town. After their arrival in London fifteen years ago, Amir had felt blessed with Kalpur, their new country and the birth of three daughters. Social and biological fate seemed to be gently smiling on them all.

Back in Kashmir, destructive troubles were hatching that he was not party to, did not understand and could never influence. Like a terrible storm, these troubles would quickly devastate his life's achievements and plans. In the North of Kashmir their two families had fallen into a primitive and internecine feud.

Kalpur, perplexedly paralysed and then controlled by the most commanding gravitational force, turned on, then ejected her husband from the family group.

When he first came to see Dr R, his distress was so raw, intense and beyond his usual vocabulary, that he could hardly speak. His demeanour told Dr R much more: his sagged, leaden gait; tearful eyes, avoiding contact, yet conveying fear and shame; a voice defeated, yet still apologetic; smart clothes, now crumpled.

From this fragile and inchoate tangle Dr R had to be delicate and patient in constructing a story – Amir's 'History' – explaining not only his immediate symptoms – his dis-ease – but also his massive losses: of marriage, fatherhood, family, home and occupation – his alienation.

After Amir's faltering and pained initial meeting with Dr R, the doctor had thought Amir's risk and distress were so high he should see a psychiatrist urgently. This was arranged with seamless rapidity. The assigned contact was more problematic: Amir later said 'they [the Psychiatric Team] just kept asking all these questions about "voices", and whether I really wanted to kill myself ... so much, so many questions! ... I couldn't really speak, or even think...' Amir refused to return to them.

Dr R thought of the old term for psychiatrist – 'Alienist' – and how this connoted a practitioner skilled in the art of healing torn or withered connections – with one's Self, Others, the world around. Dr R thought that these current Alienists were themselves alienated, at least from Amir and *his* alienation.

About a year later Amir gazes at Dr R, now with warmth, sorrow, calmness and deliberation. 'If you hadn't understood me or my situation then I wouldn't be alive now', he says with quiet, economic gratitude. Dr R experiences some glow of satisfaction. It is shared evidence, and private recognition, of his piloting such tempestuous seas. But he is also disquieted; harried by a wider concern: if he had not undertaken this, who would?

*

### 3. Clare

Clare was tormented, feared she could not understand her feelings, nor be understood. 'Am I going mad, doctor?...' Twelve years ago, her relationship with Danny had finished with ugly and menacing cacophony, leaving her alone with two small sons. Danny had always been demanding and jealous of her attention, and could not accept his new role of father, with all its compromises and deferred gratifications. Danny's second act of drunken violence decided Clare's finishing their relationship, though not her yearning or grief. After a dangerous and tangled period of threats, court appearances and injunctions, Danny retreated. Clare was left to complete the long and lonely voyage of single motherhood. Danny has not been seen for years.

Clare has heard that Danny is in prison, for another violent crime. Her sons, Sean, 15, and Craig, 17, have also heard. She has been having problems with Craig's increasing adolescent anger and intimidation; now it is worse: 'Craig's now very tall: taller than Danny ... he gets so angry, I often think he's possessed by some kind of demon ... he stands over me, his voice so loud and hard: the worst thing is that he sounds and looks to me just like Danny, all those years ago ... My feelings are so mixed-up: I become really scared, and at the same time often hate Craig, for being so like Danny ... I feel resentful and then so guilty ... How can I feel these things, as his mother? ... Can you understand all this, doctor?'

Dr R thinks this is a rhetorical question, for which she is seeking his reassurance and validation: she would not have entrusted him with 'all this' if she felt he had not understood. Dr R muses on understanding this understanding: how it has arisen from years of unstructured and unscheduled contacts, each adding to a growing bond of trusting familiarity, each enabling thoughts to be clarified, feelings to be verbalised, connections to be seen. Like a gardener, he could not use his skills to command these processes; only encourage, protect and nourish what might emerge.

*

### 4. Alf

Alf carries his 82-year-old, tall frame with remarkable uprightness, discipline and pride. He has been wearing a similar brass-buttoned navy-blue blazer since Dr R first met him in the 1970s, but it never looks worn. Despite this mien of well-kempt fortitude, Alf now looks pale and unwell. He crosses the room with slow, frail caution. As he sits down Dr R is struck by the depleted timbre of his voice, the deadness of his gaze. Alf had come with such heralding signs of depression many times and years before when, at least, his physical health was then robust.

Dr R had also known Alf's brothers. All four had a similar manner of intelligent, diligent courtesy. All had followed their father's occupation in the London Docks. Remarkably, all had remained unmarried and, at some time, all had been treated at the old Victorian Mental Hospital. Dr R can remember mechanically-typed letters from the 1960s, documenting how all (and the deceased father, and father's father, and father's brother) had suffered from 'Periodic Familial Melancholia', later 'Recurrent Endogenous Depression'. Dr R had been encouraged by how their afflictions became more manageable as the medications had improved. A fascinatingly clear constellation illustrating 'biological psychiatry', Dr R had said several times to his students.

Despite his current bleakness, it seems important for Alf to have this contact with Dr R:

'My life seems so empty, so meaningless … My brothers have all died and now I have no family at all … My Chinese neighbour doesn't speak English, or even know my name … Now I've got prostate cancer, I've never felt so alone: you're now the only person that's known me, from all those years ago ...'

He pulls himself up in his chair, his voice a little stronger:

'All my usual symptoms have come back, really badly. So, I remembered what you said last time, and yesterday increased my [antidepressant] tablets. I know there's nothing else for you to do, doctor, but I just thought you'd want to know ... Shall I come back in a fortnight, so you can see how I am ...?'

Alf, like his brothers, has never obstructed more personal exploration, though never benefited from such efforts either. Dr R has little to do but be mindful and respectful of the subtext. He ponders how apparently simple is his task, yet how important it is for Alf. Any attempt to diminish or delete this humble but subtle role would, very likely, have tragic consequences. The paradoxical skill lies in recognising the complexity of the simple.

*

### 5. Tom

Tom's normally aquiline, handsome features are shockingly obscured. His left eye is almost closed by grey and purple swelling. Above it a normally elegantly arched eyebrow has been torn, now stitched and encrusted by dried blood. A domed grey-brown bruise on his left forehead sits astride this ugly asymmetry.

Tom is unable to offer his usual playful smile to Dr R: he is hurt and hurting. 'I was Gay-Bashed ... they came from behind, four of them, maybe five: I couldn't see and didn't stand a chance ... I know who they are. The Police want my injuries recorded, and I just wanted to tell you anyway...'

A year ago Tom had come with a less visible but equally distressing pain. His father had died very rapidly from an unsuspected but evidently virulent malignancy. Tom had never had a satisfactory bond with his father: he had experienced him as critical, harsh and controlling. Tom's mother was lovingly collusive with Tom about his homosexuality, but it was never openly acknowledged with father: an unexploded bomb.

Tom, now mid-thirties, has built himself a stable and positive life: good friends, a loving partner and a meticulously orderly occupation as an Air Traffic Controller. But there is a painful gap where there was no loving father: his grief is not for the father he lost, rather the father he never had. Dr R, during Tom's fresh grief, had talked with him a few times of such things, helping him through this raw ravine. Dr R was aware of his likely role, as an older man: the father who listens, includes, accepts. The father Tom never had. Dr R thought Tom clearly realised this, though they spoke of it only lightly and elliptically.

Tom's bruised humiliation seems lightened by Dr R's inspection, witness and then suggestion that he returns in a week 'to see how things are settling'. Dr R thinks that Tom understands the meaning of this connecting and containing healing ritual.

'Thanks, Doc: you're a rock!', he says with a brave lopsided smile and an offer of affectionate banter.

*

As Dr R finished his Friday evening surgery, he thinks of Cathy, Amir, Clare, Alf and Tom – and others, too, he has seen that day – each a mixture of the universal and the unique. For each struggles for personal connection, meaning, definition, safety, comfort, recognition or belonging. Lost or foundering in the struggle, each may be diagnosed as having 'Anxiety' or 'Depression' – these are easily packaged: elementary clusters in an inevitably crude science of distress. Yet it is perceiving the uniqueness of each individual and each consultation that has most sustained, for many years, Dr R's interest, engagement and Élan Vital. This is the Art and, Dr R has long thought, the heart of healing. Here, in this fragile, often elusive but powerful space within and between persons, is where compassionately imaginative contact can grow its most prized fruit.

*

**B. The Generic – Cluster, convention and code. Start: Week 2**

It is late Monday morning and Dr R has cleared the rest of the day to attend a large professional area meeting: Plans for Commissioning Mental Health Services. Before he goes, he steels himself to read another administrative obelisk: a lengthy and didactic diktat from the National Institute of Clinical Excellence (NICE): 'The Management of Anxiety and Mood Disorders'. The format is familiar: first the awakening warning of how large is the problem and its cost in personal, financial and organisational terms; then the complex problem is broken down into functional or administrative subcomponents; finally each is delegated or despatched, via serial towers of bullet points and forests of algorithms. Implicitly it is only the parts that matter; the whole becomes an irrelevant abstraction. Dr R, heeding some internal voice of higher authority, deflects his own objections and instead disciplines his attention until the end of this document of instruction. As he does so he feels his mind constrict, his energy deplete. An unbidden childhood memory comes into his mind: an image of a Primate confined to a small bare cage in a city zoo.

What will this afternoon's meeting bring?

*

Dr S is addressing the serried ranks of higher echelon healthcare workers. His manner is courteous, amiable but commanding: a public school headmaster pep-talking his staff. He makes clear how important it is that clear diagnoses are made, so that the correct care-pathways can be followed. This can be done by filling in relevant questionnaires and algorithms that clarify, validate and quantify diagnosis: the nature and severity of the complaint thus becomes defined precisely. This yields a clear path – necessary not just for more scientific research, but also more effective treatment and then commodification. Commissioning will be expedited: more funding can be garnered. Thus, increasingly, mental illnesses will be diagnosed, containerised, despatched, streamed, managed and marketed: like procedures in physical illness now, in the new NHS economy.

The audience looks, Dr R thinks, mostly acquiescent, but not engaged: semi-slumped to obediently receive these new notions of authority. Dr R is thinking how these devices of cluster, convention and code are predicated on generic similarities, but become inimical to his personal understanding. They help him little with the complex dances he must improvise to help others find courage, heal and grow. How do we address such limitless human complexity and variation with sense and sensibility; to accurately understand each person and their maybe-similar-but-always-unique difficulties? The *Generic* is the accessible territory for planners, statisticians, economist and managers: but it is the *Idiomorphic* that often most helpfully guides the practitioner – to make personal sense with *this* person, *now*. When the Generic and Idiomorphic seem largely congruent, there may be few problems. When they are not, which is frequently, the art, skill and judgement of the practitioner are more tested.

Dr R, over decades, had attempted to repair the damage done to many patients where the generic medical or psychiatric diagnosis was expounded and executed with such unchallenged authority that any personal perspective or meaning became completely displaced. This management-without-personal-understanding was rarely beneficial and often harmful: it added to the sufferer's sense of alienation, passivity and disempowerment. Such are the perils of overusing the Medical Model. Dr R now listens to Dr S's plans for increasing the hegemony of the Generic-Medical-Psychiatric phalanx, driving its 'authority' deeper into the human wilder-ness; a realm where more fluid and delicate understanding is required. He fears not just for the fate of his patients, but his own professional integrity.

Dr R speaks out and attempts to condense his notions and concerns with courtesy but conviction. Dr S is also courteous, but appears distracted, bemused and uncomprehending. While Dr R wonders whether this is a cannily disingenuous ploy, he looks around at his colleagues. Some are looking towards him, smiling tentative encouragement. Others gaze down and away, averse to any possible discordance, especially with authority. The remainder remain immobile and impassive: bystanders. Dr S urbanely moves the meeting on: 'Any other questions?'.

As the proceedings close, several delegates approach Dr R, to offer nervous support and confederation. One is Dr T, a formally dressed, middle aged, softly spoken man. He looks over his shoulder and says, with a quietness bespeaking conspiracy: 'I'm really pleased you said all that … I don't think I'd have the courage, even if I could find the words'.

*

Forty years ago Dr R read a, then seminal, book by a maverick, elderly Hungarian psychoanalyst, Michael Balint. It was titled 'The Doctor, his Patient, and the Illness', and enriched the working lives and relationships of hundreds of General Practitioners, for a generation. Balint met regularly, for many years, with a small group of GPs, building up portraits and understandings of the personal and interpersonal subtext of their medical practice: the unexpressed or hidden world of feelings, impulses or thoughts that lay behind the diagnoses, procedures and technical utterances – the generic. This type of *qualitative* research was never officially sanctioned or funded. It has been long supplanted by *quantitative* studies, conditionally financed and committee-endorsed. But Balint's informal research path had powerful cultural and educational effects: by freeing doctors to explore the idiomorphic, Balint enabled these practitioners to find new types of meaning and understanding in their encounters with the distressed and disrupted. They found themselves more able to heal, as well as treat: most reported much deeper work satisfactions. Such were Dr R's early mentors.

But Balint's influence was in a time of unwrapping: a time of adulterated disciplines and feral philosophy: an era whose health practitioners were often insighted and incited by such creative deconstructionists as Laing, Szasz and Illich.

There are now no such luminaries to excite professional human curiosity: professional motivation is now engineered by a financially induced system of NICE guidelines, QOF points, goals and targets, and an endless rash of algorithms. Dr R is now struggling to find intellectual oxygen and human sustenance in this period of near-ubiquitous tight wrapping and containerisation. It is not just his supermarket that standardises, unit-packs, film-wraps and bar-codes natural products for managed distribution. He is working for a healthcare service that intends to do the equivalent with much higher and more sentient life forms. He thinks of Cathy, Amir, Clare, Alf and Tom …

How do we respond?

*

*'The young man knows the rules: the old man knows the exceptions.'*

Portuguese proverb

Ω

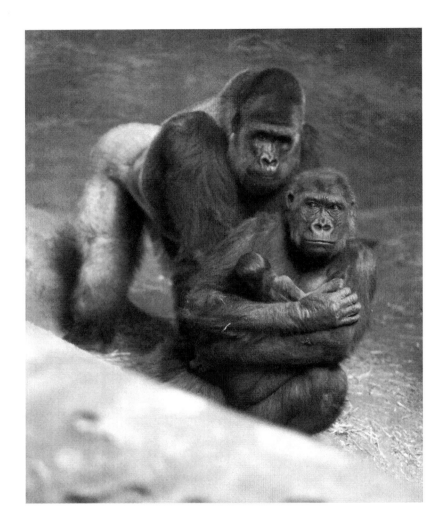

# Resolved or Abandoned?

Irresponsibly lost Transference:
a professionally embarrassed tale

## June 1980

"COME IN! ... JUST COME IN!!" My head is crowned with shampoo-lather and I shout through a haze of rising steam. I hoped that the open door would transmit my hollered voice to the front door that I had deliberately left ajar. I was expecting my teenaged stepson: he did not have keys.

The shrill ringing of the doorbell paused, then resumed. Flustered and irritated, I boomed my imperative message even louder through the bathroom steam. Surely, now he could hear.

Again, the high pitch of the doorbell drills the air. Why does he not let himself in? Realising now that direct action was needed to resolve this ambiguity, I clambered, hurried and harried, from my bath. I wrapped the closest, but small, towel round my nether regions, and, dripping and squinting, descended the twilit staircase to the half-open front door. The pattered trail of bath water was joined by thin, grey rivulets of shampoo from my mid-washed hair.

I pulled with angry impatience at the front door, to open it fully. Shouted banter at my stepson, attributing impaired hearing and intelligence, completed my unsighted greeting.

*

On the other side of the door was not my stepson. It was Elizabeth.

*

We both stared and blinked: a hiatus of dislocated incredulity. I, for forgetting (or 'forgetting') the unusual appointment time she had requested; I had agreed to this, as a 'one-off'. She, for now seeing this previously contained and impeccably professional young man in such feral and primitive disarray.

*

Elizabeth was a refined, intelligent, insighted, but painfully inhibited woman. Twenty years older than I, she had almost entirely negative memories of her Edwardian father: remote, humourless, austere, rigid, inexpressive. His barren, dark influence shadowed her life for sixty years. I, too, became an extension of that shadow. Despite my best efforts to bridge the gap, she remained ill at ease. My proffered utterances may have clarified, but did not console. She came assiduously, but I had to imagine beyond her carapace.

*

Both Elizabeth and I were struck immobile for several seconds: time to adjust our eyes, then our minds, to our respective shocks. The door had been opened: views had changed, forever.

My reaction was the more predictable: I attempted to rapidly cluster sincere apology, embryonic explanation, reassurance and a pragmatic, emergency plan – for her to return in thirty minutes, when I would be suitably attired and prepared. I improvised a pitch of tone, between professional gravitas and friendly-fallible.

*

Elizabeth's reaction was less predictable, and certainly more interesting. She laughed. First with discrete softness, but soon with raucous warmth. It was not the harsh, abrasive laughter of triumph or mockery, but the peeling, joyous, contagious laughter of shared realisation, relief and release. The laughter of unanticipated enlightenment. For her, my chaos had humanised us both. For me, her laughter had freed us both.

*

This perilously comic error had serious, yet benign, consequences. Elizabeth's dense and massive father-transference had been blown away, with a speed and finality that were probably impossible with careful, systematic therapy. The changes spread far beyond the therapy room, too. She reported a blessed shock-wave re-configuring all her important relationships.

Some months later she and I recalled these events and their surprising evolution. She drew on her background in literature and offered me an oblique observation of GK Chesterton: "Humour can get under the door while seriousness is still scrabbling at the lock."

## August 2011

This transformative comedy of errors occurred more than thirty years ago. How did it change me? On a superficial level, I check my diary more carefully: I am more vigilant to possible error. More deeply, and complexly, it opened my mind to the (often) paradoxical nature of human difficulty, struggle and change. Experience is not just a living process: it is an evolving one, too – it develops new and unpredictable forms. Hence, there is little science of the individual's metabolism of meaning.

Would I try it again, now, as a procedure? Certainly not: I am far too orthodox...

Ω

An edited version is included in *The Business of Therapy: How to Run a Successful Private Practice* by Pauline Hodson (2012), Open University Press, McGraw Hill

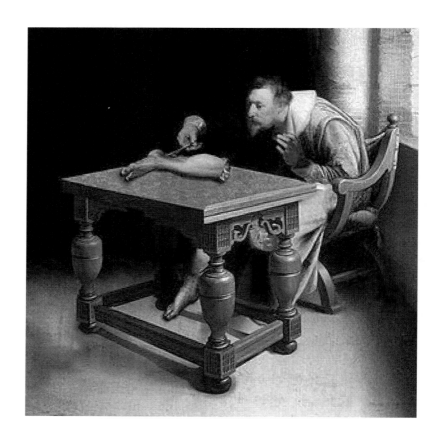

*Philip Verheyen dissecting his amputated leg* Anonymous 1675

# Sense and Sensibility

## The danger of Specialisms
## to holistic, psychological care

Increasing specialisation in healthcare is often equated with progress. Yet often, though subtly, specialisation is destructive of valuable aspects of healthcare. This article explores this theme, using the example of Specialist psychologists working with Acute Mental Illness.

*'Ten Lands are sooner known than one man'*

Yiddish proverb

## Prologue

The use of technical language and understanding to designate and remedy the entire span of distress presented to healthcare workers is partly indispensible and inevitably expands. A burgeoning of specialisms follows. Each of these, to survive, needs to develop its own distinctive language and models. The benefits of these, in some areas, have been dramatic and transformative. But such benefits become much more doubtful when problems are not primarily physical. This short essay is a response to another article proposing that the acutely mentally ill might be better served by a further elaboration of specialist services and vocabularies. The counter-argument, proposed here, is that such developments, when misplaced, often take us *away* from the kinds of personal engagement and understanding that are most likely to be healing and helpful. Neglect or abandonment of these may be inadvertent, but are insidious and growing threats to the quality and integrity of personal care.

As we get older, and when our turn comes, we are grateful for the sharp, narrow focus of specialisation. For the failing heart or eye, we welcome the territorially different skills, applied with strict topographic attention, mandating distinctions between cardiac valve and coronary artery, the lens cataract and diabetic retinopathy. We may challenge the competence of the specialist, but not his speciality.

We can call this process of progressive division of healthcare into smaller and smaller foci of activity 'Anatoatomization' (AA). This term signifies its derivation from the Medical Model (MM), a fault-in-the-machine paradigm. This, too, is based on anatomy and physiology; like foundation stones to a column of medical specialities, each successive layer becoming increasingly refined and confined.

MM and AA work so well in certain areas, that challenges rarely occur. The more anatomically located or acute the problem, the more true this is. Medical and surgical emergencies serve well as examples of near inviolability.

The *science* involved in such (MM and AA) defined activities proceeds via our conventions of clustering our observations by similarities: generic patterns. In contrast, there are other aspects to healthcare where, instead, the *art* discerns and navigates our innumerable (and less measurable) human variables; the personal and subjective – the dissimilarities that make each of us who we are. Such art and science are tensely counter-poised, but often symbiotic: an eternally recurrent test of balance and judgement for practitioners.

MM and AA, then, have well earned and well based pragmatic hegemony when dealing with physical disease: solid-state pathology. Adam Smith's doctrine of Division of Labour is here on very workable territory. But this hegemony is extended, then overextended, to other areas, and for other reasons. The language and model imply powerful blessings: for authority, definition, standardisation and measurability. This apparent conferral of clarity and control seems irresistible to planners, economists and managers. Adoption is eager and rapid. Scientifically sounding phrases then expediently bolster the language of governance: it becomes difficult to distinguish the scientific from the scientistic. Thereafter, in a cascade effect, these flow down as a kind of didactic Esperanto, instructing and defining the caring professions. The result is the 'medicalisation' of almost any problem of experience, learning, adjustment or relating. There are, too, larger cultural forces at work. For we, in our advanced industrial society, now rarely encounter the unpackaged and unlabelled. Our minds are now rendered disconcerted and distrustful by the feral and undesignated. Packaging becomes symbolic of safety.

Our medicalisation of non-anatomical problems can certainly (if transiently) seem to quell complex human uncertainties by a kind of rhetorical aura. Sometimes this is followed by real and sufficient help. Often, though, it turns specious from its assumed clarity and authority. This is because medicalised understanding is confined to generic patterns. It does not extend to individual struggle, evolution or meaning: the 'idiomorphic'. Within the ill-defined compass of Psychiatric and General Practice, in particular, practitioners who become unreceptive to the idiomorphic will miss and misconstrue much that they encounter. While 'treatment' may depend largely on objectification (MM), and thus be well-served by specialisation (AA), 'healing' runs counter to these: it requires approaches that are holistic, personal and interpersonal. Broadly speaking, treatment represents the convergence of 'science', healing the divergence of 'art' in encountering human distress.

I recently read an article: 'Where does Psychology fit in Acute Mental Health Wards?'.[2] The writing was, I thought, a solidly competent contribution to the current thinking and culture of psychiatry and medically orientated psychology. But I was struck, and increasingly interested, by a central axiom: one deriving from, and then contributing to, our increasing tendency to an errant, fragmented specialisation. It was that psychology is a naturally divisible activity from, though an optional ally to, psychiatry. This premise produces more difficulties than it solves, for such assumed divisions will seriously obstruct possibilities of holistic personal understanding and care. This poses particular hazards throughout psychiatry and medical practice. What kind of artless practice will remain if we do not include skilful address

---

[1] McGowan, John and Hill, Rosalind (2011) *'Where does psychology fit into acute mental health wards?'*. Submission to *The Psychiatrist*

of the unobvious and the unspoken? The article's designated problem of acute mental illness, in particular, represents such inchoate territory: the breakdown of an individual's functioning, integration and identity. What healing we can muster attempts to counter this with varieties of holistic reparation: good continuity and quality of personal contact are elemental and essential. To be personal, such contact must be bespoke and dextrous: this requires a wide repertoire of skills offered *in-vivo*. This kind of engagement is always a delicate dance and easily stymied,[3] for example, by any attempt to fragment personal suffering into academically abstracted sub-components, each to be sub-contracted *in-vitro*. (Presumably, eventually, algorithms would be designed to command this!)

More basically, in most of our many forms of interpersonal care, we are best served when we are imaginatively receptive. For human vulnerability usually ushers a complex of unarticulated fears and encoded needs. To meet these we will need to navigate the cryptic – often delicate questions of engagement and encounter: whether to? what? when? how? who? We can call all this 'vernacular psychology': an unschooled ancestor of current spawnings of systematic, academically-shepherded, formally packaged 'Clinical Psychology' and 'Psychological Treatments', with which most healthcare workers are now inculcated. Such vernacular psychology is guided by a quest for personal understanding, rather than any kind of 'objective' designation. Such understanding proceeds by asking questions: What is it like to be this other person, to have lived their life? What is the meaning and significance, for them, of this distress? What is the meaning and significance, for them, of me, now? What needs do I need to address that they might not (yet) be able to articulate?

---

[2] Zigmond, D (1987) *'Three types of encounter in the healing arts: dialogue, dialectic and didacticism'*. Holistic Medicine, Vol 2, 69-81

The language of such non-specialist forms of understanding can only succeed when fresh and personally meaningful. Unlike designatory language it can only be effective when our intelligence is fuelled and directed by resonance and imagination.[2] Procedural and technical language are, thus, often intrusive and antithetical to the vernacular; for languages not only communicates thought, it controls it. Vernacular psychology, with freedom of language and metaphor, seeks understanding before and beyond the shackles of our more administrative systems. When apposite it is a powerful element in the art of medicine and psychiatry. This is particularly well-illustrated in our best responses to those disabled by anguished dilemmas and unstable situations: the victims of life's shakings and tearings – the bereaved, the ravaged, the dispirited, the overwhelmed, the dying, the acutely mentally ill. These sufferers are different from those with stable and habitual patterns of distress: for such stability of distress is more likely to be receptive to our stability of approach – our reassuring and familiar structures: treatment planning, regular sessions, good-enough statistics, a premeditated and pre-packaged therapy, and so forth.

Across the wide span of palliative and curative activities, it is often vernacular psychology that best guides the kinds of empathic, compassionate approach that may enable containment and healing in the other. Being unschooled, it can be learned, by experience and apprenticeship, but probably not taught schematically: it is more the product of self-propelled education, rather than institutional training. This poses difficult conundrae for planners, managers and academics: it is easier to provide managed instruction than nurture nuances of culture.

It is worth reflecting on how important and widespread is our need for skilled, but unsystematised, psychology in our care of others. It is necessary even with the unconscious in ICU.

Shockingly, they are often much more conscious than we can bear, and they will remember.

There are many kinds of sufferers who are too dislocated and disintegrated by their distress to be able to attend to, or retain, our professionally systematised, management-modulated approaches: our 'Treatments'. They are, however, deeply influenced by sensible, sensitive understanding: communication that is bespoke, empathic, and prepared from fresh ingredients. These fresh ingredients are prepared to meet the (often) unarticulated and primitive needs of the sufferer. Rawly anguished, we all are likely to need some composite form of these: for validation, containment, comfort, encouragement, recognition, expression, understanding, catharsis or touch.[4] [5] In such encounters, each matched cluster of responses will never be exactly repeated. These intimate choreographies are thus not susceptible to standardisation or measurement; they cannot be quantitatively researched, or mass-managed. Policy-makers, managers, eventually clinicians in the current quantification-centred culture, may become expediently neglectful, then oblivious.

With high levels of chaos or distress, the acutely mentally ill are usually unreceptive, or even obstructive, to our conveniently pre-packed, management-purchased, NICE-endorsed Shibboleth Therapies (CBT and MBT were cited in the article). Aspects of any of these *may* be helpful, but only if evoked as part of a developing dialogue. Not if we administer them, as a bolus, a prescribed procedure. A maze of semiotics here awaits us, for the extremely anguished are often beyond words: our dialogue has to be finely-tuned and respectfully empirical with the implicit. To enter this ever-evanescent realm

---

[4] Frank, J (1972) *Persuasion and Healing*. New York: Shocken

[5] Zigmond, D (Sept. 2010) *'Why would anyone use an unproven therapy? Treasures in the mist'*. Journal of Holistic Healthcare. Vol 7. Issue 2 17-19

of healing art we must be prepared to be delicate with ambiguity, improvisatory with our choreography: an exquisite and disciplined eclecticism. These, in turn, must aspire to an imaginatively accurate sense of what kind of explanations, language, metaphors and dialogue the sufferer is receptive to, and can bear. Such comprises much of healing, but how do we subsume it to 'Treatment'?

To end this article we should return to the beginning, to its title and that of the article that encouraged this enquiry. Can we best encounter the acutely mentally distressed by further administrative subdivisions, by further specialisms? What happens to holism, to sense and sensibility?

Clinical psychologists are no more qualified to enter this fragile and feral fray than any other clinicians. Frustratingly and fascinatingly, this is an area of marshland where our tarmacked roads quickly sink: we must find lighter ways to traverse. Psychologists can certainly contribute to these lighter ways; they can offer their slant of analytical thinking to protean processes. Our success usually depends upon our awareness and responsiveness to the vicissitudes of human complexity and paradox. This is a difficult and different stratum of activity and thought to that executised by the prescribed, planned and packaged.

We must beware, for the discounting of vernacular psychology, then its dismemberment, then colonisation by specialities, risks impoverishing or displacing the common compassion and emotional intelligence of us all.

Tennessee Williams starkly captures what so often eludes our over-organised and presumptuous encounters with others:

> *I don't ask for your pity, but just your understanding – not even that, no – just your recognition of me in you, and the enemy, time, in us all*

Tennessee Williams, *Sweet Bird of Youth* (1959)

Ω

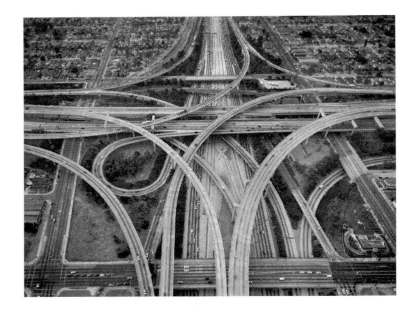

# How to help Harry

Friend or Foe?
The scientific and the scientistic
in the fog of the frontline

Standardisation of medical services – increasingly by electronic monitoring, mediation and management – has become equated with 'best practice'. This seems to offer undeniable practical benefits: clarity, uniformity, reliability and ease of transmission. But does anything get lost? If so, what? how? why? This short exploration draws from authentic situations in Primary Care: a 'heartsink patient', and a problematic professional meeting. Usual conventions of disguise assure discretion.

*We all want to be healthy. No one wants an unhealthy existence. And the job of Government is to help people live healthier lives.*
Andrew Lansley MP, Secretary of State for Health, 23 January 2012

*When you have duly arranged your 'facts' in logical order, lo, it is like an oil lamp that you have made, filled and trimmed, but which sheds no light unless you first light it.*

Saint-Exupéry, *The Wisdom of the Sands* (1948)

Dr Q inhales Harry's fatalism involuntarily. It is not just the lingering and residual odours of his staple props – his tobacco and alcohol – but his anguish-laden physiology. This continues to signal Harry's troubles, both despite, and because of, his almost unceasing attempts to chemically banish, or at least quell, his morbidly echoing memories, his shame-leeched self-prophecies. Dr Q has come to surmise that such trapped and stultified internal worlds emanate particular kinds of energies and odours: that the physical experience becomes encoded, then signalled – in our sweat, our breath and in myriad thermal and electromagnetic transmissions we are usually unconscious of. He remembers an old designation connoting something similar: the 'heartsink patient'.

Dr Q has learned to be stoic and philosophical: he can look forward to enlivening counterpoint – very different people who energise the room with an aura of faith, trust and optimism. Reflecting on this, he now recalls conversations a couple of decades ago, when there was much talk of personal 'vibes': he never explored what scientific research has been done in this area, but his daily experience reminds him with recurring and fresh evidence of its power and centrality.

\*

Harry's fatalism can be perceived more consciously, too: his trudging gait, the downcast gaze avoidant of the new or the personal, the sagging voice that has not the resolve to complete its message, his clothes and hair – clean enough – but habitually tousled, drab and dank.

Dr Q has known Harry fifteen years, and has witnessed and gleaned the story of Harry's cumulative desolation. In recent times Harry's already impoverished self-confidence was dealt a series of grievous blows: a marriage floundering from his difficulties of expression and extension, then foundering on their (his) infertility and poor employment prospects, then finally torpedoed by his wife's break-out: an affair with an 'old friend' – a confident, successful and expansive man whose attractiveness and fertility was soon evidenced by the pregnancy of Harry's future ex-wife.

In earlier times Harry conveyed to Dr Q descriptions and tales from his childhood. Of a father distant, fractious, discontent, hostile and critical. Of a mother softer, but lost in an ocean of melancholy. Her only child, she confided in him when he was old enough to 'understand'. Of the unhappy basis of her marital bond: the accidental conception of Harry in an untried relationship, ten years earlier. Of her attempts to conjure love through their Christian faith; through another conception soon after Harry – an obstetric disaster which cost mother her newborn, her womb and her future fertility.

Harry's childhood was spent trying to appease, comfort, compensate or placate those who gave him life. He could neither understand nor succeed.

Dr Q intuited something of this massive disseminated damage on their first encounter; later meetings confirmed and detailed. Dr Q's fuller portrait and biography of Harry grew slowly: piecemeal and opportunistically, for Dr Q was always careful not to encourage disclosure more than Harry could bear. Harry developed a reticent and shy trust: Dr Q sensed a flickering, bruised warmth.

Dr Q enlisted support. Psychiatrists at the times of Harry's greatest incapacity, counsellors when he could motivate himself a little more. Harry complied and they provided, at least, periodic containment for Harry and supportive respite for Dr Q. But Harry is a man of few words and little appetite for schematic enquiry: he did not respond to formal attempts at psychotherapy. His desolate view of himself and his world remains undiminished.

*

Harry does, however, entrust very limited aspects of himself to others. Now in his early middle-years, he has complied with his GP's practice screening programme. His blood lipids, checked for the first time, are found to be high. Dr Q remembers, too, Harry's response to the doctor's gentle enquiry regarding his feelings six months ago: Harry's father had just died suddenly of a heart attack. Harry had shrugged with a kind of glum defeat: 'he was never much of a father to me ... now he's not here at all...'.

Dr Q was then mindful, not just of Harry's stunted grief, but of the portents, for Harry, for such a death. His emotional tangle of recent-upon-ancient frustrations and hurts, increasingly swallowed down with self-anaesthetising doses of booze, fags and factory foods augured badly. Now with father's sudden death these portents seemed clearer still: a sharpening prophecy.

The Practice receptionist's request for Harry to see Dr Q about his lipids was a standard procedure: 'to identify, discuss and take action regarding remediable risk factors'.

At the end of the last meeting, in the fresh shadow of his father's death, Dr Q had raised those specific concerns, again. The themes were old: the clarity was new. Harry responded with a rare vein of articulation, caustic and taut: 'I know your job is about saving lives, doctor, and I'm grateful for your kindness with me, but I'm not sure I have the kind of life that's worth saving ... We can't all choose our lives and we've all got to die some time'. This quiet, courteous coda was undramatic in delivery, but arrestingly bleak in meaning. Dr Q had time only to express benign intent and tell Harry the bridge is always open.

*

Six months later, as the door opens, Dr Q knows it is Harry, booked in to discuss his lipids. These excess lipids may be the designated problem, but they represent the mere biochemical tip of a vast psycho-spiritual iceberg.

Dr Q holds his breath momentarily; he braces himself as he thinks: 'How to help Harry?'.

*

Stella has many similar meetings to address: her working days and diary are full. She has a friendly but business-like, diplomatic manner. This is reflected in her attire: trim knee-length navy skirt, cream blouse, discrete pearl earrings – a kind of uniform, smart but not alluring. Dr Q notices she is wearing her NHS Trust ID card around her neck, an emblem not just of how busy she is, but who controls her. This is a managed excursion.

Stella, though not herself medically trained, is the emissary of an expert group concerned with reducing cardiovascular disease. This committee has devised strategies and procedures which will be enacted by all relevant health practitioners. Stella's job is to brief and instruct the practitioners: to assure professional compliance for The Plan. Such compliance relieves practitioners of individual judgement and discrimination: The Plan prescribes and directs. Invisible experts decide.

Dr Q is sitting amidst his peers, local GPs. Stella is explaining the latest addition to The Plan. A new computer program is being introduced. The practitioners will feed in the relevant clinical data, and the computer will calculate the statistical chance of morbidity and mortality. This 'scientific' prediction is then shared with the patient for discussion and action. The GPs will receive an extra payment for compliance: Dr Q notices the galvanising ripple of interest and attention.

Dr Q recently attended his own GP and received the kind of consultation that The Plan spawns. Dr Y was young, brisk, authoritative. Her attention was rapt to the computer screen, where she quickly garnered and collated abstracted data. The computer prophesised favourably for Dr Q's fate. Dr Y spoke for The Oracle, as she turned from the computer screen towards him: 'That's not too bad, not too bad at all…'. She illustrated her prognostic cheeriness with some itemised statistics. Her smile seemed winsome, but Dr Q wondered who the smile was for: he was doubtful how much she had really perceived him. There had been little real discussion. Beyond medical questions, she enquired little. Dr Q did not introduce himself as a fellow-GP: his curiosity was then roused, to see what a 'standard' consultation was like. Was the smile another impersonal, though decorative, generic procedure? What is a smile to someone unseen?

Dr Q is thinking about Stella's financially-enhanced instructions, his own experience with Dr Y and how these would be templated with Harry. As he understands this, he is being paid to prime the computer, which then primes him to then say to Harry something like: 'Harry, we have fed all your available personal and family health and lifestyle data into the computer program. Your computed five-year risk for combined cardio/cerebrovascular events is 38.73%. This comprises a 14.71% mortality group, leaving another 24.02% with significant morbidity events. For your age group, this is very high risk … We can provide you with category subgroup differential analyses, if you wish …'

Dr Q is wondering how such formulaic and statisticised thinking or communication can possibly further help Harry, or many others that Dr Q sees. Dr Q's monitoring and conversations, for many years, have approached the complex issues of self-protection and self-care, but in a form and language that are personal and vernacular – not those predicated by the technical: tethered to the computer, or decided by distant expert committees.

Dr Q puts such notions to Stella. He adds that he has long-regarded what, when and how to share with each person, in each situation, as a delicate, complex but fundamental skill in Medical Practice. A good example of what anchors holistic medicine as an interpersonal art, a humanity.

Stella listens politely, nodding periodically, looking tired. Dr Q imagines her nodding represents fatigued diplomacy, rather than engaged understanding.

She reiterates how the computer program has been designed by a team of experts, and it behoves us to follow their lead. In addition, conveying quantitative information to patients, in a way that can itself be quantified, confers clear advantages to the management of practitioners, in their management of patients. 'I think you'll agree, doctor, it will make your treatment of these patients more *scientific*, and that has to be good for all of us...'

Dr Q thinks Stella is proposing this – especially her emphasised word 'scientific' – as an ineluctable summary. But Dr Q has many doubts and caveats. How to engage and interest another person in changing deeply established psychological patterns regarding their relationship to themselves, their body and their fate is often not a simple matter of data, formulation and instruction. Such complexity requires thoughtful investment in interpersonal interest, contact and understanding: activities far less accessible to quantification and science. Will not The Plan eclipse these subtle but important endeavours?

Yet Stella's declamation on the uncontentious blessings of anything that appears scientific represents a wider, currently thriving, kind of hypnotic rhetoric – a cultural ideology. The presentation of an apparent vocabulary and syntax of science becomes more important than its meaning for the participants.

Appearing scientific becomes an end in itself, a new kind of Shibboleth. Science as a posture, a garment, a cultural or status commodity becomes *scientism*.

Dr Q attempts to courteously and concisely condense this for Stella, but she is now more restive than receptive.

'Look', she says, 'you don't have to think about all that, because you'll be paid for it': a tired teacher attempting to control the end of a difficult class.

Another doctor, Dr S, turns to Dr Q, looks at his watch impatiently and offers Stella tetchy support: 'Yes, I can't see what all this is about. What won't you understand?! You're getting paid for it!'

Dr Q thinks he does understand, very well. But he remembers different kinds of meetings, twenty years ago, where they had very different kinds of discourse. He found these much more valuable. He would like to talk with them now about how to help Harry.

Ω

*Information is pretty thin stuff, unless mixed with experience.*

Clarence Day, *The Crow's Nest* (1921)

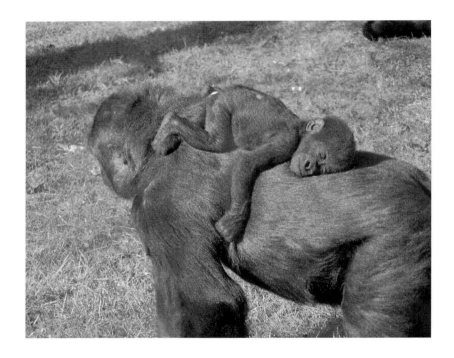

# Eric

## - diagnosis may be sometimes necessary; it is rarely sufficient

Diagnostically centred, schematic and managed healthcare has brought great benefit to the treatment of structural physical diseases. With other kinds of dis-ease its results are often much more problematic, even destructive. Current trends render this a growing problem. A true and recent story of an eternally grief-stricken elderly man serves as a cautionary and explanatory example.

# Introduction

Diagnoses – when well placed – have muscular leverage: they form the core-knowledge of most of our dramatically successful treatments for structural physical illnesses. Yet diagnoses have limitations of view; they can only offer descriptive clusters of commonality – what is generally true, the generic. They cannot tell us about the unique world of *this* individual *now*.

For this reason the generic diagnosis often fares poorly in healthcare realms where individual understanding, meaning and experience hold the key to therapeutic engagement. It is proposed here that most psychiatry, therapeutic psychology and medical encounters with functional complaints are all better addressed by a more idiomorphic approach; that the cost of not doing so is high.

Why is this important? What can happen? The following true story, about Eric, explains and illustrates.

This account is an extract from a long letter to a Director of a Mental Health Trust. The letter is written to document, and then catalyse, thought and debate about the increasingly inordinate use of the medical model – how this is leading to a complex fragmentation, and then destructive depersonalisation, of healthcare. Alarmingly this is happening especially in areas where quality and continuity of human contact and individual understanding is most important.

The story of Eric, and its inherent missed and miscommunications are a small but powerful example of a grave and accelerating problem. The letter could have been written to any similar NHS Trust. The discerned problems are now so widespread and insidious as to best be considered cultural.

The wide and complex sources of this culture are beyond the scope of this article. Yet we can begin a remedial response. Any limitation or reversal of damage must come from a countercultural ethos: I call this 'holistic compassionate care' (HCC). Some essential and guiding features of HCC are itemised in the box below.

### Holistic, compassionate care: a summary

- Personal healthcare is a humanity guided by science.
- This humanity is an ethos and an art.
- Holistic, compassionate care (HCC) requires mindful titration of art and science in ever-changing situations.
- This titration works like a carburettor: balancing opposing elements (petrol:science v air:art) in ever-changing mixtures to serve the needs of the whole (engine:person).
- Too much or too little of any one element causes suboptimal functioning and, eventually, no function at all.
- HCC is potentially important in all our encounters with human distress or dysfunction, yet always differently.
- HCC is particularly important in situations where there is not a quick and decisive physical treatment – hence General Practice, Psychology and Psychiatry are especially vulnerable to its loss.
- HCC often deals with issues that are personal, inexplicit and have symbolic meaning. Science has no access to such 'metacommunication'.
- HCC is often potent, but subtle and fragile. It is easily damaged or destroyed. Its 'habitat' needs protection.
- HCC is currently seriously damaged and impaired by an excess of 'science' and corresponding impoverishment of 'art'. [This is much like the carburettor delivering a 'too rich' mixture: the engine will have difficulties with fuel consumption, environmental pollution, power, smooth-running and starting. Healthcare analogies are obvious.]
- Thus more of something 'good' may, in fact, be worse.
- Schematisation is the opposing principle to holism. Thus, for example, excessive category-based management will

displace attachment-based personal understanding. Examples of current changes adding to this inadvertent damage: in General Practice – the loss of smaller, friendlier practices and personal lists for GPs, QOF-based remuneration; in Psychiatry – increasing subdivisions of medically-modelled care pathways and Clinical-Academic Groups; in Psychology – very similar: especially in excessive, diagnostically schematised CBT/IAPTS pathways.

- Wisdom = knowledge x reflection x experience x imagination.
- Systems that replace clinical wisdom with managerial solidarity generate very serious problems.

*'It is easier to know (and understand) men in general than one man in particular.'*

La Rochefoucauld, *Maxims* (1665)

## 1977-2010

As a GP for more than thirty years in the same practice, I have had medical responsibility for thousands of people. Eric was one of my few 'old-timers' I'd had almost no contact with. I knew what he looked like: a tall, increasingly stooped, bespectacled man, now in his early 70s, who had always dressed with neat, quiet formality and who carried a mien of discrete compliance, of well-mannered appeasement. I remembered several glimpses – spread over many years – of his visits to other practitioners. Paradoxically, I had another route of acquaintance with him that was more detailed – though more abstract – through the post: letters from specialists over many decades. Hazy memories of these were crystallised into the terminology of his disease-register and medical notes summary: 'Mature-onset Diabetes' and a 'long history of major, relapsing depression'. I remembered old letters from the 1960s: the days of outer-city Mental Hospitals, 'modern' tricyclic anti-depressants and courses of ECT. More recent letters had better news: containment and quiescence of his symptoms and punctilious compliance with prescriptions, plans and attendance. I sensed stable fragility well attended to: I had no need to intervene or understand further: if at peace, do not disturb.

*

### 2011-2012

An urgent phone call. The receptionist, Sue, correctly recognises raw and intelligent fear in the unknown woman's voice. Sue is intelligent, in response. It is not a 'good time' for phone calls, but she puts the call through immediately. Sue has an unschooled instinct for real distress, and thus accurate precedence.

'Doctor, I'm Dora, Eric's niece ... I've known him all my life ... I've never seen him as bad as this, so 'down' ... since last week I can't get him to eat, or talk, or take care of himself ... I can't really get normal conversation from him ... he's said frightening things: all quiet and intense – about his life ending, or ending his life – I can't really tell ... I can't leave him like this, but I live out of London and have young children to get back to ... I don't know what do, doctor, can you help? ...'

*

Within an hour, Eric and Dora are sitting with me. Eric's deflation, hopelessness and anguish are painfully and immediately apparent: his slow movement, enfeebled voice, depleted gaze and burdened gait all convey intense and incarcerated despair. Words – delicately baited – may later amplify or explain. Dora's presence and prescience are what I had imagined from our brief telephone contact: unintrusively engaged, lovingly watchful, fearful of tragic catastrophe.

I sense in Eric some fresh personal trauma causing this dramatic collapse: some kind of rupture; an internal haemorrhage of hope and faith. I need his words to explain: they are like frightened small fish sheltering in the darkened deep. I have to be still awhile, and patient. His words begin to surface; I lean forward, gently, to catch them:

'They've told Nancy that I can't see her anymore, that I've got to go somewhere else ... but I don't want to go somewhere else ... I just want to go back to see Nancy ...'

The words almost collapse at the back of his throat and are exhaled plaintively and weakly, as if he is dying. They choke to a halt with inhaled, silent sobs.

Dora is calmer, now she is sharing this enervated burden. I turn to look at her. She returns a knowing gaze. She does: she starts to explain:

'Uncle Eric has been seeing Nancy (a Social Worker) at the Clifton (Community Mental Health Centre) for about eight years. He's been told he has to stop. Nancy says it's due to some sort of reorganisation: that the Managers have told Nancy that what she's doing isn't what's most suitable for him: that they'll find him somewhere else ... But I know how much my uncle has been helped by Nancy: he only sees her for about twenty minutes, every few weeks. But he trusts her, and she's been kind and really got to understand him over a long time. I think that's why he's been so well for these last years ... After everything that happened to him when he was young, taking Nancy away from him now seems so cruel ...'

I realise I am dealing with broken vital connections, and a still-active volcanic personal ancient history, of which I know nothing. I must understand the essence of Eric's world, and story, very quickly.

Within fifteen minutes I have deciphered much: I am simultaneously gratified by understanding and disturbed by what I have understood.

\*

Eric was the youngest of five boys in a traditional, poor London docker's family. His mother, in her forties when he was born, ailed throughout Eric's infancy and died when he was three. He was cared for by a younger sister of his dead mother, Aunt Ada, until the onset of the Blitz. By the time his neighbourhood was shattered and ablaze, he and his four brothers and father had all dispersed, separately, away from London: Eric and three brothers were evacuated to families throughout the Home Counties, the oldest brother and father joined the Merchant Navy, hoping to stay together. They did not; father perished in an attack on the Arctic Convoy.

Eric's wartime childhood as an evacuee was abject, grief-struck and fearful. He was moved several times to different families for reasons dictated to him, but little understood by him. His experiences of care were various – kindness, affection, hostility, cruelty, indifference – but never predictable, dependable or within his control. He could not understand the difference between death, separation, abandonment or punishment. He learned to survive by appeasement, submission, invisibility. His memories of his mother and Aunt Ada brought grief that was rarely consoled: he learned, too, to appear to be brave.

At the end of The War, at the age of eleven, he returned to his orphaned family of older brothers, in the resuscitated ruins of London's Docklands. Eric's brothers were kindly and protective with Eric, though tougher than he: they had had long-enough and robust mothering. For his sense of protection and belonging, he followed his Band of Brothers to work in the Docks, soon after leaving school.

Eric's brothers and a few of his more thoughtful workmates were his social and family life, for several decades: he never made sexual relationships with women – a dangerous and painful yearning, a Bridge Too Far.

Eric's depressive breakdowns, in his thirties and forties, were possibly related to fresh abandonments: by his brothers who left him, each to move away from the Docklands to spawn their own families. By his fifties his 'family' consisted of his now distant, elderly, often ailing, brothers and a few retiring, soon-to-vanish, fellow dockers.

As his livelihood, companionship and brothers died, this vulnerable, inarticulately yearning, self-deprecating elderly man feared the waning of his solitary life, unknown and unwitnessed. Nancy had recognised this with discrete intuition, and for several years provided the kind of family surrogacy that provides humble but deep affiliation and palliation, yet has no official designation. Nancy, it seems, was guided by a basic tenet of care: that to be known to another, with intimacy and volition, is one of the most powerful balms for human distress. With evident sense and sensitivity Nancy had – with necessary professional safeguards and boundaries – contained and symbolically cradled this eternally grieving, unmothered old man. Nancy's humbly potent humanity, though, had invidious flaws: it is undesignated and unmeasurable; not part of a recognised generic care pathway. Ipso facto, Nancy should not be doing this work: Eric should go elsewhere, to a place of prescribed and recognised 'treatments'.

The consequences of this 'rationalised management'? An avoidably, yet now primitively disturbed and distressed elderly man – whose life I now fear for. What will I do?

*

What I can. My attentions to, and on behalf of, Eric have been multifarious, and for many months. My more direct endeavours have been akin, I imagine, to Nancy's – to compassionately contain, respond and guide: to comfort, palliate and help him reclaim some hope for his increasingly meagre life. Due to his feelings of unsafety now, with the Mental Health Teams, I have been seeing him every two weeks:

I accept I may need to do this indefinitely. I am sadly aware that there are now few GPs who would take this initiative, or accept this responsibility. What would happen to Eric elsewhere?

I have directed my attention more widely, too. I have wanted to understand and define the institutional misperceptions and misconceptions: how, with apparent good intent, do we deliver such miscarriages and perversions of care? I have had to be resilient and assiduous in my (re)search, motivated not only by Eric's individual and affecting predicament, but also an increasing number of other patients describing similar dislocations of human understanding by Specialist Services.

Over many months I have made numerous phone calls to various Psychiatric Teams. I have had to be patient, persistent and assertive to generate substantial dialogue. Face-to-face contact has been harder, success had been sporadic yet labour-intensive.

This Odyssey has two parallel paths – of seeking exploratory dialogue with Psychiatric Services while securing restitution of care for Eric. Both are long and difficult. This following description thus attempts salience, not completeness.

\*

I spoke initially to Nancy, then to both the Clinical Manager and the Consultant Psychiatrist at the Mental Health Team. With all three there was a layered carapace to their responses. First, wary bewilderment: why would a GP want to enter their territory with such energy of concern and enquiry? Then institutional deflection and edict: 'The Team has assessed and decided ...'. 'The Care Pathway, directed by agreed Trust Protocol ...' and other armoured phrases of unpeopled authority. With skill and patience I was able to get to the cramped and uncomfortable person trapped behind the armour.

Nancy seemed wary, weary, circumspect then relieved in her brief confiding:

'I'm sorry, Doctor … of course, I'm especially sorry that poor Eric is having to go through any of this … I'm sorry that I can't do the helpful work I know and like … I'm sorry you're having to deal with the fall-out of all this ... But I can't do anything – you know how it is with Management these days: I can't say too much …'

The others, with less direct knowledge of Eric, went through the same process of deflection, dissemblance, then confident and dispirited contrition.

Again, my tricky choreographic riddle: how to maintain respectful colleaguial relationships, while indicating clearly and strongly my wide-ranging disagreements with their policies and decisions?

My clarity and resolve – and anxious concern – were refuelled unhappily; by the accuracy of my predictions: Eric's abject misery became so uncontained that he was admitted to a Psychiatric Unit. Given his early experiences of care by strangers and the nature of current admission centres, his likely reaction was also easily predicted: iatrogenic damage was deepened. The cost to NHS resources is considerable; to human welfare much greater.

*

In my effort to keep Eric's distress closer to drama than tragedy, I contacted you in your role of Clinical Director for the Mental Health Trust. Your response was prompt, concerned and pragmatic: you delegated one of your experienced and Senior Deputies, Dr Y, who would communicate with me.

Dr Y did contact me in a way that was remarkably unremarkable: he sent me a long e-mail.

Remarkable? Unremarkable? Which?

The e-mail combines immediacy and precision of signal with remoteness of human contact: no face, no voice, no location, no touch. Yet it is increasingly used automatically, even in such humanly-demanding situations; it has become a part of our culture. But is such signalling communication? If so, what kind? What for?

Dr Y's e-mail was polite in taking control. It proceeded like an Instruction Manual, assuming that I needed his executive explanation, guidance and help. Some anomalies made this most improbable. He started by acknowledging that his reply was mostly based on his perusal of electronic records: he had never met Eric, 'but I do have a lot of experience with such patients'. As if I do not?

Proceeding to address me like a silent tannoy system, Dr Y then raised the possible therapeutic options of various psychotherapies for Eric. This line of thought seemed (to me) to assume a common simplistic notion of 'psychotherapy' as a sequestered, distilled, specialist activity that has to be designated and delivered systematically. Eric (and I would say most people I see who are distressed) do not want or need that kind of schematised activity. They do, however, want contacts that are psychotherapeutic: contacts that develop trust, hope, understanding, meaning, structure and safety. Nancy had been doing this with Eric, very appositely, for years. I could see this clearly within minutes of talking to Eric. Even Sue, my receptionist, rapidly intuited much the same. Yet various managers of Specialist Services could not, or would not allow themselves, to see this. Why? My theory: because Nancy's unschooled and undesignated therapeutic contact lay outside currently prescribed algorithms and care pathways: that which is not prescribed now becomes proscribed.

Dr Y's long and tendentious e-mail concluded, with a kind of magisterial authority, by instructing me about this man he had never met: 'Overall, the type of all-embracing care that secondary care tends to offer can often entrench such personality characteristics'. What does this mean? Like most general statements about human experience, motivation or Fate, this is a notion that is bound to be true, sometimes. But an opposite proposition is also sometimes true. The art and wisdom of practice comes from the creative and pragmatic editing and synthesis of such partial truths. So, Dr Y's statement, which may sometimes be usefully true, is now rendered hazardous by its introduction as 'Overall', which implies hegemony, like a monarch reigning 'over all'. This is not pedantry: a crucial and difficult part of our work in Mental Health is to always look for exceptions to our predicated patterns. Without skilful handling of these paradoxes, important misunderstandings will be frequent. Eric is a stark example of this, and how it happens. Dr Y's long and didactic e-mail seemed heedless of this. He paid no attention to the personal nature of Eric or my engagement with him: Eric will need some kind of innominate, but bespoke, humanely imaginative containment until the end of his life. This is not rare, yet is rarely acknowledged. Over many years of working with the mentally distressed, I see that this kind of innominate approach has been crucial. How do we assure space and resources for such unpackaged, difficult-to-measure-yet-made-to-measure, free-form compassionate contact with others? In the longer term, in contrast, I have found the currently vaunted time-limited, designated packages of care to be of evanescent interest and shallow effect.

What I wanted and needed from Dr Y was some sophistication of dialogue. What I got was a default-type of e-mail: now so ubiquitous as to be a new convention. In this culture – of screen-before-person – practitioners are now deluged by an inassimilable quantity of such signals. Few get read with good attention; even fewer intelligently discussed. Yet, if we look closely, we can see anomalies and absurdities which few would intend. This happened here: with Dr Y, myself and Eric.

*

Let us distance ourselves and look with an alien, intelligent eye. What do we see? In a highly complex arena of mental distress, where individual understanding must be key to any success, a delegated manager electronically transmits abstracted judgements and decisions. He has spoken to neither the patient, nor either of the most involved practitioners, both of whom are highly experienced, competent and intelligent. He is addressing one of them now, but does not draw on their knowledge and experience of their work or the patient. His view is, rather, distilled from absent persons' computerised records, and then submitted to 'authoritative' patterns of generic recommendations (to which there must always be many exceptions). The role of this sequestered manager is not to engage in a mutually informative dialogue with those involved. Instead, he 'posts' a long, monologous electronic signal, with intent to instruct and command. A related image occurs to me: of an Air Traffic Officer in a control tower. He is looking into a screen at symbolic representations of distant aircraft, to which he sends vectoring instructions. I have little doubt that this may be the best format for Air Traffic Control. But electronically mediated remote control for mentally distressed humans? What kind of psychiatry does this lead to?

We have here sampled what is coming.

For many years I worked in and alongside Mental Health Services where such formulaic management hardly existed, but intelligent colleagueial personal contact was abundant, welcome, even enjoyed. In all the places I worked, until recently, I witnessed the likes of Eric receiving flexible and humane care: schematic designation might have been comparatively meagre, but the human understanding and its quiet satisfactions much greater.

*

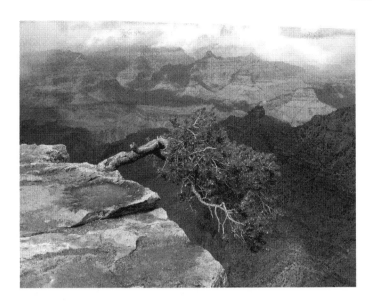

I have been striving to reconnect with – maybe even begin to regenerate – this older, more humanly-earthed professional culture. Due to my frustrations with this I contact you. But due to your business (I imagine) you delegate my request for dialogue to a trusted lieutenant, Dr Y. He, quite unintentionally (I believe) then rapidly re-enacts the bulk of my problems and discontent with NHS Institutions: he resorts to a device which short-circuits any personal contact, understanding or complexity: without further ado he transmits a didactic e-mail, defining reality to me, and for me. I don't mind this approach if I am enquiring about train times, but I want to talk about Eric. I am reminded of a Woody Allen aphorism: 'Confidence is what you have before you have understood the problem'.

Dr Y's rapid acting-out of my critique amused me as an exquisitely timed though inadvertent parody; but it simultaneously dismayed me with further evidence of the ubiquity of the problem. Yet I have hope. Firstly, that you have read this long-journeyed and thought-marinated marathon letter with good attention. Then, most importantly, I hope that dialogue will be broadened and deepened, between us and beyond us. Lastly, I hope you do not answer this with a formulaic e-mail!

$$\Omega$$

*'It is the critical vision alone which can mitigate the unimpeded operation of the automatic.'*

Marshall McLuhan, *The Mechanical Bride* (1951)

Publ. in *Journal of Holisti Healthcare Vol 9 Iss. 2 2012*

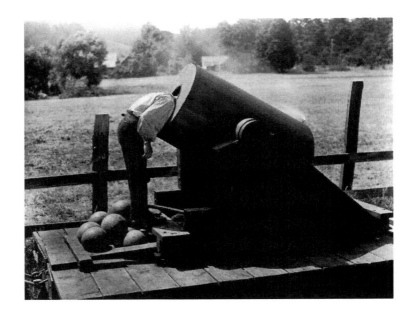

Buster Keaton  *The General* 1926

# Fallacies in Blunderland

## Overschematic overmanagement: perverse healthcare

# Introduction

For more than twenty years there have been various devices to create an internal market central to the NHS: Fiefdom-like Trusts, commercial-type commissioning, contractually defined 'purchasers' and 'providers' of healthcare are current examples. The resulting commodification and commercialisation of healthcare has become its own culture. What does all this look like at the frontline? The following authentic vignettes from contemporary General Practice provide a view. Only usual devices of disguise subtract from accuracy.

The first two tales are now commonplace and superficially trivial, but they already contain the possibilities of bureaucratic burden and distortion that make the shocking last two stories more understandable.

*

*'It is a bad plan that admits of no modification.'*

Pubilius Syrus, *Moral Sayings* (1st century BC)

*'Tis not the habit that maketh the monk.'*

Thomas Fuller, *Gnomolgia* (1732)

*

## 1. Trivial tales: serious themes

### A. The Loop

Dr T receives a letter from Mr O, an orthopaedic consultant. It is about Sheila, a healthy spirited woman of 40 who sustained a severe and displaced fracture of both bones of one ankle. She required surgery to realign the distorted bones, then plates and screws to secure them. All of this has gone well, but several weeks later her ankle remains painfully stiff. Sheila will need physiotherapy. Will Dr T please refer her?

This is not as innocent or straightforward as it may seem. A historical explanation:

Several years ago, before the fragmentation of our national service into parochial Trusts, such collateral work was usually done with speed, accuracy, ease, friendliness and very little, but essential and useful, documentation. Mr O would have spoken to his well-known Clinic Physiotherapist, Carol, and said, in effect: 'Carol, this is Sheila (and her problem) that you can help by doing "X". Let me know if there's any unusual difficulty. I'll see her again in six weeks'. Dr T may have been informed, but not involved.

Recent times and ideologies have moved to more complex procedures. Trusts now mistrustfully contend and vie, sell and buy. Mr O now has no such sensible and 'homely' arrangement with his physiotherapist (or anyone else). The commissioning health-economy mandates that fragmentation of services is introduced to generate extra revenue for his Trust. Thus Physiotherapy is now separately tariffed from Fracture Orthopaedics. Mr O must now write to Sheila's GP, Dr T, suggesting that Sheila be referred back to the hospital for Physiotherapy. Although Mr O is far better placed than Dr T to make this decision and to implement it, the new commissioning system disincentivises this. This is because the interposed administrative loop 'earns revenue' for his Trust, by 'selling' necessary physiotherapy services. This added complexity helps ensure the financial viability of the fiefdoms.

What does this mean? A short link is turned into a long loop: it is not just Dr T's professional time and attention that are distracted by this unproductive artifice – this must now involve clerks, IT coders, contract administrators, accountants, auditors. Such long threads lead to tangles, so Personnel and Contract Managers and Lawyers must be added.

The aggrandisement snowballs: physiotherapy must now present as more arcane and formidable. Mr O cannot simply make a colleagueial (if highly competent) request: such must be replaced by detailed referral forms, team referral meetings, documented referral thresholds and criteria, data collection and collation (however specious), the propagation of professional reports that illusion depth through length, and gravitas through the unnecessary elaboration of technical language.

Such seriousness must be suitably framed: Carol cannot simply and quickly decide – from her considerable experience – what to offer Sheila. Sheila must join a waiting list for a long, over-inclusive, formulaic assessment to be performed. This will be documented in assiduous and trivial detail, then sent to Dr T, though Dr T has no interest or use for this. He certainly has not asked for it. However, for the 'providers' of physiotherapy it bestows auras of completeness and complexity: devices of theatrical rhetoric and justification. A new, and now necessary, language of survival: Lebensraum.

Dr T has become an increasing though unwilling recipient of such over-laden and other-agendad communications. He now receives hundreds of e-mails every week whose purpose is not to communicate with him about what he needs to know and what may interest him, but rather to confer some kind of aura of immunity, impunity or importance around the sender.

Dr T, despite many years of diligent, competent practice, remains anxiously conscientious: he reads such letters, warding off an attrition of fatigued alienation and … resentment. He hankers for a previous era of more straightforward communications from colleagues who wrote pragmatically of what he wanted or needed to know: a culture where help came from personal connections, not a kind of commercialised totalitarianism. He sighs with unsentimental sadness and sagged purpose. He imagines restitution in early retirement.

## B. Size 13 Moonboot

Mustafa is an athletic young man, very tall and with large feet. While playing in a football away-match he fractures a metatarsal bone in his foot. He is seen by the accident doctor at the home counties hospital (HCH) who says to him: 'It's a straightforward minor fracture: your body will slowly heal it, but you'll need a Moonboot for several weeks to get around. You've got very large feet: unfortunately we don't have any size 13 in stock. But you live close to the large London hospital (LLH): they are bound to have some. Just go along to their accident department and they will fit you up. It will be quite straightforward …'

That was true until recent years. It is now very different.

Mustafa goes to the accident department of LLH. After a long wait he is curtly told that as this is not a fresh injury he will need a referral from his GP, Dr T. Mustafa sees Dr T, tired at the end of a morning infiltrated and obstructed by such bureaucratic formalities and ritualistic documentation. Dr T writes a clear request for the Moonboot and a routine follow up, with an equally clear and concise account of the background problem. Until the recent past this would have been responded to in kind.

Not now.

Mustafa reattends LLH accident department with Dr T's letter. A triage nurse peruses it briefly before consulting a Manager. She returns to deliver an accurate slow-spinner: Dr T is bowled-out with her first ball: 'Your doctor and HCH obviously don't understand the system. We can't just give you a Moonboot. You have to be formally referred to Orthopaedics, and then a proper assessment has to be made by a Specialist...'

Dr T had not really understood the concepts of a 'purchaser/provider split', 'Commissioning' and related notions to focus and facilitate healthcare. He is learning now as Mustafa's agent, in these shuttlecock exchanges between Trusts: through these frustrations he is becoming familiar with the procedures, language and protocol.

What he has not learned – what he cannot see – is the value of all this to his patients, or his own efforts on their behalf. Amidst his many conversations – seeking to clarify the benefits of such systems – he talks with Dr Q.

## 2. Absurd but true: A corrupt cadenza
   ## – how the schematic becomes perverse

Dr Q is, like Dr T, a stalwart member of an older but dwindling species: a single-handed, vocationally-motivated, psychologically-minded family doctor. He is a quiet man of understated but sustained and sustaining warmth and laconic humour. Professionally close, in both geography and ethos, Drs Q and T meet for companionable support, ventilation and experienced guidance. Dr Q listens, and identifies with bemused and increasing frustration: he has experienced his own varieties of The Loop and Moonboot.

'I've got one to appal and amuse you ... Yes, both! ... But I have to be careful who I tell ...' says Dr Q, teasing gently with competition and conspiracy.

He talks of one of the many institutional directives attempting to raise the standards of practitioners and practices. Most such devices are now measured, scored and complexly linked to remuneration. He is describing one yoked to substantial (written) complaints from patients. Each practice must now show evidence of how it responds to the complainant, and then turns this to positive reflection, learning and changes in their procedure and organisation.

Dr Q slowly unravels his tangle of frustrations: 'Of course, I agree with the better philosophy behind all this: listening, looking, thinking from another's viewpoint; not being too busy, proud or fragile to reflect on, or share such variations.

'So far, so good – but from here it gets worse, for me anyway. You see, I've spent a working lifetime really interested in these complexities. Probably because of that I haven't had any substantial complaint for about twenty years. That's an achievement I'm happy with, but the absurdity is that my practice has lost substantial income through being unable to complete the exercise. For the last few years I have been financially penalised because no one has complained about me!

'Well, my Practice Manager, Muriel, has many abilities but I hadn't realised how she is also a Mistress of Dark Arts. She quietly conjured a miniature masterpiece: she forged a fictitious letter of complaint; invented a practice meeting to respond to this with discussion, reflection and action plans; provided minutes of the (non) meeting, and a summary report for the monitoring authorities. The result of all this? We invent a complaint, because we don't have one, write a long bogus report for an authority that doesn't read it, and then claim the same money as everybody else! Is that a good way to spend doctors' time or NHS money?' Dr Q expresses his rhetorical coda: 'Righteous fraud!', he laughs sharply, a kind of self-parodic cymbal-clash.

But now a cross-current of doubt, more hesitant. He clears his throat: 'That's not the way I normally behave, is it? ... I mean, what would you do?'

Dr T has not expected this earnest question. He shrugs self-consciously, while attempting awkwardly to combine expressions of fraternal collusion with innocent bewilderment. This is difficult: finding the right formula of words impossible. He shelters behind an enigmatic smile.

### 3. Absurd but tragic: When Care Pathways obliterate care

'I don't think I can do it any more, doctor. I think she needs to be looked after somewhere else ... I'm not as strong as I used to be ... I can't lift her, especially if she falls. And now she's much more confused and gets upset in ways that I can't reason with her about ... It's so hard, doctor: I think it might kill me ...'

Dr T thinks he is not exaggerating: it might. Cyril is aged nearly ninety, Iris is ninety-four. They married seventy years ago, a wartime marriage. As a twenty-year-old signaller with the Royal Navy protecting the Atlantic Convoys, his hunger to marry Iris had been talismanic as well as romantic: he somehow believed that ritualising the strength of his love would protect him, help him survive. He had, and forty years later he had described to a young Dr T his then-unspoken war-time terror, and the transcendent power of his faith-in-love.

Iris had been a very attractive younger woman, but ravaged by primitive anxieties: severe early losses and cruelties had been semi-healed by Cyril's loving devotion, but her wounds were shaken open by a late miscarriage. The subsequent birth of a son assuaged but did not resolve. Dr T remembers reading the unusually neat fountain-penned notes of his predecessor, referring to her 'numerous functional complaints' and her 'polymorphous anxiety'. From the 1980s Dr T would help guide Iris through this hazily mapped, apparently endless, medical wilderness. His patience and imagination were his most important resources, but Cyril was his most important ally. For more than thirty years Dr T witnessed the finest manifestations of loving devotion, *Agape*: indefatigable support, humorous affection, practical containment. Cyril was happy in his role of loving protector: Dr T was appreciated for his professional support and guidance. There followed a long period of eddied stability, until the onset of Iris's dementia.

\*

As so often the dementia was first signalled insidiously and ambiguously, in her ninetieth year. Unsighted by retinal degeneration and unwilling to wear her hearing aid, this frail and slight old lady became increasingly difficult to contact. Her confusion of place and persons was distressing. Her shards of insight even more so: with angrily tearful eruption she would rage at her humiliated disintegration: Cyril tended her with quiet, soft tears of sorrow.

When Cyril developed his increasingly untreatable heart failure he knew that his tide, too, was running out. 'I just want to be able to look after her long enough, doctor …' he had said with characteristic, stoic courtesy.

*

When Cyril – looking haggard, exhausted and afraid – talks with polite deference of his inability to cope and a premonition of his death, Dr T has no doubt about the need for urgent action. Iris needs immediate respite care. He calls Social Services.

*

Many years ago Dr T recalls a similarly abject and acutely disintegrating situation, and his similar request. He remembers his meeting and conversations with the Social Worker, Phyllis, a thoughtful, sensible middle-aged woman with maternal warmth and grand-maternal wisdom. Phyllis had been quick and seamless in her understanding and intelligent actions. Dr T had thought that such dextrous and humane holistic engagement had transformed a painfully tragic situation into one with a kind of elegant pathos. He had felt grateful, moved and proud to be associated with such unglamourised expertise.

*

Now, in 2012, it is very different. Dr T is phoning the duty-desk Social Worker, Vanessa. He is trying to convey, with intelligible rapidity, the nature of his problem with Iris and

Cyril: a brief history and his urgent recommendations. This is turning out to be very difficult. Vanessa clearly has another agenda. Her voice sounds young to Dr T. She transmits it with manicured, polite cautiousness. She explains a protocol which must be adhered to: preliminary screening questions must be completed. Existing Social Services' package? Home OT Assessment? Number of falls? Mental competence? Screening blood tests? Complete Medical and Psychiatric history? Most recent Social Services assessment? Yes, yes, yes … and YES! Dr T attempts to tell Vanessa that a colleagueial dialogue can get to the important points more accurately and quickly. But Vanessa is well briefed and disciplined: she sticks to her prescribed course. At the end of her formulaic collation, Vanessa (who has never met Iris and Cyril), informs Dr T (who has known them both well, for thirty years), that respite care can only be considered after she has been assessed and reported on by 'appropriate' specialist clinics: specifically and separately for her falls, her dementia, her mood instability and her age-related medical complaints. No, there cannot be exceptions. Dr T – almost incredulous, certainly incensed – asks to speak to Vanessa's manager.

There is a delay. When the manager, Marjorie, calls Dr T she seems to be listening diplomatically, but then, equally diplomatically, seems not to have heard or understood. Yes, No. She understands (?) but must support Vanessa in her correct responses: that is how these situations must be managed. Yes, she can understand Dr T's frustration: 'I'm sorry'.

Dr T does not accept defeat. He makes further phone calls. He will shake some senior sense from Social Services, but is told that the regional Director of Social Services is away for two days. He then phones Cyril, whose voice sounds weaker and more short of breath. Dr T asks him about this: Cyril is resigned, self-abnegating, (again) disarmingly accommodating. Dr T refers to administrative delays with respite care: he does not elaborate, but apologises and makes clear he is active in trying to make things happen. 'Yes … Thank you for everything you're doing, doctor … I'll manage somehow.'

But Doctor T does not feel good about this. It is Friday afternoon.

*

On Monday morning Dr T hears. The carer had gone in the previous day and had found both old people on the floor. Iris was moaning with hunger, confusion and soaked underwear, unable to raise herself. Cyril was beside her, but still and silent: grey-mottled and dead. He had probably been trying to lift her.

Iris was immediately taken into care by Social Services.

Dr T feels immersed in an ocean of sadness: for our human frailty, fallibility, folly, pride and evanescence. His surgery is due to start; he dries his eyes.

The whole is more than the sum of its parts.

*

*Plans get you into things. But you got to work your way out.*

Will Rogers, *The Autobiography of Will Rogers* (1949)

Ω

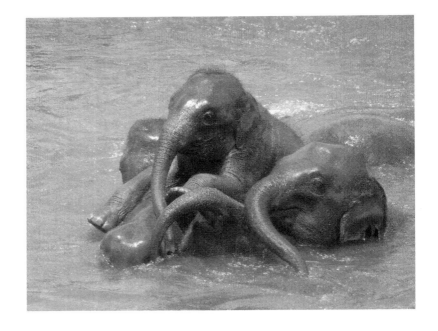

# From Family to Factory

## The dying ethos
## of personal healthcare

For more than 40 years I have worked as a frontline NHS doctor, mostly as a psychiatrist and GP. With other newswatchers, I join the surges of angry moral revulsion when hearing of the latest exposure of gross neglect of care, or even darker cruelty.

Yet my outrage, sadly, is not shocked: I have long considered such events almost inevitable. For in our eagerness to exploit the efficiencies of industrialisation we have carelessly sacrificed the caring human heart of healthcare. We see 'treatments', but people become invisible. This is – at least sometimes – the price we pay when we create a culture that excessively objectifies and commodifies the complexly human.

I remember a different ethos. At the start of my work in the NHS – before our hermetic rhetoric of measurement, quantification, computer-coding and managed goals and targets – I thought of my working milieu as a (mostly) good-humoured, well-functioning family. Complex tasks were shared across disciplines with welcoming courtesy and cooperation. Roles and experience were sensibly recognised and respected, but rarely rigidly enforced. Likewise inter-professional boundaries: we usually accurately understood others' competence and responsibility and adjusted our activities and encounters accordingly. There was often considerable overlap of skills and practice: this would now be regarded as 'untidy' and inefficient, but actually was usually to everyone's benefit – we could provide a more seamless service: it was easy to refer patients across to colleagues whose work and language we understood, and who were often personally known to us. Although one practitioner might be best suited to a particular task, others could expediently temporise and substitute themselves when necessary: like well-functioning families, where good-faith prevails, this would be guided by open dialogue – by sense and sensibility. The result? Patients rarely got lost within or between systems: personal attachment and knowledge guided a sense of continual care. Practitioners, too, enjoyed this broad conviviality. We can see these principles operating in well-functioning families: the healthy resilience both of the entire group, and its individual members, depends on an ever-changing mixture of structure and flexibility.

In human families there are essential jobs to be done: the 'infrastructure' for the security and welfare of all. But beyond that families exist to play, provide nourishment, pleasure and meaning for one another – and then create new life that transcends and may surprise them all. These life-affirmations all had their equivalents in my first two decades of NHS work. I felt part of a large 'organic' network of care – colleagues then seemed like relatives of many kinds, who also ranged in familiarity, seniority, wisdom and power. There were other subtle fruits from this family-like network of care: we knew and understood real families far better than we do now. I remember many helpful conversations with 'family doctors', helping us understand the struggles, yearnings and sorrows of the ailing within their patients' families. Within this family-sensitive, vast, sprawling NHS 'family' I had myriad and mostly good contacts with my healthcare 'siblings'. I appreciated then – more now – that I was part of one of the best, and most workable, kinds of 'Confederate Socialism'.

*

It was not to last. For the last two decades we have seen a progressive dismantling of this family ethos. Successive think-tanks, management consultants, specialist committees and then briefed-politicians have adopted the mindset of the engineer, the industrialist and the market-economist. Healthcare is now forged as a kind of Civic Engineering or, even, a project for Venture Capitalists. Some forms of healthcare submit well to these approaches: the elimination of Poliomyelitis and the spur to advanced pharmaceuticals are respective examples of clear successes. The treatment of certain well-defined physical illnesses – for example, a the surgical remedy of the blocked coronary artery or opaque eye lens – are now routine 'products' of these approaches.

But we must beware of losing our balance: for our new managed healthcare culture is now evolving more like an insect colony than a human family: roles set rigid, repetitive, prescribed, and dictated. Skills become narrow and executed without either consciousness or view of the whole. Care is reduced to a complex system of interlocking, algorithmically proceduralised tasks: an Airfix Kit of (non) human engagement.

In contrast, a healthy human family is like a garden: growth is facilitated, protected, tended – never coerced. Relationships are nourished and encouraged as ends in themselves, not for any external 'product' (though often this may be spawned). How different this is to our insect-colony-like healthcare factories where all human conduct is mandated and managed by the group's circuit-board. Relationships and communications are subsumed to a strict division of labour – rarely are they ends in themselves. Individual variation is likely to be perceived as subversion. The group's totalitarian function commands all.

Clearly the ethos and activities of the family and the factory both have essential – yet very different – places in our complex lives. This extends to our healthcare. An important task needs to be discerned: the necessity for wise and flexible judgment as to how to balance these opposing principles in all our important human projects. Failures are common. For example, attempting to 'manage' family life by uncompromising parental authority will not work for long: eventually myriad forms of unhappiness, subversion and defiance will obliquely countermand.

Yet, as we have seen, our factory-industrial approach has procured us massive benefits, otherwise unreachable. But, when overused, this approach can alienate, erode and destroy important human bonds and understandings. In healthcare we must be vigilant, for these conundra and complexities demand our endless capacity for fresh and creative compromises.

\*

Our factory-type healthcare will deal poorly with those many human ailments that need different kinds of personal engagement for their relief and transcendence. These require healing encounters that mobilise the sufferer's internal resources for immunity, growth and repair. These are subtle and delicate activities and – importantly – cannot develop in a factory culture, whose structure and function both depend on rigidity (like a vehicle chassis). They can only emerge and thrive in a family-type milieu where structure and function and strength are linked to flexibility and elasticity (like a tyre). The general principle for healthcare is that while factory-type management may be best for conduction of less psychologically demanding tasks ('Science'), it is much less suited to socially and psychologically complex situations, where subtle, imaginative induction is required ('Art').

We need these kinds of inductions for any successful attempt to understand personal experience and meaning. For these there are no adequate plans or maps – for while personal experience and distress may contain universal themes, they are always – in some ways – unique. The factory cannot recognise such important discriminations and thus can only hinder us. Yes, our ideas of faulty biomechanics are essential in many of our healthcare encounters but we will often need, also, other approaches of flexibility and imagination. We need some understanding of this person's life, experience , struggles and relationships: holism and semiotics – this is that as well as this. In a culture that is less industrially rigid and driven, the power and meaning of personal attachments will extend far beyond procedures. This is what happens in 'good' families.

*

The price of short-circuiting all this is high: it is what we have now. I am told there is much academic, systematic research into such matters. In my realm – a veteran frontline doctor – what do I experience? I now inhabit a world much richer in precise, high-technology interventions and informatics, and much safer from evident rogue or incompetent practitioners. Yet it is a world more humanly impoverished: of human connection, knowledge, understanding, affection or enduring personal concern. I now attend many meetings with harassed, dead-eyed, fatigued, dispirited doctors. They say: 'I do what I have to', and talk of earliest-date retirement – despite being better remunerated than ever before. Our meetings are pressure-cookers of abstracted management: Agendae, Goals and Targets, budgets, performance indicators, Care Pathways Exception Reporting, Integrated Care – a new lexicon of depersonalised management. It is many years since I sat together with colleagues to better personally understand and develop our frequent and inevitably flawed, fragile and evanescent human work. The factory has driven out the family: I am frustrated and sorrowful. I still have some cohorts: displaced older members of a now-homeless vocational family. We commiserate.

*

What of patients ('service users'!): what do I hear? Those most satisfied – I fear transiently – are those plucked with timely and efficient specialist intervention from cardiovascular or malignant catastrophe: the life-saving coronary artery stent or hemicolectomy. Well-managed factory-healthcare does well here: these beneficial matchings must be acknowledged and continued.

But I hear many more stories of another kind: of vulnerable, fearful people (all of us, sometimes?) feeling personally insignificant, unknown and unanchored in a large, complex, indecipherable system. There is a new kind of anomie in our healthcare: I hear it routinely from intelligent, conscientious, alert people – that they do not know the name of their GP ('The Surgery is so big and busy: I see somebody different each time.'). Likewise the elderly or mentally anguished ('No, I can't remember the name of the clinic or the doctor: there are so many ... They said they'll send me another appointment. Yes, I'll do what I'm told ...'). From older patients I hear laments for the loss of smaller, friendlier practices and the hospital general physician who saw them through many travails ('Dr X and his staff knew me and my family: I didn't have to explain ... I felt understood and cared for ...'). Wanting to continue my ethos of family doctor, I frequently extend my interest and the interview, to develop better personal understanding. Younger patients are surprised – positively and appreciatively ('No one before has shown the interest to speak with me like this.'). As a family doctor this was easy: it is much more difficult as a 'primary-care service provider'.

*

The ennui and fractious demoralisation of our NHS has become a constant back-drone in our national life. Periodically we can expect interruptions: startled shrieks from many more sickening healthcare atrocities. These will usually occur within forests of managing regulations and procedures. In the shocked tumult, listen for the displacing, buttressing countercharge: 'Inadequate resources!'.

I do not usually believe this. The impoverishment is of another kind.

*

Healthcare is a humanity guided by science.

Ω

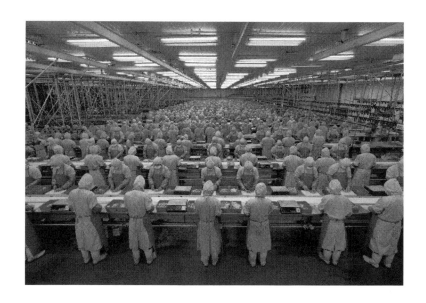

# Understanding the Other Four Elemental Questions for Therapeutic Psychology

## A personal view

Psychology in healthcare faces a conundrum. By entering an arena dominated by the Medical Model it adopts particular types of language, theories and schemata. This it does to be able to 'trade' within the dominant medical 'currency'. Yet such attempts to designate and objectify often displace views and contacts that are more personal, naturalistic, holistic and effective. Thus, the overly academic and technical will frequently miss *this* person and situation. The following, written by a veteran frontline NHS doctor, offers a brief introductory analysis and restitution.

For more than forty years I have had long and short-term responsibilities for myriad forms of human distress presenting to the NHS: as a psychiatrist, psychotherapist and General Practitioner. Throughout this time there has been no shortage of schemata – analytical or interventive – to explain, designate, guide, sometimes enforce. These have changed with the era and the healthcare sector. At times I have wished to pursue and explore these; at other times I have been instructed or commanded, a reluctant recipient. All the mental health schemata have had partial and conditional truth: such fragile connections with human complexity may offer help in attunement, but folly (or worse) when ill-judged. How, then, do we decide? Again, there is no shortage of experts offering more schemes, to direct our decisions. Superficially, this may seem reassuring. Yet I do not think our best judgements readily emerge from such 'authoritative' attempts to objectify and systematise. Our creative discretion is often better served by other perspectives: those that are both more holistic and – simultaneously and subtly – more flexibly personal, more imaginatively bespoke.

What are these perspectives, and how to they escape subsumption to pre-packaged, designatory psychologies? What else can guide our understanding of others and their distress? In my working lifetime I have found the following four questions[1] primal to any likely successful engagement:

- What is it like to be this other person, to have lived their life?
- What is the meaning and experience, for them, of this story and this distress?
- What is the meaning and experience, for them, of me, now?
- What do I need to understand of their needs that they possibly cannot yet express, or even think about?

---

[1] Zigmond, D (2012), 'Five Executive Follies: How commodification imperils compassion in personal healthcare.' *Journal of Holistic Healthcare* Vol 8, Issue 3, December

These questions lie behind and beyond all systematic therapeutic psychologies. They are more fundamental: if a scheme or intervention cannot answer these questions, my engagement is unlikely to be therapeutic, though – paradoxically – it may bring me consonance and belonging among my colleagues. Conversely, sometimes schematic and systematic psychologies can help answer the four questions, though not schematically!

The four questions are 'naïve': unlike our schematic or designatory psychologies, they assume little. Because of this they are more likely to lead to personal understanding that has vernacular qualities, rather than the generic and abstracted nature of more conventional, objectifying psychologies:

*'T has never recovered from the childhood terror and sorrow of his experience of father's raging cruelty, brutality, then final desertion. T's life has been spent yearning for, but mistrusting, male support, esteem, affection and affiliation. My lateness for his appointment seems to stir in him intolerable ancient residues of vulnerability, uncertainty and abandonment. His response to my greeting is staccato, flushed and tense: he seems angry and afraid. I sense a conflation of fight and flight and I think, again, of his wounded early childhood.'*

Contrast this with:

*'T has a long history of recurrent agitated depressive illnesses with anxiety/panic reactions. He had a poor record of maintaining work and long-term relationships. He also has problems with anger management: this was evident to the Clinic Staff when I was unavoidably delayed. This inconvenience was clearly explained to T, who nevertheless was unacceptably angry and rude to the staff in response. It is thus likely that T also has a Personality Disorder.'*

The first account is guided by the Four Elemental Questions, the latter by currently conventional designatory notions. Both have their strengths and uses. Optimal practice often comes from a skilful blend. Throughout my decades of practice, though, I have usually found the former to be the more illuminating and helpful. Disturbingly, the necessary engendering ethos – of evocative personal understanding – is now increasingly imperilled: our excessive attempts to standardise and industrialise NHS healthcare have led to a culture where the designatory will thrive and the resonant will perish.

More than a century ago, well before we had become so lost in our forests of systemised abstractions, here is Mark Twain: 'One learns peoples through the heart, not the eyes or the intellect.'[2] Evidently this is only partially true and from another age, but there is pithy wisdom here that is probably more urgently relevant to our times than his. The message in this ancient and folksy voice could help us reclaim our collective sense.

Mental healthcare is a humanity (sometimes) guided by science.

Ω

---

[2] Twain, Mark (1895), 'What Paul Bourget Thinks of Us.' *North American Review*, January

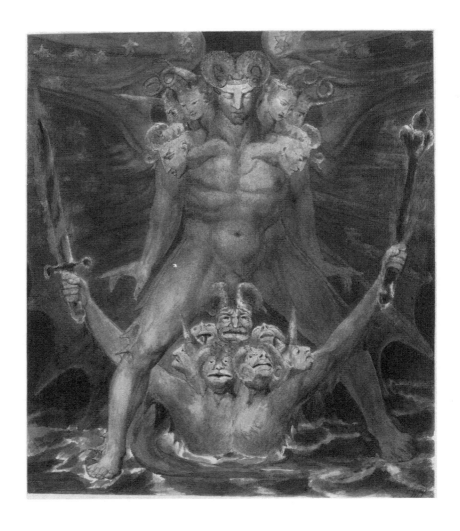

William Blake *The Great Red Dragon and the the Beast from the Sea* 1805-10

# Words and Numbers
# Servants or Masters?

## Caveats for holistic healthcare
## Part I

Holism's fuller engagement with realities is an aspiration and ideal. It can never be complete, and in practice, there are many obstructions. These range from our use of language to our highly managed and industrialised culture. How does this happen? What are the consequences? This is the first of two articles.

## Prologue: caveats for holistic healthcare

Holism (and its lack) may be easier to recognise than define. It is more readily communicated and perceived by stories, rather than data or abstract formulations. This presents problems: holistic mindsets are now becoming harder to access and maintain, for our culture is now one that increasingly conceives and conveys in packages: food, fuel, news, entertainment, even thought are all likely to be coded, metered, monitored, measured or packed. This causes fewer problems when our encounters are with inanimate or less complex life-forms: the production and distribution of eggs or detergents cause fewer ethical and social conundrae than the industrialisation of complex welfare activities (though even our simpler activities eventually confront us with wider ecological – ultimately Gaian – consequences).

We thus have an insoluble handicap. It is always easier to think in parts than wholes: language, analytical thinking, our micro and macro economies … all tend to fragment our perceptions and activities: 'this is this, and that is that'. In contrast, holism's tenet of infinite and often hidden interconnectedness tends to erase boundaries and conflate territories: 'this is that as well as this'. Such thinking largely eludes schemes, packaging, academia, economic analyses. Our use of language, too, struggles to convey any sense of holism without serious loss or distortion.

The following two articles present a collage of notions illustrating, very partially, the extent of our difficulties and task. The notions themselves are presented without usual conventions of academic thoroughness or cohesion. The first article presents the skeleton of the view: the second provides further illustrations and variations. Overall, they represent some unsystematised, though summative, personal reflections from one practitioner's decades of working in human healthcare – a chimeric and often paradoxical world. Philosophical contention is ever-present. We are accelerating our mandates for factory-like language and procedures to service increasingly complex healthcare: human nature and predicaments remain considerably more ambiguous.

## 1. I've got a measurement – it must be a fact

## The rise of data and the curse of scientism

*'Nothing vast enters the lives of mortals without a curse'*

Sophocles (c 496-405 BC)

There was life and technical success before computers, yet these are rapidly becoming harder to understand. Some examples: the manufacture of antibiotics, the D-Day Landings, Man on the Moon, Concorde – all of these were achieved with minuscule or no computer-power – things we could not manage now in our 'progress'. We have become empowered but deskilled: in healthcare, as we shall see, these subtle discrepancies lead to grievous losses.

Before the widespread use of computers, the harvesting and collation of measurements – data – was manual, labour-intensive and therefore slow. It thus required much deliberation and discrimination and – relative to today – its volume was tiny and consequently much more manageable.

The electronic unshackling of these activities has freed them from the constraints of our individual capacities for engagement, assimilation or understanding: data has multiplied exponentially and is now pumped and piped at us like gas or water – public commodities.

Measurement, the blood-brother of data, has thus been conferred pre-eminent status in many humanly-complex activities. Numbers are the most easily digested 'food' for computers, and computers are now essential to the functioning of any public service. Existence of people and their activities must be continually monitored and broadcast in a form that can ensure their organisational recognition, management and survival. The virtual world now defines and commands the real: measure or perish. Once started, this is difficult to slow or stop.

So, our institutions are now electronically held together by computers, computers need data, data need statistics, statistics need measurements; ergo: measurement becomes the basic language and activity.

What does this mandatory measurement mean for healthcare? The consequences vary greatly with the type of activity. Sometimes the effect is facilitating and benign. For example, with activities that can be easily and directly measured, standardised and proceduralised: here the measurement culture can be applied with relative ease and evident benefit. Laboratory services, vaccinations and cataract extractions all serve as common examples. All have in common a clear, circumscribed physical basis, little variation in technique or human response and a high completion/success rate. In short, they can be easily humanly 'mechanised'.

But much of healthcare does not offer this kind of simplicity for measurement, and then the effects often depart widely from the benign and facilitative. Measurements are at their most competent with physical objects or phenomena: a blood-count is far less problematic or contentious than a mood-rating scale. This is because attempts to assess, measure and code other people's experiences must be derived from something else: self-reports, or other people's perception being the commonest. All are subject to massive contention, contamination and compromise. What does this mean? Here are some personalised examples:

**Ms B** is in dispute with the Department for Work and Pensions (DWP)[1] over her Disability Living Allowance. Ms B claims severe symptoms and invalidity from Depression, but her invalidity seems invalid to the DWP assessor: he asks the GP, Dr F, for his opinion. Dr F[2], in a complex but rapid judgement, agrees with the assessor. This 'objective' assessment is stymied by Ms B's continually high self-reported, but quantified, depression scores. 'Something's wrong' they all say in different ways. 'Only the wearer knows where the shoe pinches' says an old adage, but when is this untrue? Who decides? How?

**Kenny** is sixty-two years old, a single, lonely man, appeasing and self-deprecating in his manner. Harsh and neglectful parenting left him with impoverished self-esteem. A working lifetime as a road worker has riddled his lower body with degenerative arthritis. He left school at fourteen: his intelligence exceeds his words. After several years of courteous wariness he is, with Dr F's gentle encouragement, beginning to talk of his burden of fear, loneliness, shame and longing. The ancient story behind it is poignant and powerful. Kenny has great faith in Dr F, but continues anguished in his small and crumbling world. Dr F asks for help from NHS Psychological Services, to help Kenny occupy his limited life more positively. Kenny returns to Dr F a fortnight later, fearful, tearful and trembling. He nervously indicates the immediate cause of his distress: a tightly-stuffed, freshly opened envelope. It is from the Psychology Services. Dr F surveys several detailed questionnaires[3] aiming to define diagnosis, severity, disability and numerous personal and demographic details. In addition are various bureaucratically prolix letters and documents explaining 'The Service', a Complaints Procedure and instructions for the Service User. No one has spoken to him

In his frightened and faltering language Kenny conveys to Dr F his sense of bewildered humiliation and abject inadequacy: 'I don't understand all this, doctor … I just can't do it … I just want to talk to someone – like I do with you, doctor.

The doctor remembers many years ago reading of Heisenberg, an early 20th century physicist. Heisenberg found that it was impossible to plot simultaneously the velocity and locus of an electron without changing these in an indeterminate way: the observation changed the reality. Dr F as a young man could not identify how this was relevant to his meagre knowledge of physics. Many years later he is seeing clearly how personal observation – when formulaic and non-bespoke – can adversely affect people he knows well.

**Philip** is eighty-six and Dr F is visiting him at home, the week after his discharge from hospital. He had taken a first-ever overdose of his medication to end his life. An earlier than expected visit from his carer had found him collapsed and vomiting.

Philip now looks tired and Dr F again senses immense melancholia beneath the mask of rigid discipline, of understatement. The doctor knows some of Philip's recent trials and sorrows: his wife's gruelling and fatal malignant illness, followed rapidly by the sudden death of his beloved son, their only child. And then the increasing impoverishment of his own Parkinson's Disease, a gathering bass-note.

Dr F had premonitioned Philip's trapped but mute anguish and its possible tragic fruition, and had asked for help from his mental health services. Their (non) engagement proceeded by asking Philip to fill in detailed mood and anxiety questionnaires. These indicated mild, stable disturbance – measurements meriting merely a brief psychological care package from a Low Intensity (skills?) Worker, and a routine, templated report of all this, electronically conveyed to Dr F.

Dr F's perception is discrepant. He shares his unease with Philip, whose intelligence and insight survive his ravages of grief: 'I don't like to tell anyone my troubles, doctor … I wasn't brought up like that. I have my pride, you know … It's different with you: I've known you years, and I don't have to say much, for you to understand. But answer all those questions for a stranger? No.'

Dr F thinks of Philip's formative years: a harsher, crueller, braver world of much greater trials, losses and endurance; a black-and-white world where contained and stoic fortitude was a social essential. Dr F understands this with few words, and Philip understands that he understands. But a questionnaire?

Yet Dr F now inhabits a professional world in thrall to designated experts who are keen to quickly code and quantify the distress of Philip and Kenny, as well as Dr F's ministrations, and then to instruct them all. Dr F's understanding can seem piecemeal, slow and never finished: features of the intersubjective, one-person-and-situation-at-a-time. By contrast the questionnaire has slick allure: its 'objectivity' may be specious, but it is quantifiable and can be given to all – a demotic science. Dr F is thinking of the distinction between the scientific and the scientistic: which is which? He is thinking, too, beyond his own professional end: who then will be speaking to the Philips of the world, and what kind of conversations will they be?

*

## 2. I've got a word – it must be real
## The trap of reification

*'In the Beginning was the Word'*

John 1:1 (date uncertain)

Language does far more than merely 'communicate': words first contain, then command and control our experience, and then our influence of others. The implications of this for healthcare are subtle, powerful and rarely discussed. A brief linguistic analysis will help us understand these.

All words are there to package and convey a description of, or notion about, human experience. All ultimately come from our perceptions, then our constructions. The basic components of language are: adjectives, describing qualities of experience (what something is like); verbs, describing activity producing change (what something does); and nouns, which attempt to capture a more static state, a 'something', from which these other two emanate (what something 'is'). For example, I describe a small vertical platform supported by four vertical supporting posts: someone comes and sits on it – it is a 'chair'. Generally, we think such 'real' things endure and we attribute them by nouns: adjectives and verbs are more the flux of experience

In our usual waking life this may present few problems, with nouns seamlessly providing apposite bridges and anchors for the rest of our sense-experience, and those of others. But potential dislocation is ever-present.

An example: I am at a friend's table, eating an unfamiliar dish. I do not recognise the texture or flavour of the meat, although I enjoy both. I enquire what 'it' is.

1.  I am told: 'It is lamb'. I am mellow with appreciation for my sensations, my friend and the cosmos.

2.  I am told: 'It is Alginon, my ginger cat. She was very old and was dying anyway'. What is in my mouth now triggers an explosion of nausea, and retching. I jump up with disgust and mistrust. My friend and the cosmos turned malign.

The 'actual' experience is transformed by the idea of the 'real' source-object (lamb v cat). This noun now determines my subsequent experience and action: the adjectives (pleasure or revulsion) and the verbs (sitting and eating v jumping up and retching). All this happens despite my never seeing the putative lamb or cat: they are abstractions rendered powerfully 'real' by the noun. Such is the power and gravitational force of nouns.

Nouns work with greatest clarity and efficiency when applied to physical objects: the words 'table' or 'television' rarely cause problems except to a foreigner, a lawyer or certain kinds of academic. We generally accept these object-nouns as 'real'. Elsewhere the use of nouns is more problematic and more interesting: God, democracy or love may sound like (sacred) 'things', yet are essentially variegated ideas. Innumerable stories from world or domestic histories show how little clarity and consensus the nouns manage here, yet how real they are to their believers.

There are striking analogies in healthcare. One working definition of medical diagnosis is the organisation, then transformation of adjectives (a) and verbs (v) into professionally conferred nouns (n) which then determine explanation, therapeutic action and prediction for others. With afflictions that are predominantly physical – 'structural pathology' or disease – we can call this type of noun a 'Substantial Diagnosis'. Here is a simple example:

**Tommy** is six. Last night he became listless (a), pushed away (v) his favourite supper, complained of soreness (a) in his throat and abdomen and then started to shiver and vomit (v). Dr Y is now with Tommy and his mother. His job is to find and then confer the right organising noun, or diagnosis. When he sees Tommy's much enlarged, reddened tonsils, flecked with creamy pus, he has the precise constellated noun: 'Acute Pustular Tonsillitis', though he thinks 'Tonsillitis' sufficient for his verbal communications. The formulation and conveyance of this word are beneficial for all: Dr Y knows what to do and what to expect, Tommy will almost certainly get better, Mother is comforted by this and the containing, reassuring clarity of this noun – the Substantial Diagnosis. For all, this process is helpful and uncontentious: the doctor's knowing and naming the 'thing' of Tonsillitis is a cooperative and shared blessing. Importantly, Dr

Y's diagnosis also relieves the sufferers from having to search for their own explanation, meaning of, or influence on, events.

In other areas of healthcare this hegemonic use of nouns runs into many more difficulties. This is particularly so where the doctor is dealing with bodily dysfunction (functional disease) in the absence of the evident structural changes of bodily disease. Equal difficulties are encountered with disorders of behaviour, appetite, mood or impulse (BAMI): the core of psychiatry and clinical psychology. The results here are more mixed: our medical-noun type diagnosis may sometimes bring evident clarity and relief to these physically non-fixated forms of distress, but often it will not. Then the professionally conferred noun – the diagnosis – is conveyed, but the benefits do not follow. In these situations the diagnosis may be 'correct', but clarification, relief or prediction remain poor. The doctor has – by convention – done his job, but none of the participants are gratified. We can call this a 'Nominal Diagnosis'. Here are two examples:

**K,** a tense, conscientious, sensitive woman of twenty-six years has seen several doctors over several years with benign abdominal and bowel symptoms. All have agreed she has Irritable Bowel Syndrome (IBS) and prescribed the usual medications, always with little or transient effect. Dr T realises that a wider vocabulary is needed to differently understand and influence her complaints. In his endeavour to do this, he learns a lot about her unhappy childhood home and how this has led to her guarded perfectionism and her painful ambivalence about close relationships. The long-term effects of this widened dialogue and vocabulary were slowly gratifying for both K and her doctor.

Here the conventional noun-diagnosis of IBS was relatively ineffective and – probably – obscuring or obstructing more helpful personal understanding: it thus proved to be a Nominal

Diagnosis only. The idiomorphic understanding she developed with Dr T proved much more helpful.

**Maggie**, fifty-five years, has collected a variety of diagnoses from her many years of faltering contact with psychiatrists and psychologists: Generalised Anxiety Disorder, Agoraphobia, Panics, Emotionally Unstable Personality Disorder with Cyclothymia, Recurrent Depressive Disorder, Bipolar Affective Disorder. All are documented in the usual formalised language of designatory healthcare which then rhetorically confine and define Maggie by Nominal Diagnoses. These conferred nouns may superficially appear to offer real therapeutic understanding, leverage and prediction, but actually do not. None have offered Dr V. greater personal understanding of Maggie.

Dr V. decides to create a larger and different kind of space for Maggie to talk. This dramatically changes not only Dr V.'s view and understanding of Maggie, but also Maggie's behaviour: her symptoms become much quietened.

How does this happen? Dr V. wants to know Maggie's story, not for a Management Plan, but so that he can better understand. Her story has obscurely disturbed her for decades and it will disturb Dr V. now.

Twenty-five years ago she was married – happily she thought – with three children. She experienced her husband as kind, attractive and funny, but a bit feckless: he drank a lot. She suddenly has unmistakable evidence of his alcoholically hazed, repeated sexual contact with their ten-year-old daughter, Amanda. In a volcanic eruption of mixed and primitive feelings, her marriage and family are destroyed. Years later the ruined landscape of her life is still littered with explosives. She tells Dr V. of a current torment: Amanda – now a tough, cynical, sexually alluring, drug-abusing, spiky thirty-four year old single mother – has restored affectionate contact with her father and his second wife, and takes her children to see them.

Maggie's feelings towards her daughter are raw, kaleidoscopic and irresolvable: 'My mind goes crazy with it, doctor ... She was only ten: I should have known, should have protected her: but she knew, and she knew that I didn't know ... She was a child, but was – I didn't know then – a serious sexual rival. Now she is stronger and healthier than me, and has more of a family – mine is destroyed. I love her as a mother, but hate her for what she did, what she does, what they have all done: but can I blame her? ... Has she triumphed over me? I feel crazy and terrible for having just said all that, doctor, yet it's such a relief that I can say these things and that you can understand ...'

Dr V. has a bespoke and ongoing dialogue with Maggie about her tragic story and her responses to it. Her distress often exceeds her capacity for words, yet words and ideas are what they exchange and they are many: guilt, shame, loss, rage, hate, love, contrition, resentment, despair, despondency, alienation, disconnection, blame, humiliation, revenge, sorrow, defeat ... All touch on part of Maggie's poisoned cauldron, but only part, and only transiently. Maggie now talks less of her symptoms and Dr V. does not much offer his vocabulary of diagnoses or treatments. As their language has changed, so has the nature of their exchange, and then the pattern of Maggie's distress. Maggie, so long burdened and defined by her multi-diagnoses, is now freer to suffer with her unique and humanly-understood tragedy. Dr V., too, though distressed by her story, is also touched and, paradoxically, nourished by such candid and courageous contact – the staple of compassion.

Others have asked: what is 'really' wrong with Maggie? Is there a word: is it 'Depression'? What is the 'correct treatment'?

> 'Language is, by its very nature a communal thing: that is, it expresses never the exact thing, but a compromise – that which is common to you, me and everybody.'

> Thomas Ernest Hulme (1923), *Romanticism and Classical Speculations*

This article continues in chapter 2.17 *If you want good personal healthcare see a Vet.*

*

## Notes

[1] DWP – a UK nationwide governmental department that administers and manages state pensions, sickness and welfare benefits etc. Assessing disputed levels of distress and disability is a task it currently often subcontracts to other agencies.

[2] The doctors, patients and situations throughout this article are real but anonymised. The examples of doctors' encounters will be relevant now to many other types of healthcare professionals, especially those working for the NHS or large corporations.

[3] Detailed questionnaires are now being vaunted and proceduralised throughout most NHS Psychology and Counselling Services. This is explained by authorities as making the services more scientifically efficient. This is contentious, at least. In this author's view it leads to specious science, dehumanisation, and a healthcare cult of Scientism. The obstructive and destructive effect of these is extensive and subtle. See my articles 'How to Help Harry' (Zigmond, 2012) and 'Sense and Sensibility' (Zigmond, 2011a).

## References

Zigmond, D (2012) *How to Help Harry – Friend or Foe? The scientific and the scientistic in the fog of the frontline*
Zigmond, D (2011a) *Sense and Sensibility: The danger of Specialisms to holistic, psychological care*

Ω

Publ. in *Journal of Holistic Healthcare Vol 10 Issue 3 2013*

# If you want
# good personal healthcare,
# see a Vet

## Caveats for holistic healthcare
## Part II

The over-explicit and over-schematic can block our perception of larger and more subtle realities. This second of two articles explores further how this happens, and what we may be left with.

*The fairest thing we can experience is the mysterious.*
*It is the fundamental emotion which stands at the cradle of true art and science.*

Albert Einstein (1934), *The World as I see It*

## 1. Never invade Russia!

This was Churchill's droll, jesting yet ominous response to an enquiry about his most crucial guiding military maxim.

Napoleon and Hitler are the best-known examples of Churchill's warnings of epic folly: maelstroms of shocking, humbled hubris. Both launched their expeditions fresh from success in easier campaigns and fuelled by specious optimism. They were driven also by rhetoric for the rightness and feasibility for the possession of new territory. Both started with startling triumphalism, then slowed, then succumbed: exhausted by the vastness and strangeness of a climate, terrain and people they had poorly understood.

There are useful analogies for some of our current enervating endeavours and conundra in healthcare. First, our expectations have been primed and inflated: Life for millions in the Twentieth Century was positively transformed by applied science. Biomedicine has had spectacular success in countering, even eliminating, many infectious, inflammatory and degenerative physical diseases. In all this industrialisation – mass-production, standardisation, quantification, speed – has been essential. Such successes have led to a long flush of optimism: surely we can gainfully apply similar schematic, industrial-medical type thinking and interventions to *all* our other sources of distress and pain – our human dis-ease, our polymorphous anguish, our inevitable (yes, still!) decline?

It is here that our invincible march founders, for ailments of our metaphorical heart are proving far harder to locate, define or reverse than those of our anatomical heart. Human motivation, meaning, communication and (un)consciousness yield very meagre territories to objectifying science. Beyond is our vast hinterland, navigable (sometimes) by other kinds of knowledge and influence.

Our reluctance to heed this accounts for many of our most curious and (superficially) indecipherable healthcare follies. In our thrall to measurement we neglect more important unmeasurables. In our urge to treat we do not pause to heal. In our (often unnecessary) compulsion to convergently image the part, we become blind to the divergent – the whole: *this* person, their story and networks. When we define, we also often confine – ourselves and others – to a tunnelled vision and selective deafness. For language, perception and action are tightly linked. If the language of our culture becomes restricted to the technical, the commercial, the procedural and the defined, then our patients – people, like us! – are seen as merely biomechanical problems to be controlled, managed, traded or disposed of. The abstract becomes hegemonic: the real become abstract.

Hyperbole?

Even in 'straightforward' physical care our over-industrialisation is producing shocking calumnies. Consider the following story recently widely reported in the media: [1]

A man is admitted to a London Hospital with a rare but well recognised physical complaint (Diabetes Insipidus) which renders him particularly and hazardously vulnerable to dehydration. He knows this and can usually communicate well. He is seen and assessed by a succession of healthcare workers, some of them specialists. In their complexly successive, jigsawedly interlocking, brief contacts with him they do not heed this increasingly desperate requests for water, which culminate in his calling 999 from the hospital ward. Only after he dies does it become clear that all these algorithmically-managed practitioners had been effectively deaf to his voice and blind to his demeanour. Hospital spokespersons' public comments are woven with grave contrition and confusion. The former might need construction, the latter does not. The Hospital used to have world-renown for its standards of medical practice, teaching and academia; emblematised also by its historic, stately architecture. Relocated now in an undistinguished, unloved, ugly, airport-like, sprawling conurbation, the containing architecture expresses with unintended accuracy the healthcare culture – a hive of hired healthdroids.

That a highly-funded, well equipped and specialised *medical* unit can so misunderstand and depersonalise someone with a *physical* complaint can only bode poorly elsewhere – especially for those who require yet more personal and thoughtful kinds of listening and understanding. This is the case, but often less obvious. With non-physical complaints our failures of care and communication are less dramatic: a slow slide into lonely and dislocated oblivion will gather no headlines. Living silently with a broken-heart attracts no crowds; an untimely death from a heart attack does.

Our current healthcare is in increasing thrall to a Scientistic folly: that generic formulations can be mass produced for all individual distress – that human dis-ease can thus be easily subsumed to impersonally managed forms of civic engineering. Such is contemporary healthcare's Invasion of Russia: grandiose but flawed in assumption, then unsustainable, impossible and incurring vast casualties.[2]

Healthcare may be guided by our science, but science must rarely eclipse our humanity.

*

## 2. If you want good personal healthcare, see a Vet

*'I like peasants – they are not sophisticated enough to reason speciously'*

Montesquieu (1689-1755), *Variétés*

When Dr F takes his dog to the Vet, Mo, he is simultaneously disarmed, comforted, ashamed and envious: Mo has a guileless and effortless rapport and liking for the animals she is handling. Dr F wants to know more of these unaffected and unbookish skills: he asks to sit in with her.

What Dr F witnesses is humbling and radically refreshing. After asking the owner a few questions, Mo stands back from the animal, scanning it with her eyes, listening carefully to its breathing and other sounds. Then she makes active contact with the animal, the approach being based, Dr F thinks, on some kind of 'holistic mind-set' that she senses the animal is now inhabiting. Dr F notices how different her approaches are: with one she gazes at its face with unwavering directness while speaking in a firm and commanding voice; with the next she averts her gaze, softens her posture and lowers her voice to a soft reticence. Sometimes she quickly and directly grasps the nape of the neck with decisive dominance, a wordless control. At others she is slow and light of touch, gently stroking the flank while humming; a trans-species fraternalism. Dr F wonders whether Mo's accuracy, range and speed of rapport with these different creatures is somehow akin to inducing hypnotic states in humans. He asks Mo:

'Oh, I don't know about hypnosis – I'm not that clever. Nor do I know much about humans: they talk too much for me to be able to understand them!' She curls a playfully commiserating look at Dr F. 'My furry friends here can't say much, but I have to understand them quickly: are they frightened, hungry, confused, in pain, angry, unloved? ... Yes, really! ... Do they need to feel they still control their territory, or do they need to know I am dominant? All such things I have to get right without much delay, otherwise I cannot get docility enough to do my job ... Yes, I'll get scratched and bitten, too. With larger animals it can be more serious: you can easily become lunch or squash!'.

Dr F leaves Mo that morning with a deeper gratitude than he is easily able to express. With little psychological scholarship, theory or instruction, this open-hearted, open-minded, freshly-instinctive woman is able to resonate with, and thus 'read', the mind-set of these (humanly) mute creatures. What natural gifts we (all?) may have!

He thinks of the cumbersome, academically conceived, elaborate-yet-clumsy devices healthcare workers are being instructed to use, to inform all about the experience – the 'mental state' – of others. He thinks of the obedient but hopeless Scientism of giving detailed questionnaires to Kenny and Philip[3]. He then thinks of Mo: her almost wordless, seemingly magical, rapid and affectionate rapport with very different animals. He wishes he could be understood like that, and laughs to himself. His laughter diffuses to a smile at the contrasted memories: Mo has inspired him to retrieve some fresh depth and contact in his work. He will reconnect with himself too, before and beyond words.

*

## 3. In difficult encounters, think about sex

### The tyranny of the explicit

*'Every person's feelings have a front-door and a side-door by which they may be entered.'*

Oliver Wendell Holmes Sr, *The Autocrat of the Breakfast Table* (1858)

Dr Y is thinking about sex. It is not the first time, but now it is different. He is thinking professional thoughts about how our thinking and behaviour around our sexuality could greatly enlighten our healthcare.

More specifically, Dr Y is thinking about a very delicate, complex and evanescent interweaving – of the implicit and the explicit: how these have to be rapidly and accurately discerned, deciphered, jointly understood and then responded to. All of this happens on a second by second basis. And choreographing this medley of meta-communications is essential for any kind of sexual competence – let alone deeper unifying satisfactions. We have to have a (usually) unspoken sense of what the other is desirous of, receptive to, 'on' for, and when and how. We must quickly sense error and redirection. Mostly, in better sexual congress, this can happen by dextrous implicit exchanges: the explicit may sometimes then be added potently and sparingly – a mutual aphrodisiac. If the explicit is necessary, the exchange is faltering. If it is necessary for long periods, the relationship is in serious trouble. If the explicit is used by one, without implicit desire by the other, the exchange becomes embarrassed, self-consciously clumsy, possibly abortive. Many such misattunements doom a relationship. Seriously regarded, they can become work for lawyers.

Dr Y is amusing and confusing himself with how weighty and complicated are the responsibilities of this ancient[4] and near universal activity. How do most of us ever (think we) get it right?

These implicit-explicit dances are certainly at the heart of our sexual contacts, but extend throughout our important relationships. They depend on our being able to seamlessly interchange the implicit and explicit, by 'tuning-in' to the other. We want (and expect) our partner to understand what is troubling us, without our having to name it (yet?): soon after, we want them to now be receptive to the beginnings (or resumption) of the explicit. We want, now, to be able to talk. Yes, directly.

Familiar?

Dr Y extends his thinking to how important such exchanges are in healthcare. He remembers Maggie's[3] long story and considers how any success he has with her is due to his being mindful of such delicate dances: he had been patiently implicit with her before she trusted him with the explicit. And then, with gratified relief, her healing reverted to the implicit. Maggie had told Dr Y of earlier psychiatric interviews and how they had become too explicit too rapidly. She had retreated to the shelter of the implicit, but had not been understood. The implicit locked.

Dr Y remembers well the kinds of discussions he used to have with colleagues, at the beginning of his career. He recalls many years of interrupted-but-never-finished, free-wheeling explorations of our complex contact with others. The concepts and vocabulary were rich and wide: influence, confluence, identity, boundaries, encryption, territory, projection, surrender, escape ... The notions and vocabulary were plastic and uncompleteable, yet each alightment could enrich – differently in different conversations: subtly or evidently, with immediacy or incubation, with implicity or explicity.

Dr Y now rarely has such polychromatic and rewarding exchanges. The computer has predicated a new healthcare language for the 21st century: a restricted and restrictive machine-mandated vocabulary. Healthcarers communicate now – almost entirely – in dull narrow administrative, technical words: of conventions, clusters and codes; of quantifiable procedural activity and description; of conduction but not induction – all designating the objectively generic but excluding the humanly variable. Computer compatibility may thus build some bridges to our outer lives, but very few to our inner. What remains has little room for the nascent, the semiotic, the metamorphic, the ambiguous – all the subtle hues that we must mindfully respect to provide nourishment and meaning for our important relationships. The explicit now burgeons beyond our needs, understanding, tolerance or stamina: the implicit ails and dies.

*

Its passing takes much of us, too.

*

The whole is more than the sum of its (explicit) parts.

*

Healthcare is a humanity guided by science.

*

Humanity may be commanded by the explicit: its best understanding is often implicit.


*'The water in the vessel is sparkling; the water in the sea is dark. The small truth has words that are clear; the great truth has great silence.'*

Rabindranath Tagore, *Stray Birds* (1916)

## Notes

[1] It is hard to gain statistics about the human and economic cost of inflexible, officious practice and uncompassionate – if 'correct' – depersonalised care. What correlates does one measure? Who is going to fund this? Although quantitative research may be difficult to set up, vernacular evidence is plentiful and ubiquitous. See my articles 'Five Executive Follies' (Zigmond, 2011b) and 'Love's Labour's Lost' (Zigmond, 2010). Also letters to Clinical Directors of Mental Health Services.

[2] Kane Gorny, age twenty-two, died on 25 May 2009 of dehydration as an in-patient at St George's Hospital, south London. The inquest in July 2012 revealed the facts recorded here. The story is only one of several similar in recent years, eg see also reports of Mid Staffs and West Midlands NHS Trusts. All have been met with convulsions of outraged incomprehension when made public. The fact that they come clearly to public view reflects well on investigative journalism but – of course – seriously damages confidence in NHS care. This is rendered more confusing when such episodes occur in institutions deemed to be 'performing' excellently by other, measured criteria. The responses of managerial gravitas, concern and contrition seem real enough. Some sceptics have averred that these conceal some kind of collusion, albeit unconscious. The latter possibility is easier to cite and sense than see. If true, this is cultural: powerful, but difficult to tether or examine, except by inference.

[3] Kenny, Philip and Maggie are all real but anonymised victims of over-schematised and over-explicit mental healthcare. Their encounters with Dr Y are described in the previous article 'Words and Numbers: Servants or Masters?'

[4] The activity itself is much older than many people realise. For example, this author – together with many of his generation – believed they were its initiators in the 1960s. However, since that time there has been increasing evidence from many sources, indicating that it far predates that period – possibly even prior to the birth of this author's own parents.

### References

Zigmond, D (2011b) *Five Executive Follies: How commodification imperils compassion in personal healthcare*

Zigmond, D (2010) *Psychiatry Love's Labour Lost: The pursuit of The Plan and the eclipse of the personal*

Publ. in *Journal of Holistic Healthcare* Vol II Issue 1 2014

# Democratic Fatigue - Information Overload

So, few people seem interested in electing a Police Commissioner. Soon after, the media parade for us politicians, academics and pundits – all expressing perplexity or concern. One recurring salvaging explanation is that citizens do not have enough information to make a choice.

As one of these unengaged citizens, I do not share these puzzlements, concerns or notions. My mind and life are overwhelmed by choices and information, and I cannot cope with more. There is a great difference between wanting to have an individual voice and access to dialogue, and submitting to governmentally initiated and designed choice of other people's packages. I may want the many authorities in my life to listen, but I do not want, necessarily, the responsibility of having to vet or choose who all those authorities might be. Evolved democracy is very different from democracy by government prescription.

There are interesting parallels here to our current healthcare commissioning. As a senior GP I know most of my peers have little enthusiasm for their freshly bestowed mantle of authority: Clinical Commissioning Groups. Yes, we want managers to listen, but we do not want to have to do their job. Putatively democratised devices to commission Welfare Services appeal to certain kinds of politicians, academics and tank-thinkers. But those with long experience on the frontline usually have much less confidence or enthusiasm for these demotic initiatives. The nature and delivery of our complex human activities are often very protean. Such formulaic systems of presentation and packaging, however well-intentioned, will serve them poorly.

Solutions? There are none. We can offer only our wisest compromises. In the past, I think we understood this better.

Ω

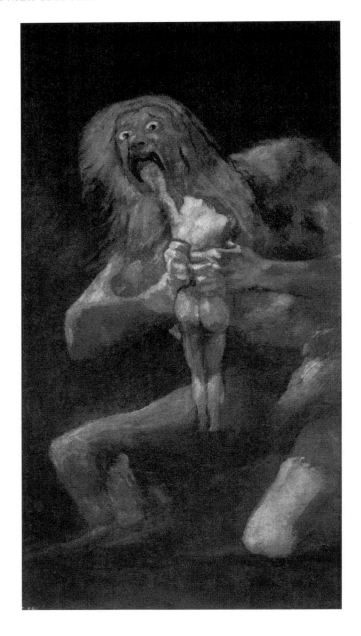

Francisco de Goya *Saturn Eating his Children*
1819 - 23

# Institutional Atrocities

## The malign vacuum from industrialised healthcare

Flagrant neglect or abuse in our care of the vulnerable within our advanced Welfare State seems shockingly perverse. How and why does this happen? This article argues that excessive industrialisation and schematisation are speciously alluring, but then alienating. Restitution of any culture of more compassionate care is like an organic process: it must develop from milieux that have receptive space for attachment, affections, and containment.

So, from the tide of depersonalised healthcare we have netted a flagrant and demonic example of maleficent neglect at Mid Staffs and, now alarmed, subject it to forensic analysis. Understandably we want to know: how could this happen? Who is responsible? Who can we blame? Government? Inspectors? Policymakers? Regulators? Practitioners? Administrative Managers? Clinical Managers? Almost immediately we have rhetorical cries for justice and resolution: More trainings, inspections, management! Professional eliminations! Clear and strong leadership! Show-trials for public pillory!

All of these responses have relevance or truth yet seem, to me, to miss some deeper understandings about how advancing technology is changing not just our thinking, but also our configurations of human connection. Like our banking and economic systems, our problems extend far before and beyond our crises, or our judgements of villainy or technical incompetence. These events are grotesque aspects of Zeitgeist: we are all in this together. We are all easily, unwittingly, victims or perpetrators; we have much to understand.

In my exploration I have come to some different, though contiguous, ideas. At their centre is this: that healthcare has become too beholden to the objective, technical, systemic and informatic; that the unmindful excesses of these have driven out interpersonal understanding, attachment and, thus, instinctive and gratifying caring. We have ignored – at great cost – an omnipresent paradox in our care of others: that is, impersonal treatments and formulations (science) tend to countervailance with personal engagements and holistic understandings (art). Our contemporary healthcare thus requires a vigilant balance: to offer our best skill, effectiveness and humanity, we must be able to combine these opposing principles – to weave and titrate them – differently with each encounter.

Four decades ago I was mentored by doctors who, generally, had a canny awareness of the importance of such complex balances. Successive generations have lost this sentience in our cultural rush and thrall to the impersonally managed, measured and procedural. In our increasingly push-buttoned world we are increasingly uncomprehending or intolerant of anything else.

I recently watched a BBC Newsnight programme: graphic descriptions of cowered, helpless people dying of dehydration on soiled sheets exampled our problems. The fractious lobbyists and pundits exchanged recriminations and accusations and never-again contritions. Several talked of inadequate or incorrect training, assuming that it is training that prevents a gravitational drift to blatant inhumanity. My view is different. Such omissions of care and connection are not a matter for adding specialist training, but of retaining or reclaiming our common humanity. How have we lost this, and on such a massive scale? How do we repair this, and in a way that will be sustainable?

In answering these questions it is important that we first acknowledge the blessings from our accelerated industrialisation of healthcare, for these have certainly brought us dramatic benefits alongside the insidious losses we are exploring here. The benefits are greatest for complaints that are primarily physically localised, and then are speedily and decisively resolved by procedural expertise. Clear examples are timely interventions in cardiovascular disease and some cancers. The way we systemise deliveries of such blessed interventions can be thought of as being like a factory.

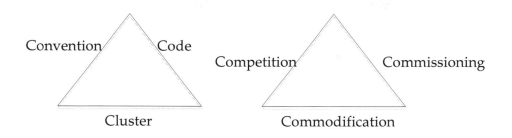

**Figure 1:**
*Generic ordering of structural illnesses*

Easy to measure and subject to 'factory' processes

Impersonal

**Figure 2:**
*The current boost of industrialised healthcare*

Designed to optimise management, measurement and 'factory' efficiencies

Impersonal

Yet the modelling of healthcare solely on this illness/procedural intervention paradigm is hazardous: when our suffering or its causes are not easily despatched, we need a culture that encourages something very different –attachments, affections and containments that develop between people. This enables personally anchored understanding and care: these offer not only comfort, but also the subtle inductions of healing within the person: of immunity, growth and repair. These activities cannot be schematic, but they are vital and vitalising. Notably attachments, affections and containments are at the heart of any healthy kind of family.

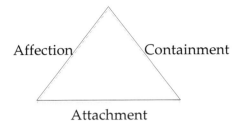 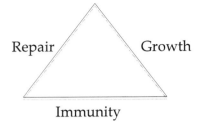

**Figure 3:**
*Interpersonal healing inductions*

The 'family' ethos of well-fared welfare

Difficult to measure

Personal

**Figure 4:**
*Intrapersonal healing inductions*

The 'family' effects of well-fared welfare

Difficult to measure
Personal

While factory and family healthcare paradigms both have irreplaceable functions, their coexistence is not straightforward: for our best benefit can come only from ceaseless and careful choreography between them. Failure to understand, respect and achieve this delicate balance leads not just to ineffectiveness, but then to inhumanity or hazard. This is our current nemesis: our healthcare has become factory-rich but family-poor; informatics and scanner-sighted, but humankind-blind.

We have erred through our indiscriminate and thus excessive use of systematics: objectification, coding, planning and atomisation into managerially proliferated and boundaried specialisms. This may be a good way to run a robotic factory; it is definitely not a good way to raise a (healthcare) family.

Many will regard the Mid Staffs' debacle as criminal; I think it is more true, and more instructive, to think of it as cultural – Mid Staffs is thus a severe symptom, a warning sign, of our collective and collected errors. It is, of course, a severe event, but also one of many and now everyday examples of our healthcare anomie and human disconnection. This has happened both despite, and because of, our ever-increasing welter of commissioners, statutory bodies, dividing and divisive specialisms and competing autarkic Trusts – all these have led to a kind of healthcare that may look good as an architectural model, but is not good to live in. The worse the economy, the more impressive the economists.

I used to work in a much more heterogeneous NHS: the worse was worse, and the better much better. What was that 'better'? For the professionals working hours were longer, but morale was higher. Official Regulation was less, but vocational conscientiousness greater. Physical treatments were simpler and cruder, but personal care more sustained and sensitive. Electronic signalling non-existent, but conversational dialogue much easier. The pay was less, but the human reward was more. Didactic training facilities were meagre, but educational discourse richer. Most of my older mentors passed on loving care for their work, now my younger colleagues attempt to control others by formalistic Personal Development Plans.

And what of the patients? In the earlier, less technocratic NHS the better clinicians understood the importance of attachment, affection and containment in healing: we assured time, flexibility and imaginative space for these. We knew that such subtle interactions were often our best offerings of care for those conditions not easily cured – probably the larger part of our healthcare (yes!): our ageing, our mental distress, our tangled, troubled reactions to life's vicissitudes. For these our best efforts are more imaginatively pastoral than procedurally technical. Here the professional's integrity and judgement need personal enlightenment and nourishment, yet these are now often driven out by further technical management and training. The stark inhumanity at Mid Staffs is what happens if we do not understand and then neglect this delicate ethos of human connection; it is not about the kind of competencies that can be quickly and easily trained and regulated. The realisation of this may be an awakening, to reopen our eyes, hearts and minds.

This schematic desiccation of human connection in NHS healthcare is thus seminal to many of our serious and widespread problems. Over the decades I have observed this previously humanity-rich but imperfect organisation become more and more machine-like. People in the NHS I now work in, have a steadily declining personal knowledge or understanding of one another. In this ex-human vacuum the computer now sits, like a glowering, increasingly obese and enthroned emperor, appropriating the impersonal hub and frontline of administrative and informatic continuity.

What does this lead to? Anomie and depersonalisation. Few people can now name their GP, hospital consultant, or even the name of the specialist clinic they attend – mostly the computer will bid and book them, and mostly they will comply. GPs are increasingly working in large conglomerate practices where they offer little personal continuity of care, do not know families, neighbourhoods or even the names of their own receptionists. The receptionists, in turn, are disconnected from their (many) doctors and increasingly from the patients – 'reception' is now often done by a computer screen, leaving the receptionist 'free' to tend the computer with other tasks. Those other tasks often involve some kind of electronic data-collation, which will be necessary for the doctor to have on the screen, when he is having a procedural (non) contact with a patient he will never really get to know, and does not look at (because he is instead looking at the computer screen) … Get it?

In hospitals this anomic haze is even worse. In my local airport-like hospital I have seen consultants doing ward-rounds with rota-directed junior doctors they have never met before, attended by nurses who do not know their own colleagues, the patients or any other ward staff. This consultant, clustered with strangers, then attempts quickly to evaluate a complex (for we are) human/technical problem in a patient he is seeing for a first and (often) only time. Such a symphony of fragmented depersonalisations has been orchestrated by successive layers of 'improvements' to logistics and efficiencies of healthcare's training, standardisation, procurement and delivery. Examples? Amalgamation of medical schools, the dispersal of hospital nursing schools to universities, standardised modular trainings (rather than apprenticeship-type education), the encouragement of subcontraction, the abolition of GP personal lists, autarkic powers of NHS Trusts, payment by results, the fragmentation of 'Psychological and Psychiatric Care' into complex speciality-based streams, the European Working Time Directive, and, of course, the 3 'Cs' (Commissioning, Competition and Commodification) ... all of these exampled initiatives – plotted and hatched by experts – have added to the remote-control complexity of our healthcare machine and the human inaccessibility for its operators and operatees.

*

Authentic caring is not a commodity to be traded or a skill-set to be instructed. It is an ethos, a metaphorical effusion of the heart. It is a benign, often relayed, human transmission that tends to mirror, then amplify, the incoming signal. It is a similar, but opposite, process to the contagious relay of cruelty, bullying or intimidation. For caring we need holistic imagination – to perceive or conceive more than is explicit or apparent. In contrast, cruelty requires us to see in a person or situation less than is clearly there. Cruelty is a kind of reductionism. Yet out current systems of management will urge us to the simplistic, formulaic and formalistic. Trust-employed healthdroids are now paid to look only at one prescribed part of complex problems, and in the Trust's officially prescribed manner. This is usually influenced significantly by the Trust's interests of autarky or economy.

Caring for others also depends on our own morale: whether we feel cared for, embraced by human connection and value. This, of course, will depend much upon our milieu: as health carers how do we perceive our working and employing culture? What kind of 'factory' or 'family' do these represent for us, and in what kind of ratios?

The quality of how we care about our care of others depends on ensuring receptive and imaginative mental space and time to make possible personal attachments. From these may develop affections: the investment of bonds with discernable feelings – for now we become significant, then important, for one another. This establishment of affectionate attachments then makes possible another and essential aspect of compassionate care: containment – we bring comfort, calm and often understanding to others when we receive, hold and share what they can no longer bear alone. Again, this is often a relay effect: the sufferer is helped to contain their suffering by feeling contained by the helper, who can do this much more readily if he himself feels an equivalent caring containment in his environment. Caring containment is thus passed on in successive relationships, like Russian Dolls, one within the other. It is important, so reiterated, that the opposite experiences and effects – of indifference, fear, cruelty etc – are passed on in a similar way. Thence come our dysfunctional or hostile families and institutions. Was Mid Staffs such an example of discontainment?

So, caring and containment can be best assured where attachment and affection can develop. As we have seen, this is unlikely in an NHS in which the ethos of the 'factory' has largely driven out the 'family'. Consider, for example, an undramatic and very common scenario: the process of a hip replacement in 1983 and again in the more industrialised/ schematised 2013.

## 1983. A technical task: personal continuity

Ali is 65-years-old and already crippled and housebound by his hip arthritis. He goes to see Mr O, an orthopaedic surgeon. Mr O hears Ali's story and complaint: Ali tells Mr O of how his life has been diminished and disempowered by his infirmity. Mr O recommends a standard hip replacement and sees Ali several times before and soon after the successful procedure, and then for longer-term follow up. The two men develop a low-key but cordial and discernable affection. Ali expresses his gratitude for a much restored life and feels encouraged by Mr O's interest and advice early in his recovery: he talks of him warmly as 'my surgeon' – this is affectionate, not presumptuous or possessive. Mr O is grateful, too. It is good for him to see the human effects of his technical intervention, to hear from Ali about a life restored. Mr O's work is often difficult and stressful: such human contacts nourish and sustain him, too. One of his young and idealistic students once tried to interest him in a conversation about Holistic Medicine. Mr O had replied that he'd never really understood what the term means; he was 'just a surgeon'. For Ali he was more: Mr O knew this, but did not speak of it.

## 2013. A technical task: a production line

Ali is Ali's son: he, too, has succumbed to a similar disability at a similar age. Ali attends the same hospital as his father had, but its inner workings are now very different and Mr O has long retired. There seems to Ali no equivalent or replacement for his father's surgeon, for he sees someone different each time he goes to the hospital. He does not know if the stranger he is talking to is a nurse, a doctor or a physiotherapist and he does not feel he should ask. Nor does he remember the names of the different clinics, but takes the appointment letter with him to ensure his accurate destination. He is seen by different practitioners for orthopaedic assessment, preoperative assessment, surgical admission, surgery, surgical recovery, and post-surgical follow up. He does not know the name of any of his attending clinicians or who replaced his hip. Ali thinks his technical care was 'probably alright', but confusing. He was afraid in hospital, but told no one. He found recovery painful, lonely and difficult: he had no quietly affectionate professional relationships to encourage him, and no smile of gratitude to bestow. 'Job done', true enough, but no human connection or deeper satisfactions for Ali or the anonymous 'Teams'. And the innominate, unknown hip surgeon – Mr or Ms O2 – what sustains them? What gives their tiring job human value and meaning?

*

## Vernacular maxims: no statistics

After more than four decades as a frontline NHS Doctor I have mounting sadness and fear for the human and philosophical impoverishment of my profession. If I live long enough I, too, will have a serious role as a patient. The Mid Staffs exposure may shock many: for me it is merely another shard of disheartenment. Every working day I encounter similar, if lesser, systemic human disconnections. I look back over the rolling eras of errors, and management ideologies, and the hundreds of collegueial conversations I had trying to make sense of them. In all of these I am searching for general caveats and motivational principles – the kind that might better guide institutions to enable, rather than stifle, imaginatively compassionate healthcare. Like the work itself, my compilation is flawed, never complete, and must always be revised:

- If we like our work and find it interesting, we will do it well and willingly.
- Such liking and interest often involves the gratification of seeing our work's longer-term evolution and personal effects. Deeper satisfactions, too, are often personal and holistic: conversely, fragmented, short-term work offers little of these.
- Encouragement to draw on our experience to make intelligent creative decisions is likely to engage and develop our best qualities. Submitting to endless committee-designated diktats does not.
- We thus prefer flexible and collaborative working arrangements rather than those that are rigid, competitive and divisive.
- If we get know people well, we will be well-motivated to care for them. The more you see of someone, the more of someone you see.
- If we do not know people it is far easier not to care, or even to collude with harm: History has innumerable examples prior to Mid Staffs.
- People who feel attached, interested and positively personally engaged need relatively little disciplinary or motivational management.
- In contrast, it is very difficult to get good work from people who do not enjoy their work, feel attached or positively, personally engaged: these are primary deficits, and no amount of regulation, management, training or financial incentive will rectify them.

**Figure 5**: *Imaginatively compassionate healthcare – some guiding caveats and principles*

If large organisations, like individuals, can have breakdowns of spiritual and emotional integrity, then the NHS is set for an epidemic. This is largely due to our disinvestment of natural and positive attachments. Mid Staffs is but one early, now publicly flaunted, casualty.

*

The whole is more than, and different from, the sum of its parts.

Healthcare is a humanity guided by science.

That humanity is an art and an ethos.

Ω

Published in: *Journal of Holistic Healthcare*, Vol 10, Issue 1, Spring 2013

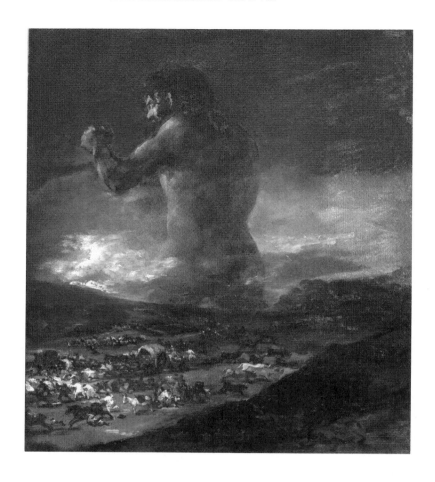

Francisco de Goya  *El Coloso,* 1808-1812

# Beyond Orwell

## Healthcare's hollow governance

Our smallest difficulties with others are often rich in political complexity. What does this mean? Two apparently trivial examples from healthcare administration are explored.

*'Totalitarianism spells simplification: an enormous reduction in the variety of aims, motives, interests, human types, and, above all, in the categories and units of power.'*

Eric Hoffer, *The Ordeal of Change* (1962)

*'Men reform a thing by removing the reality from it, and then do not know what to do with the unreality that is left.'*

GK Chesterton, *Generally Speaking* (1928)

## Prologue: Brave New World

My formative years working in healthcare occupied a kind of pre-industrial world. The now ubiquitous and centre-staged rhetorics – to measure and manage – were then minor, quieter players. Like all industrialisations the transition has brought gains through losses: technical treatments are better, but personal care often worse.[1] The most parlous practitioners are now detected and removed earlier; but the pre-emptive management required to do this is often at the cost of our finer personal vocational identifications, devotions and initiatives: these often ail and then perish.[2] Healthcarers' technical errors may be less, but so too is vernacular human understanding. In forging such industry, we change the culture: a vocationally conscientious 'family' of practitioners has been steadily replaced by a 'factory' of centrally programmed and managed personnel: healthdroids.[3] A new term has been invoked to legitimise all this: governance.

The official intentions are sloganned into allures of healthcare improvements and entitlements to be delivered by ratchets of efficiency, equity and vigilant policing. [4]Increasingly these are procured and corralled by computer-compatible – thus electronically mediated and standardised – forms of surveillance and control.[5] While all this may work well with simpler tasks and scenarios, it elsewhere leads to perverse incentives and squandered resources.[5] Alarmingly, such

525

surveillance and control then develops hermetic and ineluctable qualities: no-one claims ownership or the authority to intelligently divert or discriminate.[6] Matters of subtle and sensitive welfare become rapidly and automatically delegated to new kinds of cybernated servomechanisms.[3,7] The complex galaxy of human needs and meanings must now submit to a culture of computer-templated compliance solely beholden to its own consistency and completion: a Frankenstein's Monster of non-humankindness, Technototalitarianism.[8] The following two apparently prosaic examples from General Practice are commonly endured though resented; rarely (as here) explicitly disclosed or discussed.

*

## 1. 'We've all got to do it. We've got to feed The Beast: that's the way we get the money.'

Eddie's distress is raw and naked: it is stark and disturbing and needs no further evidence for Dr T to know that Eddie needs much compassionate containment and guidance. Eddie's wounded sensibilities far exceed his meagrely educated capacities for articulation. His tremulous tearfulness bespeaks awakened shock from the past. This has conflagrated a subterranean arsenal of long 'forgotten' childhood memories: a leaden legacy that, til now, has wordlessly crippled his life. The force of this awakening has blown aside his frail defences: Eddie is now unable to stem the erupting intensity. His sense of fear, shame, humiliation and sorrow has accelerated beyond his words. Now, with Dr T he struggles to have a personally disclosing conversation for the first time in his life: his vocabulary is sparsely stocked. The doctor knows he must pay careful attention to these highly-charged but inchoate utterances. He will need his imagination, too, if he is to make much personal and systematic sense of this cloistered, encoded and intense drama. If he has any success Dr T will need much other help in his efforts to help Eddie: he starts the necessary contacts.

*

Eddie's first contact from the Psychology Service brings him bewilderment and alarm: he receives through the post a densely packed envelope. In it, amongst the legally required (but rarely requested) information documents and leaflets, there are many questionnaires. These firstly ask for wide-ranging personal and demographic details, and then there are those asking for more precise disclosure of the nature of his 'complaint'; its history and the severity of his disability. None of these make any sense to Eddie, who has needed all his courage to trust his few and difficult words with Dr T. He left school at 13: he is semi-literate. His level of distraction and distress make impossible the process of self-objectification required to competently complete such forms. More inadvertent though meaningful complexity emerges, for exposure to the questionnaire has itself worsened Eddie's fear of inadequacy and rejection: the 'science' pre-requisited as essential for the therapy has itself become countertherapeutic (and can offer only a contaminated vagary of science).

*

Dr T wants to procure psychological help for Eddie, yet he must also protect him from such procedural thickets he finds impassable. Dr T doubts that these complex routines will bring to Eddie any timely benefit. Yet to get this fragile man Diplomatic Immunity from the Psychology Department's Informatics Scanner is proving difficult. Dr T starts an escalade with their office staff and then Manager: their responses are polite but tethered – they have their instructions to instruct others. No, they are sorry they cannot accept exceptions. Next he tries a Senior Practitioner, SP, who baulks at what she considers Dr T's presumptive 'diagnosis' of Eddie. She attempts to explain to Dr T that 'psychological treatments' are now much more scientifically based and accurate: for Eddie to receive the benefits from these it is necessary for him to submit to these procedures – it is for his own good. Dr T wishes to demur and dissect, but SP instead wants him to submit to instruction, correction and compliance. He diplomatically disengages: he will try to recruit higher powers.

The Clinical Director, CD, another older practitioner, listens carefully to Dr T, who is relieved by CD's sanguine manner and open intelligence. His interest in people and their complexity seems still fresh and compassionate, but he now talks with a tired, stoic cynicism of the larger picture, of the vast, increasingly industrial NHS service to whose upper ranks he has been promoted.

CD is looking at a pencil which he taps on a note-pad, a discrete becalming rhythm, as if slowly Morse-Coding to unseen sympathisers. He raises his gaze to Dr T and smiles, a mixture of vicarious apology and conspiratorial sentience. His sigh is emphatic, a wished-for exhalation of greater difficulties.

'Yes, you and I both know how obstructive and redundant all this is, but it's the way we've got to do it. The way the System works now requires us all to produce the right data and statistics for our managers and Commissioners. We've all got to do it: we've all got to feed The Beast, otherwise the money doesn't come through and we don't get fed ...'

\*

## 2. 'Don't ask questions: just do it!
## That way they make it easy for you.'

The week is a hard one for Dr T and his defence of any autonomous or vocational homeland: he is due for an Annual Appraisal, his ritualised submission to governance. This year it is with a much younger colleague, Dr YC.

Dr T's difficulties are mounting. For as successive appraisals have increased their demand for rigid format, formality and itemised detail, so has Dr T's difficulty in conforming to them. He is increasingly aware that the committee-consensused mindset and ethos come from a very different world of values and intent to his own. For decades he has been sustained by warmth and nourishment in his work, by a culture of unengineered and yet (mostly) mutually affectionate and respectful contacts with staff and patients. By assuming the primacy of such quiet attachments, other things have followed naturally: keeping curiosity and engagement fresh and alive; learning by his own enquiry, rather than others' protocol. His understanding of people, too, has been kept vernacular and fluid: he has avoided the crystalline solids, the public convenience-packs of devitalised psychiatric and social diagnoses. Essential to maintaining this engaged stamina is an enjoyment and wonder of our shared – yet often denied – human complexity – of ambiguity, paradox and semiotics. For behind the evident almost everything is also about something else. What? When is that useful? Who decides? How?

Dr T likes such questions, not for any clear or definitive answers, but because the process of questioning suffuses his mind and work with interest, light and life. If people become personally interesting they are much more rewarding to care for. Such questions have thus helped him start each of his thousands of working days with alertness, imagination and curiosity: for alongside our commonalities each moment, each individual, each encounter is unique. Such is the Art of Medicine.

But the new culture of governance, and thus its many employees, are now increasingly if unmindfully countervailed to such philosophy and holism, such semiotics and humanism. The language and format has consolidated as a commonality of schedules, items, boundaries, lists, measurements and prescribed plans.

*

Dr YC has a friendly manner and face. Her handshake is warm and reciprocal. Dr T is encouraged, but also wary of a brisk convergence in her movements and speech: she is a multi-tasking young woman and Dr T senses her bristle with delay.

Her survey of the voluminous obligatory documentation is more to identify anomalies and deficiencies than to pursue creative enquiry. She asks why Dr T has not filled out the section on his Professional Development Plan more fully and cogently. Dr T replies that he cannot: in more than forty years of exemplary medical practice and senior academic work, he has achieved a great deal, but has never had a private or public plan for any of it. His record has clearly been long, fertile and excellent, but never had governance. Dr YC draws in a breath and offers a brief mock-puzzled smile: 'Yes, I can see that – but it's not what is required now…'

Dr YC finds another failure: the selected Audit Project is not up to date: the Practice's documented and templated analysis of a defined area of prescribing is last year's. Dr T had not even been aware of his bureaucratic lapse. He is frustrated by being technically compromised about something that, beyond administrative formality, has little other value or meaning. What do they learn about him from such an audit? That he can think clearly? Can collect, collate and analyse data? That he can organise his staff? That he is mindful about prescribing? Surely, Dr T is surrounded by evidence that he can do all of these things. He also knows that such ubiquitously harvested audits are hardly read by anyone: they are perused and inspected, to see only if they pass muster. Usually they are then quickly cybertised for an oblivious eternity. Why, then, are thousands of doctors, throughout the land, having to spend time on projects that have no evident benefit or interest to anyone?

Dr T has a view: that such requirements of governance are rituals of hegemony, demonstrations of roles of dominance and submission, and shibboleths of acquiescence. They indicate – in diplomatic code – who is in control and who will obey, who is the definer and who the defined, who decides language and meaning. It also implies the spectre of professional extinction for non-conformists. Like an electric-fence for cattle, it may itself have flimsy structure, but its sharp, hidden signals quieten and control vast populations.

Dr T thinks this cattling of professionals raises important matters of integrity: not just his own, for he has seen the effects throughout the Welfare Services. He tries to interest Dr YC, but her cordiality is timed-out and is evaporating to irritated fluster:

'You may be right, but I have two children I must soon collect from school: I simply don't have time to talk about that kind of thing...'

She looks at her watch with tensioned resolve, and then toward Dr T, as if throwing him a line:

'Look ... a lot of us know that most of this is nonsense, but we've got to do it, so we do. My advice to you is: Make Things Easy For Yourself. Don't ask so many questions. Just do it! That way they make it easy for you...'

\*

## 1984 in 2013: Epilogue in dystopia

Dr YC's brief attempt to rehabilitate Dr T awaits fruition and formal process. While his fate and intent remain doubtful he has an impulse to look again at George Orwell's 1984, a book he first read well before that date. Then the book was prophetic; now it occupies historic prophecy.

Dr T is unsure of the origin of his urge to return Back to The Future, but he thinks it is something to do with his encounters with CD and Dr YC. He thinks now of his early life, shadowed by relics and prophesies of totalitarian malignity. Bomb-wrecked, hollow buildings; shuddered, fresh fragments of tales of Samurai or Nazi atrocities; revered and mantle-pieced photographs of the keen-eyed, young deceased; silently or expletively despised images of the violently fallen, ogrous, totalitarian dictators – these picture his 1950's memories. That era gradually gave way to a quieter, more insidious, totalitarian menace: the Great Bear's Communism and the long Cold War. The fear and evidence of The Enemy at the Gate became less visible; the communal experience was less clear, more of an undertow. It was at this time that Dr T first read the, then, prophetic 1984.

As Dr T revisits Orwell's world, he notices his disparate reactions of gratitude and gloom. The harsher, barer aspects of Winston Smith's Oceania are mercifully absent: the endless war, the dreary physical deprivations, the mortal hazards of exposed dissent, the ubiquitous transmitted images of the nation's salvation and nemesis, of Big Brother and Goldstein.

But he has also ominous awareness of less flagrant similarities. He thinks of Oceania's omnipresent television screens and loudspeakers endlessly streaming public information, statistics and diktats, of the screens that spy as well as transmit. He thinks of Oceania's Doublethink: then thinks again of CD and Dr YC – how they must also fork their tongues to keep their jobs.

Dr T thinks of other subtle and geared-down similitudes. In the last decade he has seen his previously benignly-spirited, if sometimes heterogeneous, profession become drilled into a cowed, dispirited, orderly hive of healthdroids – of obedient supplicants or prescriptive commissars. True: there is no Room 101, yet Dr T has seen colleagues' fear – how anxious they are to show evidence of conformity: how their professional behaviour and speech then becomes a self-conscious, imitative, stilted carapace. There may be no party uniforms, yet such uniformity of thought, conduct and vocabulary have successfully completed their tasks: uniformed attire becomes unnecessary. Much of the conformity is anchored and assured by Technototalitarianism:[7] the now requisite pathways, algorithms, templates, key-words, codings and procedures. How and what to think or say is decided by unseen authorities. Thought and dialogue outside prescribed agendas, boxes or codes becomes increasingly irrelevant, uncomprehended and eventually subversive. Independence implies dissent; dissent is a precarious perch: there is unemployment beyond.

Dr T has glimpsed the faint, secreted, spectre of procrustean murders – the quiet expedience to remove any obstructions to the industrialisation of Welfare Services. He has seen the constructed and fatal undermining of well-respected and liked colleagues who failed to demonstrate timely enthusiastic alacrity for the new colonising trusts and plans. It is The Plan that must endure: individuals can be airbrushed from the picture. For the survivors, disquiet is quiet, murmured and brief – survivors have gratitude for their jobs. That gratitude turns fragile and nervous.

*

Dr T is talking to another senior survivor, Dr S. This sixty-year-old cohort may be assumed to be more secure and comfortable in this driven and industrialised culture, for he is a long-established advisor to government: a citizen in the citadel.

Dr T tells his old cohort first of his recent experiences and then of his tangled thoughts and feelings: he wants a thoughtful and experienced view from the other man, not quick and expedient commiseration or collusion. He is encouraged as Dr S seems intently attentive and sympathetic, nodding and softly ahaing. Dr T takes care, and whatever impartiality he can muster, to convey clearly his knotted frustrations.

He thus curbs his urge to overtalk and pauses, leaving a short, silent rest for his weltered thoughts. Dr S sits quietly too, as if in meditation, separating then gathering his thoughts. From this brief hiatus Dr S gazes and speaks. His directness has a soft, slow deliberation; he has clearly been incubating his thoughts well-prior to this encounter:

'Yes, I am of a similar inclination and generation to you, so I am sympathetic but, alas, not effectively so as I am beleaguered and outflanked by factors beyond my control or – and this is both alarming and deeply depressing – anyone's. Sometimes we introduce administrative or regulatory devices, believing they are sensible and helpful, only to find later that they are difficult to stop, and that their overgrowth has become more of a problem than the one we are trying to solve in the first place.

Sometimes the overgrowth spreads and roots rapidly: these devices, planted on the surface, leach into the subterraneum to produce culture; both our consciousness and unconsciousness change – we cannot easily rescind such things. We now live in a world that expects speed, standardisation, convenience and clearly labelled packaging. We've set that up in healthcare, and it's initially certainly brought us some advantages, but now we can't stop … so we continue to try to turn all healthcare problems into computer-compatible data, mass-produced processes and then a complex economic system that commodifies and trades in these. This speeding juggernaut is now difficult to brake: we now have hundreds of thousands of NHS staff whose salaries, status, homes – whose livelihoods, even identities – depend upon occupying a role in this healthcare emporium. And then the people who are likely to do best in all this are those most surrendered to the culture: those who most believe it...'

'So it's just like Orwell's 1984', says Dr T, offering what he tritely thinks is a pithy summation.

'Oh, no! This totalitarianism is much more refined – and probably durable – than our fictional 1984', Dr S quickly retorts, a slightly acerbic and ironic taint to a residually courteous manner. 'Our system doesn't need endless wars, flagrant scapegoats, monolithic and ever-present leaders or a life-threatening Secret Police: our system now largely runs itself: that's one definition of culture. There isn't really anyone in charge! Even at my level many of my colleagues seem – to me – unaware of how much they have bought into the package and thus speak the language. In my meetings with them I try to influence quietly: with patience, stealth and diplomacy. But I'm careful to stay in The Tent: if you're outside The Tent you have little influence, and you probably won't be heard...'

Dr T protests against his own agreement with this: his interruption intends reason, but is soured by concealed, petulant grievance:

'The problem with that is if you stay in The Tent long enough you lose your own voice and vision, and end up talking there like everyone else.'

Dr S sidesteps the beginnings of this angry charge, like a seasoned and taciturn matador:

'Well, in my case I hope that is incorrect. But I have more than myself to hold onto: my wife and family ... my mortgage is not yet paid off, and I have two teenage children still to put through university…'

Dr T is quiet again, but differently, now gently melted with fresh and protective contrition.

All is not what it seems. Citadel? Yes. Citizen? Yes, but also hostage.

Dr T imagines a conversation he would like to have with George Orwell.

*

*'Everything begins as mystique and ends as politics.'*

Graffito, Wall in Paris, Student Protest, 1968

**Ω**

## Further reading

[1] Five Executive Follies: How commodification imperils compassion in personal healthcare

[2] Further NHS Reforms: inevitable and unintended consequences. Letter to BMJ

[3] From Family to Factory: The dying ethos of personal healthcare

[4] How to help Harry – Friend or Foe? The scientific and the scientistic in the fog of the frontline

[5] Fallacies in Blunderland. Overschematic overmanagement: perverse healthcare

[6] Bureaucratyrannohypoxia. An open letter to Mental Health Services Director

[7] Words and Numbers: Servants or Masters? Caveats for holistic healthcare Part 1

[8] Edward: shot in his own interest. Technototalitarianism and the fragility of the therapeutic dance

# Language is not just Data

## it is a custodian of our humanity

Computers and informatics have become central to NHS healthcare. All experience and activity are now subject to official technical designations. This changes our communications: language becomes increasingly lackeyed to the computer's requirements. Much else is lost. What?

*'If language is not in accordance with the truth of things, affairs cannot be carried out to success.'*

Confucius, *Analects* (6th century BC)

I suppose I was lucky, but then – at some level – I chose them, too. Beyond that, and more importantly, we were all part of a culture that could accommodate – even foster – such things. My first mentors in General Practice and Psychiatry – galvanised by the just departed 1960s – were all nourished, enlivened, then enlightened by literature and philosophy. Such proclivities were not ponderous or self-conscious postures, but pursuits that were shared with a mien of quiet and unaffected pleasure. I remember many conversations where, in order to understand others better, we made wefts of contemporary pragmatic practice with illuminated threads from drama, philosophy, literature or mythology.

The then-fresh Balint movement, too, encouraged us to step up and out from our scientific base of standard diagnoses and treatments; while we recognised that these certainly helped us, they could do so only with generalities. So grounded, we were spurred to thoughtful experiment: to engage with the humanly speculative and imaginative – for these could help us, instead, with the individual: this person and this situation. To do any of this we needed to draw from a panoply of human thought and testament. Imaginative understanding of others is a kind of 'play', and for any successful foray into play we must encourage an expanded, rather than constricted, language. For sometimes it is an unusual word, simile or metaphor that catalyses greater understanding and then rapport.

Even at the most pragmatic levels of service this previous broader and richer language was more likely to capture and convey the uncodifiable untidiness of real life, the crucial vicissitudes of Practice. I recently had an unexpected reminder of this, and it is a good example. While seeing Matthew, an amiably direct, stalwart and unnervously jocular thirty-five-year-old, I rummaged through his old manual records. I found there a mechanically-typed letter from a hospital Casualty Department. It was written to me in 1980 about a toddler, Matthew. Here it is:

*"Dear Doctor*
*Matthew P, age 2 years*
*This delightful little boy was brought here on Sunday morning by his very anxious and solicitous mother. Mother was worried by an alleged fever and cough of two days' duration. Matthew himself was alert, bright-eyed, active and playful. He had no signs apart from a very mild catarrhal cough, which he didn't seem to notice!*

*Mother seems a sensible and intelligent woman, but inordinately anxious about Matthew's minor symptom. In talking to her it came to light that her own sister has recently been diagnosed with Acute Leukaemia. Understandably this has shocked and shaken the family. I had a long discussion with Mrs P in which I told her that Matthew is perfectly well apart from having a slight cold, and that her very real anxieties about her sister have unintentionally spilled over onto Matthew. I hope I have been able reassure her. I have taken the liberty of asking her to see you for follow-up.*
*Yours sincerely*
*Dr TS, CSO"*

All these years later I remember a couple of phone conversations I had with Dr TS – a warm, friendly, bantering Northern voice that conveyed intelligent pleasure in his work, its people and their welfare. Reading this letter, more than thirty years later, brought me both joy and sorrow.

The joy was humble though clear; it was the memory of such quiet, subtle suffusions of personal interconnectedness: here Dr TS had shared with me his brief connection with – but growing understanding of – Matthew, Mrs P and all her family. Matthew's slight catarrhal cough was thus given much greater human – and thus healing – meaning. This sent a gentle benign ripple across the whole matrix: we all felt better about ourselves, one another and our work. This is well-fared welfare.

But then came my sorrow, for the massive yet little-voiced loss of such things. For it is almost impossible that I would receive such a letter now. Both because of, and in spite of, the endless blizzard of electronic, data-particled e-mails transmitted from my local airport-like hospital, I have with them almost no conversations enlarging my understanding of people. Dr TS's personally sentient letter would now be replaced by an anonymised electronic, templated format. This would machine-gun me didactically with tabulated impersonal data itemising myriad aspects of the (normal) physical examination; the healthy child's measurements of oximetry, temperature and respiratory rate; the immunisation status; the social status of the child and whether Social Services' involvement has been triggered ... This surfeit of (usually) unedifying administrative detail would have neither space nor vocabulary for the brief glimpse of the importantly unobvious; the human story that gives this (non) medical scenario significant and compassionate meaning. We have lost both the personal language of healthcare and its colleagueial discourses.

Such losses coalesce, then anchor. Eventually a restricted language and format will not merely confine description, it will – hypnotically – limit our thinking and actions too. Language, thought and action are often less divisible than our analyses of them. Expansion or contraction, encouragement or proscription, nourishment or impoverishment – influence one and the others will probably change in a parallel way.

The more complex the human activity, the more this matters. We have seen, with Matthew, how language can service or disservice a relatively simple, yet humanly-complexed, medical problem. Let us take a more intricate and chronic problem. Geoff is a troubled dis-eased man in his mid-30s. Here are two accounts from an encounter he has with a psychiatrist.

## A. Patient as object. Language as designation

*G has a long history of agitated depressive illnesses with marked anxiety/panic components. Although his questionnaired depression scores were high, they were discrepant from the MDT staff's assessment. He has a poor record of maintaining work and long-term relationships. He also has problems with anger management: this was evident to the Clinic Staff when I was unavoidably delayed. This inconvenience was clearly explained to G, who nevertheless was unacceptably angry and rude to the staff in response. It is thus likely that G also has a Personality Disorder.*

## B. Patient as person. Language as understanding

*G has never recovered from the childhood terror and sorrow from his experience of father's raging cruelty, brutality, and then final desertion. G's life has been spent yearning for, but mistrusting, male support, esteem, affection and affiliation. He wants comfort from others, but fears betrayal, so disguises his needs. My lateness for his appointment seems to stir in him ancient residues of imperilled dependency, uncertainly and abandonment. His response to my greeting is staccato, flushed and tense: he seems both angry and afraid. I sense in him a conflation of fight and flight, and I think again of his wounded, early childhood.*

*

If it were you that was distressed, which doctor would you wish to tend you?

*

One definition of the success of a Specialty is that it replaces vernacular language with its own vocabulary. Thus specialisation both colonises and short-circuits common speech, replacing this with its own distillate. The losses involved vary greatly: the dehumanising potential of 'Megaloblastic Anaemia' is negligible, that of 'Depression' considerable.

Archimedes' notion of displacement is instructive far beyond the physical world: it often operates in the realms of human culture and language. The overgrowth of the technical and the schematic can all too easily – without malign design – extinguish the organic and the human. Our world of ever-increasing mass-production has many hidden taxes. There are hungry conundrae, too: how do we safeguard literature in our language, art in our (medical) science and heart in our practice?

*

*'A man is hid under his tongue'*

Ali Ibn-Ali-Tabib, *Sentences*, (7th century)

Ω

Published in *British Journal of General Practice*, March 2014

# Post Mid Staffs:

## A Plenitude of Platitudes

Mid Staffs refers to the Mid Staffordshire NHS Trust in the UK, which has been clearly exposed, in numerous cases, of flagrant and gross neglect of care of vulnerable, usually elderly, hospital in-patients. Many of the examples far exceeded privation or indifference of care, and had qualities of active cruelty, even sadism. There is much further evidence that such abuse is widespread throughout the UK NHS, though Mid Staffs may be an extreme example. While individual responsibility must always be important, the Mid Staffs debacle has raised gravely important questions about the nature, direction and ethos of UK NHS healthcare culture.

Can the harmful excesses of depersonalisation in healthcare be usefully addressed by further redesign of systems and management? Or do we need a different kind of thinking and vocabulary?

**The worse the economy, the better the economists.**

Likewise, Post Mid Staffs, we are now blessed with a tranche of experts who talk confidently of management designs that can lead us quickly to the clear, Sunlit Uplands of healthcare.

In the last week[1] we have heard, for example, from Nick Seddon,[2] Geoffrey Robinson[3] and Lord Ara Darzi.[4] All talk in a similar revelatory manner from a common stock of maxims and metaphors. Here are some: 'Greater transparency', 'opening up the cutting edge of practices', 'celebrating and rewarding success; identifying and rooting out underperformance', 'turbo-boosting quality', 'putting measurement at the heart of safety culture', 'improving workforce by enforcing links between pay and performance', 'zero tolerance of failure', 'centralised systems of reporting and review': all these sound-bitten imperatives are late seedlings of Jeremy Bentham's Prisons' *Panopticon*[5] and BF Skinner's behavioural carrots and sticks. This history of attempts to systemise and control human behaviour is instructive: limitations are evident.

What these pundits seem not to consider are the aspects of caring that involve ethos and vocation: imaginative empathy and compassionate attachment. Their offerings seem devoid of

---

[1] The week beginning 18/2/13. The quotes are taken from newspaper articles and media interviews of that week.

[2] Nick Seddon. Deputy director of Reform, an independent think-tank.

[3] Geoffrey Robinson. Businessman, management guru and TV presenter.

[4] Lord Ara Darzi, chair of the Institute of Global Health Innovation, Imperial College, London. Previously a Minister of Health.

[5] Jeremy Bentham (1748-1832) was a philosopher, jurist and social reformer. His Panopticon was a design for prisons, enabling the jailers to have constant view of all their prisoners.

any philosophy of pathos or ethos: how and why should we care for one another? What motivates altruistic transcendence?

It is such psycho-spiritual considerations that seem, to me, glaringly absent from the current debate and – most importantly – from the system we have created – the culture that then creates such dissociated, alienated atrocities in healthcare. Perversely, our pundits then offer us yet more depersonalised thinking to counter depersonalisation.

For all its more primitive technology and heterogonous management, I found my previous decades of work in NHS healthcare far more personally imaginative, responsive and respectful.

In our impatient quest for Welfare Services efficiencies, we have compressed our welfare to behave like object-spewing factories. Such industrialisation has expediently jettisoned our human attachments, connections and understandings. Offered here is an alternative assortment of maxims that can help us re-route our culture, so that we may re-root our humanity in healthcare:

## Imaginatively compassionate healthcare
## – some guiding caveats and principles

• If we like our work and find it interesting, we will do it well and willingly.
• Such liking and interest often involves the gratification of seeing our work's longer-term evolution and personal effects. Deeper satisfactions, too, are often personal and holistic: conversely, fragmented, short-term work offers little of these.
• Encouragement to draw on our experience to make intelligent creative decisions is likely to engage and develop our best qualities. Submitting to endless committee-designated diktats does not.

- We thus prefer flexible and collaborative working arrangements rather than those that are rigid, competitive and divisive.
- If we get know people well, we will be well-motivated to care for them. The more you see of someone, the more of someone you see.
- If we do not know people it is far easier not to care, or even to collude with harm: History has innumerable examples prior to Mid Staffs.
- People who feel attached, interested and positively personally engaged need relatively little disciplinary or motivational management.
- In contrast, it is very difficult to get good work from people who do not enjoy their work, feel attached or positively, personally engaged: these are primary deficits, and no amount of regulation, management, training or financial incentive will rectify them.

Looking back, I can see that it is such notions that sustained and nourished my generation of better practitioners over long, gratifying and appreciated medical careers. Such ways of thinking of, and relating to, others used to grow naturally from certain kinds of culture and education. They fare far less well in our current forced march to homogenised and hegemonised management or trainings.

Sticks, carrots and panopticons are often poor motivators for the more complex aspects of human care.

*

Healthcare is a humanity guided by science. That humanity is an art and an ethos.

*

We must beware.

Ω

# 'GPs know their Patients, Families and Communities'

## – Really?

GPs are increasingly employed as task-directed, upper-echelon *healthdroids*. They are losing the pastoral skills that depend on holistic views and vernacular understandings. Why is that?

During the first week of the new GP-led commissioned NHS, a televisioned young doctor offered this GP-led soundbite: 'GPs know their patients, families and communities.'

Really?

My experiences as a long-serving GP, and as a recently signed-up patient, are very different. Your GP is now likely to be part-time, short-term and serving in a multi-doctored practice where *personal* continuity is increasingly rare. You are thus likely to see a doctor you have never seen before, and when you see them they may see even less of you, as they will probably spend more time looking at the computer screen. Commuting to work, they are unlikely to have a personal home or roots in the immediate neighbourhood. They may develop some knowledge of one of your 'conditions', but almost none about your nature, story, family or life-milieu. They are most unlikely to know your kin. The better among the previous generation of 'Family Doctors' responded well to all of these. They mentored me; I witnessed this, just as I now see its disappearance.

There are many causes for this loss of more personal healthcare. Among some of the avoidable causes are: the managerial hostility to small practices (favouring large impersonal conglomerates), the abolition of Personal Lists (thus devolving the interested responsibility of a particular doctor to a large, generic 'Team'), the sub-contraction of Out of Hours services to agencies (that are unlikely to have any personal knowledge or bond at times of greatest vulnerability and need), the increasing use of shorter-term, sessional, commuting staff (who have no vernacular knowledge, roots or interest in the locality). How can doctors working in these conditions develop personal and holistic understandings of any length and depth?

Doctors are not unique in this disinheritance. *Postman Pat* used to be a reassuring hub of the community; a fount of local human and geographic knowledge. Alas, our postman now is often only recently employed, a new immigrant, and himself, lost and asking for directions…

Marketisation cannot buy or commission the kinds of bonds, understandings and communities that constitute the human heart of healthcare. But marketisation can destroy them.

Ω

# Hello, Health Commissioner. Goodbye, Family Doctor?

## The new healthcare reforms and their threat to personal doctoring

The idea, now diktat, that GPs should lead the complex provision of healthcare for localities may subtract more than it adds to overall health-welfare. How and why could this happen?

*'Simplicity is the most deceitful mistress that ever betrayed man.'*

Henry Adams, The Education of Henry Adams (1907)

Today, the first day of the new era of GP-led NHS commissioning, I saw a young GP on the television. She was interviewed to sample a voice of professional support and enthusiasm for the just-hatched, reformed regime. She spoke with an authoritatively quiet manner and an assured economy of phrase. She said: 'GPs know their patients, families and neighbourhoods.' A think-tank pundit, later in the programme, said much the same. Their views sounded solidly sincere, weighted with the calm dullness of uncontentious fact. On reflection, though, what I heard was specious – optimistic and plausible sounding, but substantially misleading: for GPs' personal knowledge of patients is increasingly short and shallow.

Yes, their assertion was once true, yet even then only selectively so: of the better and more vocational GPs, until about twenty years ago. I was mentored by that kind of doctor: they mostly served smaller (than now) practices, full-time, often for several decades. This combination of smallness of scale, ethos of vocation and length of time-span made much easier certain kinds of personal bonds and understanding: these were dyadic (the doctor and his patient), familial (the patient and their family) and vernacular (their particular world, beyond the family boundary). So, yes, it is true that those kinds of doctors and their patients, in that generation, could more easily develop an informal and often inexplicit understanding of one another. Certainly I witnessed many times how these could, with quiet and subtle patience, lead to gratifying and healing encounters. For about three decades these natural nexae of healthcare developed – were fuelled by and then created – a vigorous culture of person-centred discussion and literature. The Balint movement was a good example of the flowering of this and its subsequent neglect.

The dissolution of this humanly networked healthcare started, then accelerated, from the beginning of the 1990s – the time of the first substantial computerisation and attempts at (internal) marketisation. This rationalisation has had many effects that few had anticipated or intended.

What has this led to? To healthcare far more able with generic management than with personal connection and understanding. True, this is variable and most evident in large (as most now are) hospitals. It may be less true in General Practice, but still a serious and growing problem: doctors and patients are increasingly personally unknown to one another.

What does this look like? Often now, GPs do part-time, shorter-term work in ever-larger centres. These populous, busy conurbations are more like the milling milieux of a contemporary airport then the personal refuge of an erstwhile Family Doctor. In these large health centres doctors engage a world that has turned increasingly computercentric: in the waiting room in many surgeries the patient is not now greeted by a receptionist, but by electronic self-registration on a touch-screen. Then, in the characterless consulting room, the doctor is incrementally yoked to centrally-determined, computer-designated impersonal tasks and an endless incoming tide of e-mails: in this cybersurgery colleagues and other staff become more accessible to electronic signalling than natural conversation. This computercentric abstraction and anomie leaches to patients, too. Consultations often rapidly default to an administratively correct form of data-harvesting or officially despatched response. The patient's unique voice is not really heard, the unspoken not imagined, their face not remembered. The computer may provide images of the abstract that too easily replace other realities.

We now have little literature, or even talk, of the vagaries of *relationships* in medical practice: the very real and fertile, yet so-often-elusive, heart of our work: three decades ago such personal understandings were regarded as essential staples, or vital keys to therapeutic contact. But such notions cannot be easily measured, standardised or mass-produced: they have been bulldozed aside by notions that can. The result is an unstoppable data-blizzard, an errant sophistication that will often blind our view of people.

The infusion of commercial and industrial maxims into healthcare is thus wide-ranging but unequally obvious. The previous example considered the problems arising from abstracting complex human problems into formulaic forms of quantifiable data. This has become nearly universal and thus cultural: easily seen and expediently accepted. Other, more particular aspects, are more easily overlooked: the little recognised yet massively influential abolition of GP Personal Lists is a good example. This little-consulted measure – to ease administrative facility and tidiness – has been widely destructive of person-centred GP bonds. It has led to an anomie where doctors and patients increasingly become strangers to one another. We lose the myriad and humbly unique personal understandings and investments – and then the gratifications and therapeutic possibilities that can emerge from these. The system may look tidy, but people feel lost … and it is not just the patients.

*

So it is a sparse but diminishing truth that most GPs 'know their patients, families and neighbourhoods'. The reality is starker and harder.

*

Yet more trouble awaits us. For the contentious suitability for GPs to *lead* the commissioning will become more knotted (and notted) as it evolves. In previous times GPs' personal knowledge of people and their networks made them a valuable resource to be *consulted* for planning and management: paradoxically this was then little used. Perversely, now that GPs' special sentience has almost been destroyed, these semi-blinded, administratively-weary GPs are now commanded to *manage* the planning and management. Whatever little attention and interest GPs are now able to pay to the personal aspects of care will be further displaced and eroded by these new managerial demands. For the more doctors' heads and diaries are crammed with meetings, e-mails, action-lists, data, agendae, pie-charts, flow-charts, deadlines and algorithms, the less creative and personal attention they can pay to the people who come to them (or themselves).

The GP who is caught in hostile and litigated negotiations about tendered tariffs for hip-replacement surgery is far less likely to perceive or understand the significance of the recent death of a cat to a childless, lonely, elderly widow whose husband died last year. Such is a typical scenario from the near-future. Care needs certain kinds of imaginative receptivity. The time and space for these are easily crowded out. How do we ensure that the Healthcare Commissioner does not finally asphyxiate the Family Doctor?

*

Healthcare is a humanity guided by science.

*

We must beware.

*

'Seek simplicity, but always mistrust it.'

Alfred North Whitehead (1861-1947)

Ω

Publ. by *BMJ Group Blogs*, 7/6/13

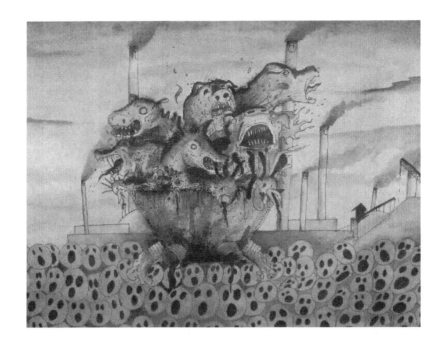

W. Hayemann – *Factory Farming*

# Our Welfare is ill-fared by yet more strictures and structures

Surely, all Welfare professionals should forever be more strictly appraised and registered? Here are some reasons why not.

Tristram Hunt, Shadow Education Secretary, recently vaunted a policy to improve our state schools: that all teachers should be regularly and strictly appraised and licensed, as is now routine in the medical profession. This may seem overdue and briskly sensible. Yet wider experience shows that such plans and their consequences are often bewilderingly discrepant. This is a brief survey of that discrepancy.

We can probably all agree on our starting point: a wish for our Welfare professionals to have good personal, technical and ethical standards and skills. The crystallising rhetoric is always appealing and easy to construct. How to foster and assure these human qualities proves considerably trickier. What goes wrong, and why?

As a long-serving GP I have been increasingly witness and subject to this process: to managerially quality assure all NHS doctors. The results often turn paradoxically perverse: the laudable intent rapidly degrading into a bureaucratic maze of procedures, passable only by 'correct' statements of compliance. This rapid transition from aspirational to bureaucratic is now a common welfare anomaly and leaves a long wake of leaden consequences. For our consequent coagulations of acquiescence then obstruct the possibility of any more searching or authentic dialogue. Most doctors expediently practise recitation of the required protocols, shibboleths and submissions: this is called 'Preparing for an Appraisal'. The appraisal itself is usually undertowed and subtexted by compounds of fearful obedience, pragmatic stoicism or concealed resentment. In such a coercive charade how can anything real or useful be exchanged between practitioners and their governing bodies?

So, such formulaic attempts to govern welfare turn heavy, blunt and blind. Their success is restricted, possibly, to the most egregious or wilful failures of standards: the obvious ones. Our public safeguards have thus frequently relegated themselves to mere theatres of hegemony. This is an excellent current example of how, with good intent, substantial NHS time and resources are squandered. Goodwill is an early but lasting casualty.

Longer-term damage accrues insidiously: it is now wide and deep. For excessive and clumsy hegemony begets fearful compliance – and then the human terrain turns barren; our personal habitat becomes unable to nourish or sustain creative spirits of personal vocation and its gratifications. This is important because our best Welfare evolves from a delicate blend of self-responsible freedom and inner discipline. Clearly this kind of inner growth and balance cannot be simply conjured by yet more external rules.

Throughout Welfare our planners and politicians have lost sight of an important natural and human principle. It is this: people who like their work, generally, will want to do it well, and will need relatively little management. Conversely, those who do not like their work will be inveterately resistant to all management initiatives – be they payments, inducements, trainings, threats, goals, targets or deadlines. In Welfare particularly the nature of our human input cascades and amplifies: so, an increasing plethora of remote controls and formulaic edicts will produce demoralised and officious practitioners. Throughout education and pastoral healthcare, our positive influence comes more from attitude and morale than technical compliance and qualifications.

In NHS healthcare such principles are often disregarded in the stentorian 'driving up standards': the price we pay is akin to a stress-related internal haemorrhage. For example, we can readily adapt the imperative to eliminate the small number of severely substandard or rogue practitioners. But how do we do this without an even greater loss amongst the remainder: of morale, trust, goodwill and empathic vocation – the natural springs of professional humanity, colleagueial beneficence and thence good Welfare? For those doubting the seriousness of this question: look at the statistics about Welfare services workers –

these indicate clear and rapid rises in sickness, intrainstitutional litigation, career abandonment and early retirement. These are the human costs of disregarding such questions. Hence it is that the excess and heaviness of our management is ill faring our own welfare.

This wide range of evidence converges back to an observable truth that should now be a truism, but in our hustling business we have become heedless to. It thus merits reiterating: frustrated and etiolated Welfare professionals are unlikely to work well or to stay long. Our mounting healthcare debacles are yet another alarming reason for us to revisit and restore our investment in human connection and understanding – for this is the provenance of any wholesome realm of human care. These lessons may be currently sharpest in healthcare, but are seminal throughout our Welfare services.

To understand and nourish one another better in our indefatigably industrial world we must know when to take our hand off the ratchet and our foot off the accelerator.

$$\Omega$$

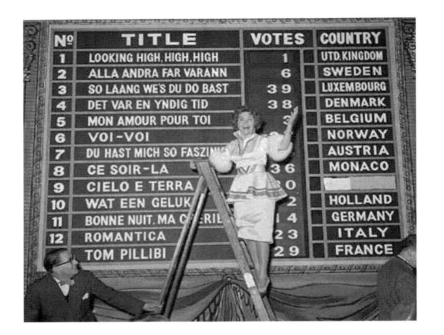

# Bingo!
# Majoritarian Healthcare!

## Early auguries for GP Commissioning

Transparency, Accountability and Democracy can seem like a protective triumvirate for public decision making, but these can easily turn shallow, demotic and false. Here is a small example of what is coming.

*'We do not wish ardently for what we desire only through reason'*

La Rochefoucald (1665), *Maxims*

## I have seen the future, and I want to go back to bed.

Recently I attended the first working meeting of our GP Clinical Commissioning Group. At the end of a working day, many dozens of GPs sat with, mostly, fatigued and bovine obedience as we were guided through some power-pointed-slick but humanly-dull portrayals: first of our barren yet hazardous current financial terrain, and then the administrative and constitutional complexities of the organisation we have been corralled to devise, our Clinical Commissioning Groups. The obedience was due to an unspoken ultimatum: manage or perish. The new commissars – like emperors' messengers – did their best to sound determined and positive. But their efforts sounded, to me, like staged postures of will rather than currents of real enthusiasm. The complexity of the topics was more than most of these tired GPs could readily engage with or assimilate. Deadened eyes and slumped postures indicated bodily presence but mental absence. Be present or be disappeared.

\*

After being given this map of the new order we were set our first task: to decide on which local healthcare problems we should prioritise. We were all sat at round tables of about ten doctors; each table had a predesignated leader. Each person was given the same paper-list of thirty healthcare problems with brief explanatory notes as to their putative importance. All groups were instructed to peruse and discuss this list and then, individually, to choose the four we considered more important, and then rank them. Each person then clicked buttons on issued electronic devices to silently transmit their ranked choices. A giant electronic smart-board very quickly collated and summarised these ranked, and thus top four, collectivised priorities for all participants. We were given twenty-five minutes to reflect on, discuss and decide from among these thirty healthcare problems.

*

I was uneasy with this, for in my experience, and to my mind, *all* of the problems had interesting and hidden complexity, and also unobvious connections. To any one of them I could extend many hours of exploratory thought and discussion. But this is agribusiness, not organic farming; and our professional tables have become like cattle-pens. Quick herding and milking is what is required. Intelligent discussion is an irksome and irrelevant procrastination: prompt and quantified results are the goal. I demur, attempting to point out that this ingenious and rapid mass-choreography is very discrepant with the subtle complexity of the tasks. But I am sidelined as an eccentric anomaly because by now the computer is proclaiming the GPs' collective decision. And the chairman – an affable, gracious and intelligent man – now has a nervous stage-smile as he constructs some kind of blessing for us all and our new project.

*Bingo!* We have Majoritarian Healthcare.

*

I understand the chairman's attempted glow of beneficence. He had carefully planned and completed this first step onto the new staircase to locality democracy: one based on transparency, accountability and democracy. Yes, I respect the intent behind this, but doubt what it yields. For these tired and over-multitasked GPs are slewing into speedy, whimsical, expedient decisions – responding to a mandate and under time constraints. They are making such judgements, and in such a manner, because they are told to, not because they want to or have felicitous wisdom. Also, importantly, they want to go home. The depth, form and rapidity of evaluations reminds me of the *Eurovision Song Contest* (ESC): I fear our collectivised wisdom will make a similar quality of contribution to healthcare culture as the ESC makes to Music. I share this as a comic yet serious comment: many look (or pretend to look) perplexed, a few laugh with joyous relief and release, more speak to me afterwards: 'I'm really pleased you said that ... I really agree, but no, I don't want to step out of line ... I have to safeguard my job...'

Everything has its price. Sometimes we do not want to see the bill. Yet someone will have to pay.

*

How did our Health Service work before such attempts at internal markets and local autarkies? In the older, more federal, more macro-socialist system – say thirty years ago – who decided priorities and payments? And how? It seems to me that few knew then, and far fewer know now. As a young practitioner I had a few glimpses that formed an impression that has since been subject to decades of decay. Yet some recent archaeological research supports my memories. My recovered impression is this: the NHS was run by wise Mandarins. These were usually experienced, older, intelligent, thoughtful, little-known Civil Servants. They were unideological, though principled; unpartisan though committed to their task; non-specialist though could quickly understand the different assumptive worlds. They often provided high quality diligent service for a working lifetime in a world not yet insistent on visible indices of transparency, accountability and democracy.

Such an opaque, inscrutable and unelected system lasted for decades: it should have been a scandal. And yet it now looks as if such a potentially incompetent and corrupt regime managed their smaller world with quietly competent beneficence, and with much smaller resources.

For me this earlier mandarin-managed service was – compared to now – a blessing of stability, sense and sensibility, pragmatic flexibility and accessible authority. It certainly was not perfect and there were some stupid or bad practitioners, but the *systems* were not stupid or bad. The systems now are frequently both, stymying even the better practitioners' competence, efficiency and humanity.

\*

We are now driven by systems with good moral rhetoric but poor human understanding and connection. This is a fascinating and cruel paradox. How do we account for it? Here we must enter the world of speculative, motivational and group psychology – an exploration beyond this writing. The following though – a seemingly unlikely parallel – may be edifying. I present it as a question: Why are Northern European elected republican presidents so often corrupt or criminal; by comparison, why are Northern European unelected constitutional monarchs usually so diligent and respected? If we understand this we can perhaps understand a little more of what is most unstraightforwardly important about humankind.

\*

*'The truth is rarely pure and never simple'*

Oscar Wilde (1895), *The Importance of Being Earnest*

Ω

Published by *Open Democracy*, 2013 as 'NHS Decisions, Euro-vision-style'

# Form Devouring Essence

## When brokered services
## tend broken hearts

Our healthcare rhetoric of data and systems has largely destroyed our capacity to make the kind of personal bonds that understand and heal human dissonance. Stephen and his plight serve to illustrate and explore this.

## 1. A Prologuing Parable

*'What would you like, Dali?' says Ali, from behind the Pizza Bar.*
*The Dalai Lama squints and marvels at the long list of offered combinations.*
*'I want One with Everything!' he replies, throwing his arms wide in rapture, to suggest Infinity.*
*Preparation takes Ali some time and the box is made up specially, the largest he has ever used.*
*To pay for it the Dalai Lama gives Ali the largest banknote he can procure and then waits, patiently at first.*
*'Can I have my change, Ali?' he asks eventually.*
*Ali sighs softly and shakes his lowered head slowly, with muted sorrow and disappointment: 'Oh! Dali! You, of all people, should know not to ask for this; that all Change must come from Within.'*

The Tibetan Book of the Dudes 7th century BC, upgraded and rebranded version, 2014

## 2. Form devouring essence

Stephen's origins fifty years ago were chaotic and prophetic: an accidental conception by a young, brief and impulsive coupling. The unreceptive conceivers hurried to expediently jettison their conception: father rapidly for oblivion; mother bridled until Stephen's birth, then passing him to her own parents for care.

Stephen's early childhood was thus repaired and reprieved for a few, and the most, secure years of his life. Mother then met another partner and thought the omens were now right to start a more deliberate family. Through contention, then acrimony, then litigation between mother and her own parents, Stephen was removed from his grandparental loving home and returned to his parental and capricious source. Fate was not kind to any of the converged players in this new act: mother never had another live birth, and stepfather's geniality of promise turned to a sullen resentment of envious disappointment. The knot tightened and darkness gathered: indifference turned to sarcasm, slashing words conflated with beating fists and bodily shakings. Stephen shook, retroflected and planned escape. For her own security, mother colluded with power. Stephen left home age fifteen looking for some predictable and protective influence. He soon joined the Army.

Stephen never really found the peace or inclusion he craved. In his early adult life he lost himself in sports, macho banter, the consoling hazes of alcohol, drugs and thence to sexual deliria, with little-known partners. A brief marriage first absorbed such continuing assaults, then listed, capsized and sank, leaving a vengefully confused ex-wife adrift, huddling for comfort and buoyancy with their two sons. Stephen's growing awareness of how he was, in many ways, re-enacting his own abject beginnings was more than he could bear: he sought further escape through the only routes he knew – from the comforts that drew in his nemesis …

In his forties Stephen's life is slowing and he is beginning to see more clearly the pattern of his personal carnage. He tries to rebuild, but finds that this is akin to footholding sliding shale.

By his late forties his old defences are in terminal decline. His distress can no longer be distracted or buttressed and far exceeds his vocabulary. His signalling becomes urgent, intense, scrambled and uncontained. Dread, rage, guilt, fear, grief, shame, contrition all jostle to inhabit his confused and alienated loneliness. His offered quanta of anguish are inchoate and polymorphous: insomnia, panics, overwhelming physical symptoms – without – signs for the doctors, the sense that his mind and body are sometimes exploding and other times imploding and then colonised by others, consoling or persecuting superstition, bleak and suicidal despair, his fear of harming those that venture care or closeness: all are presented to A&E departments, Walk-In Centres, Out of Hours call centres, thence to Psychiatric Services and, finally, his new GP, me.

*

Stephen enters my room and my life for the first time seeming turbulent and adrift. I fine-tune the signals: I think I discern a mistrustful yearning for affection, inclusion and reassurance. An unbidden image fleets my mind: of a storm-tossed, mast-broken caique limping into the shelter of a small harbour. All of this is communicated to me wordlessly and will-lessly: I have intuition for his story – history – but this is not yet tethered by details. When disclosed, such details coalesce to warn of the difficulty of our task: we will need to offer Stephen several capacious and flexible containers – hearts, minds and diaries – to quieten, nourish, and heal him. Now, forty-five years after the disintegration of his brief exposure to wholesome family life, Stephen will need the best kind of family surrogacy our Welfare Services can muster. Such belated balm for his ancient wounds will not cure him, but slowly, from outside-in, it may awaken Faith, Hope and Charity* – *Agape* – the heart of healing.

*

Who will provide such supportive and guiding scaffolding? As his GP I can play a small yet important part, but I will need much help, particularly from psychiatric services. Yet here, where I am needing easy access to a bridge, I look out instead to a chasm: there is no 'family' to receive him, just a succession of placements.

To reify the metaphor: in one year Stephen was seen by many boundarised and separate Teams. Specifically: Hospital Liaison (3), Emergency Psychiatric, Home Treatment, In-patient, Community Mental Health for Mood Disturbance, Community Mental Health for Psychosis (his protean disturbance made distinctions only administratively meaningful), Psychology: Cognitive Behaviour Therapy, Psychology: Behaviour Activation Therapy.

Very significantly Stephen does not know the name of any of the Teams and cannot recall the names of any of their practitioners.

This anomie does not daunt the sharply missioned (now commissioned) Teams – for all, it seems, have an agenda to 'cure' him or, at least, to ensure brisk progress along a relayed 'Recovery Pathway'. This process, it seems, attempts to short-circuit more primal, powerful needs: these, through personal attachments, can create individual understanding and thence a growing, deepening capacity to create positive meaning and gratifying bonds.

Over many years an underlying principle – now increasingly disregarded – has become clear to me: that desired change comes often by an indirect route. Symptoms then dissolve not through direct countervailance, assault or ablation – what some like to confidently call 'management' – but by certain kinds of attuned and resonant apposition; the deliberate fostering and protection of certain kinds of *relationship*. Such constitute the inductions of *healing*, which contrast with the conductions of *treatment*. As a young psychiatrist in the 1970s I was engaged with many such personal projects. It was humbling and unglamourised work, but had quiet, slow, deep satisfactions. It was impossible to standardise and very difficult to measure, so we did not. This did not matter then because, in healthcare, we had not yet entered a world so tightly managed and systemised. The recently emergent healthcare realms have subsequently attempted to subsume all human problems and activities to standardised codes, procedures, quantifiable data and generically packaged Care Pathways. These ensure computer-compatibility, but there is a costly undertow: Technototalitarianism.

In my early years of practice the difficult work of looking after Stephens was much more possible: I had around me a colleagueial extended 'family' for synergy and support. Often these people got to know both the patient and myself, sometimes over many years; we developed a well-fared web of personal familiarity: welfare.

Such longer, personal, confluent contact has become almost extinct. My contact now is usually once-only with a sharply-boundaried, specifically-tasked duty-desk worker or Team Leader. Like Stephen, I feel my family has gone. My work has become homeless.

*

For the last decade, since the disintegration of my colleagueial family, I have been trying to understand the riddle of our increasing personal disconnection in healthcare. This is happening both in spite of, and because of, our mandates for 'efficiency': our increasingly resourced, ratcheted and managed systemisation. How and why have we created a culture that is less able to care for Stephen than forty years ago? What do we need to reclaim?

## 3. Re-anchoring essence

I think much can be explained by a little discussed, but seminally important, shift of axioms in planning, teaching and academia throughout pastoral and mental healthcare. We have abandoned the previous flexible equilibrium between *phenomenology* (a description and clustering of how things *are*, or appear) and *semiotics* (a speculation of what things might *mean*).

The significance of this needs a little elaboration. Phenomenology is more compatible with objective and scientific discourse and explanation. In contrast, semiotics is necessary for imaginative human understanding. So, phenomenology is more concerned with treatment, while healing must draw largely from semiotics. It is the thoughtful balance and dextrous exchange between the two that makes *holism* possible. The art of medical practice and compassionate care are mostly impossible without the broad, flexible intelligence of holism.

In the last dozen years there have been influences destructive to the fragile habitat of such holism. This is largely due to an accelerated coupling of computer use to projects aiming to standardise and industrialise all healthcare. This leads ineluctably to a reductionist healthcare rhetoric: to displace semiotics (an unmeasurable art) by phenomenology (in mental and pastoral health a proto-science, easily and speciously overdeveloped).

Such projects can readily turn to follies. Indiscriminate and overzealous attempts to forge a science of manipulation will risk extinguishing the art of understanding. This becomes much more likely as our NHS services are designed to be brokered – this is now implemented by such devices as autarkic and competing Trusts, Commodifying Commissioners, Payment by Results and competitive tendering. The consequent follies thus turn what should be artful science into a cult of *scientism*: hermetic systems of technical language and data which develop like monoculture farming and become inimical to wider questions and dialogue. Commercial and organisational interests almost always will be allured by such streamlined production and tamper-proof packaging. Hence form devours essence.

What we are losing are anchoring principles: *Healthcare is a humanity guided by science. That humanity is an art and an ethos.* How do we retrieve them? We must re-establish the more fragile art of healing alongside the now oligarchic science of treatment. We must create head and heart-space for the rich vicissitudes of human bonds and understandings. We must understand and respect the fact that the heart of many of our most precious experiences and activities cannot be directly codified and measured: they require conservation of different kinds of language and thought. When we have seriously understood these we might dare to take our hand off the ratchet and our foot off the accelerator. We might then care for one another in more natural, imaginative and wholesome ways: with more sense and sensibility.

*

*Men reform a thing by removing the reality from it, and then do not know what to do with the unreality that is left.*

G K Chesterton (1928), *Generally Speaking*

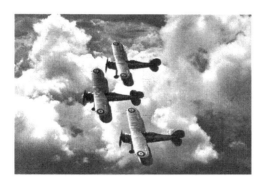

**Note**

\* *Faith, Hope* and *Charity* were the names given to three obsolescent RAF Gloster Gladiator fighter biplanes that were the only aerial defences of Malta at a crucial stage in early World War Two. Due to the skill and heroic resolve of the pilots, these three old planes warded off the vastly more numerous and modern attacking Italian Air Force. Malta occupied a pivotal position for massive opposed forces: the surrender of air-supremacy would have changed world history radically. This remarkable respite created a hiatus sufficient to shift the balance. The full significance of *Faith, Hope* and *Charity* only became clear much later: timely small acts and events can have exponential consequences. Likewise, healing also often needs opportunistic hiatuses into which faith, hope and charity may be both transmitted and take root.

Ω

Essay for mental healthcare colleagues and managers South London and Maudsley NHS Trust 2014

# Autoasphyxiation

## The doomed brief of
## GP Clinical Commissioning Groups

The corralling of GPs to design and commission health services cannot counter the inherent disintegration and depersonalisation of Marketisation. A glimpse from the frontline.

Our new GP-led Clinical Commissioning Groups (CCGs) will fail: they will be strangled by their own matrix. Here are two recent and prophetic inter-professional encounters to illustrate.

Last night I attended a CCG meeting. The genuine interest of these many GPs lags far behind their attendance record. They know the unspoken rules for survival: the human energy in the room is fatigued, desultory and acquiescent.

An executive officer is addressing us with well-worn competence. His messages are clearly sound-amplified and Power-Pointed onto the screen behind him. He is vaunting yet another, again rebranded, initiative for Integrated Care, as if an arcane group of scientists had made an exciting discovery. He profiles the many dislocations, replications and retroflections as if we do not know: we do, though not his statistics. The standing managing expert speaks: the many sitters mostly look blank – it is hard to distinguish listening from vacuous passivity. The executive winds up with authoritative courtesy: 'Any questions?' There is an inert fugal silence, like waking from a light anaesthetic. I want to galvanise my individual consciousness, so I raise my hand. I am given nodded assent to speak: 'I think you (and we) have long had good intent about these matters. But we cannot counter the massively divisive and fragmentary influence of the NHS Internal Market that embeds and commands us. This – and then its subsidiary procedures of Competition, Commissioning and Commodification – make better kinds of holistic integrated care almost impossible. All experienced, thoughtful older practitioners – who served well before the Internal Market – recognise this fact and hold this view. This toxic burden is spoken of frequently privately, yet not publicly. Can we please do so now?' The executive looks discomfited, repeatedly shifting his weight from one leg to the other as if testing his most solid posture. He clears his throat softly: 'Um ... I don't really think that is an appropriate topic for this meeting...'

He looks toward the chairman who nods support. I have little voice now, so I want to have the last word: 'So, we have no forum now where such discussion is deemed "appropriate". That is the size and nature of the problem: the official policy is of level talk and democracy, but somehow the translated reality becomes oligarchic, and then, as here, our range of discourse is controlled and prescribed.' There is a rustle of further awakening among the sitters. The chairman parries my democratic heroism with apparently effortless and deft alacrity: 'Thank you. Any more questions?'

\*

I need to loosen my tangled mental processes and re-establish blood flow to my periphery. I leave the hermetic conference room to stroll in the spacious lobby. There, a smartly attired woman is gazing into a small mirror from her handbag while finalising her make up. Jocelyn looks up at me in friendly recognition. She is another CCG Executive. I ask her what her prepared entrance is about. 'Oh', she says with diplomatic cheeriness, 'in a quarter of an hour I have to talk to all you GPs about how we can cut down inappropriate and excessive Accident and Emergency attendances. It's costing the CCG an awful lot of money, you know.' She says this, I think, with a faint tinge of accusation: that if people like me tried harder, this profligacy would be stemmed. My already streaming thoughts about the Internal Market have primed me for pre-emption: 'Jocelyn, there's only so much GPs can do. Yes, of course, we must give our best to be accessible, competent, friendly and imaginative. And then give patients timely and correct information about the correct use of Services. But to further change the pattern, we must have a very different quality of relationships within our enormous and increasingly divided Health Service. Our current system makes genuinely collaborative and cooperative work almost impossible. We certainly need to retrieve such colleagueial confederation in what you're about to talk about...'

Jocelyn looks openly and genuinely puzzled: 'In what way?'

I was expecting the question: 'Because the Internal Market is divisive, and division is the opposite of integration. Yes, we want to "save money" by keeping patients away from hospital A&E departments, but the hospitals want to "make money" by treating "our" patients there and then charging our Trust for their services. So in this commercialised, competitive healthcare system all the Trusts have to pour in money and professional time, attention and guile to stop the competing Trusts gaining advantage and control. In this kind of endless tug-of-war how can we assure our better qualities and energies? How can we perform our subtle, longer-viewed human welfare work? Welfare is not business. Providing people with good urgent care and advice often depends on making good, trusting relationships not only with them, but also between us – the healthcarers. We're doing increasingly badly with the relationships...' I pause. 'The Internal Market is ill-faring our Welfare', I summarise with, I think, pithy bombast.

'Oh, *that*!' she says, as if irritated by familiarity. 'You can't change *that*. We're much too far down the line to do anything about it. You're right, but nobody's going to listen to you. The system is far too entrenched and massive...' Her voice wearies, she looks away and her shoulders sag a little.

'Well, the Soviet Communist system looked pretty formidable for six decades, and then it rapidly crumbled...' I venture, trying to regain her interest or alliance.

Her shoulders rise and her voice sharpens. Her look is direct, strong and warmly ironic: 'Six decades might be rather long for me. I have a family, a home, a job, and I want to keep them. With my work I'll do what I can, but there's no point my destroying myself trying to change what I cannot.'

My democratic heroism limpens.

Jocelyn with stalwart expedience enters the humanly packed and brightly lit conference hall. I escape in the opposite direction: a fugitive, alone and into the dark, humanly vacated and silent car park.

This time, with Jocelyn, I do not insist on having the last word. She knows what I want to say: it would be clumsy and churlish.

Ω

Published by *Open Democracy*, 2014

# Neglect in NHS Healthcare?

## We have turned families into factories

The dissolution of family-like configurations in healthcare staffing has impoverished the health and welfare of staff and patients alike.

In December the Daily Telegraph published a letter by eight senior surgeons, which was disturbing in its wider importance (*Surgical teamwork*, 14/12/13). They wrote of how the quality and competence of NHS surgical care has been stymied by successive moves to fragmentation and devolution. Equally significant, they refer to the resulting widespread practitioners' work frustration and dissatisfaction.

Their arguments are pertinent to all areas of NHS healthcare where problems are not simply and speedily resolved: for it is here that personal continuity and investment greatly help accuracy and sensitivity of response. My own areas of practice – as a long-serving GP and Psychiatrist – have witnessed a similar degradation of personally connected and responsible culture.

In their letter the surgeons hark back to now extinct clinical 'firms' which better enacted now-imperilled values: of a personal healthcare ethos. The consultant-led firm, then had its own designated staff, clinic and ward, and was responsible (with rare exceptions) for the total arc of care from initial diagnosis and assessment to surgery, recovery and follow-up. Within this system patients felt more identified, understood and cared for; professional staff shared this, too, in deeper, subtle work satisfactions.

The good surgical firm was like a well functioning family, where the consultant had both directing and nurturing parental functions. This had parallels elsewhere in the NHS: for example, with Medical and Psychiatric firms and the erstwhile small practice family doctor. In all of these, personal investment, responsibility and connection were anchoring professional principles.

In the last two decades – apparently in the interests of mass managed efficiency – we have first not recognised the merits of such 'familial' systems and then pushed them aside in favour of more industrial and commercial modus operandae. We have replaced the spirit of the *family* almost entirely with that of the procedure of the *factory*.

Most veteran doctors of my generation take a similar view to the eight senior surgeons. We see that most of the layers of NHS reorganisation have been expensive follies, both humanly and economically. This is true especially where competition, commissioning and commodification are used to subcontract and devolve. This almost always fragments and depersonalises care.

We have little influence on demographic changes and, maybe, European Working Time directives. But there are other destructive factors we can abolish or substantially revise. Among these are primarily the NHS Internal Market, and then such subordinate devices as autarkic Trusts, Commissioning, payment by results and excessively numerous and boundaried sub-specialties.

Most of healthcare – even surgery – is more of a human interaction than a manufactured commodity. Industry and commerce can only provide very restricted guidance in our complex care of others: Welfare. Our heedlessness of this principle lies behind the broad span of our healthcare malaise: from disgruntled senior surgeons to our Mid Staffs nemesis.

It is the family ethos of Welfare that must command the systems – efficiency of the factory. Not the other way round.

$$\Omega$$

# Section Three

# What we may do

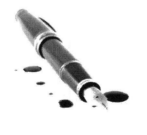

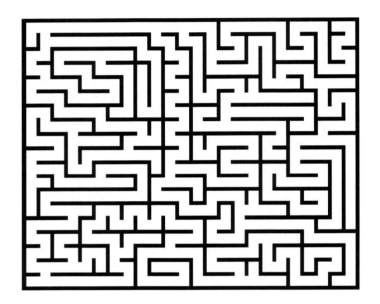

# Bureaucratyrannohypoxia

## An open letter to
## Mental Health Services Director

Dear Director of Mental Health Services

**My experience with an urgent psychiatric problem: an instructive example of current institutional complexity, rigidity and unresponsiveness. Bureaucratyrannohypoxia**

In a recent phone call, I described briefly a fresh episode to you. It seemed (to me) a good example of the rising tide of depersonalised, procedural complexity. This burgeoning is burdensome: obstructive to sensible, sensitive, attachment-respectful care. It is often confusing, frustrating and disheartening for professionals, patients and possibly (even) managers. It is very expensive.

Before time submerges memory, I want to record this episode, and some of my thoughts about it. The episode is one of many: I choose just one, for focus and dissection.

My detail is very deliberate: please take your time.

## 1. The Prelude

Early one afternoon (in June 2010) I am telephoned by the mother of a 39-year-old woman. The mother herself is clearly fearful and distressed by convergent difficulties gathering around her daughter: "Ellie is crying all the time … she won't eat and yesterday got drunk (again) … she was doing so well until she foolishly and briefly tried to get back together with Omar (ex-partner) … Just one night, but she accidentally got pregnant … She was shocked and realised it was a terrible mistake. She had a Termination, but when Omar found out, he 'went mental' with rage and broke her arm so badly she had to have complicated operations, and now cannot use it … She can't look after her little boy (Sam, age 4), so my sister is looking after him … Ellie says her life is so useless and painful, she'd rather not have it … I've got a disabled husband: I can't stay with her … She doesn't want to go into hospital, she's had bad experiences there … Can you help us, Doctor? …"

*

Ellie joined my GP list three months ago. I had seen her twice for routine appointments. She told me she was a 'refugee' from an acrimoniously broken relationship with Omar, and had moved across London to create both distance and defensible space. My more psychiatric questions clarified a pattern of several years' fluctuating Reactive Depression and spasmodic alcoholic consolation. She told me of her failed attempts to make a durable, loving bond with a man. Each ended with a variety of hurt, abuse, betrayal and derogation. It needed little prompting for her to talk of the developmental roots of this: her descriptions of a charismatic, powerful but sarcastic and alcoholically violent father; a cravenly collusive and melancholically abstracted mother. Her manner was naïve, warm, submissively apologetic, distressed and affecting. She was tearfully and copiously grateful for my interest in her current dilemma and its history, both recent and ancient. I realised how important quality and continuity of personal care would be for her. While re-prescribing her established anti-depressants, I communicated this to her: as her GP I offered her both periodic anchorage and guided-support across her Sea of Troubles. I talked with her of possible help from longer-term Counselling and Alcohol Services. We conjured and glimpsed future possible scenarios from a rebuilt life. She left me, both times, with a moist-eyed smile and a proffered, warm, firm handshake.

*

My urgent visit to her revealed rapid disintegration. Having retreated into her bed and nightclothes, her chaotic and spasmodic speech was rent further by anguished sobbing. Her physical needs and safety were provided by her mother, now buckling under the heavy contagion of distress. Despite the intense level of emotional disturbance, I was able to establish sufficient recognition, communication and alliance with Ellie to calm and contain them both. I held her hand, to gently push out a fragile bridge to the small island in Ellie that could think and speak clearly. We established that she was so overwhelmed by her life-events, and her distress, that she could no longer competently care for herself and would need supervised care, until recovery. I told them I would try to arrange this for her, at home. I then returned to my surgery, to record a diagnostic formulation that would be required from the Mental Health Team(s).

'Acute Severe Schizoaffective Reaction/Agitated Reactive Depression (choose either). Risk to Self only (probably undeliberate). Co-operative/motivated to help. Previous binge-drinking. Needing immediate supervised care (at home, if possible). Complex and chronic emotional/family/relationship problems: will need much reconstructive psych. work later.'

That would do.

## 2. Complex Times: The Institutional Response 2010

On arriving back at my surgery I ring my Community Mental Health Team for contact details and procedural advice. I am given these, and contact the Crisis Team Manager, after much delay, via a Paging Service. The eventual telephone contact is one of a unilateral pro-forma interrogation (of me), rather than any kind of colleagueial dialogue. Her questions are formulaic, and I have the sense that the questioner is guided more by institutional rules than relevant experience. At the end of her questions she tells me that a member of her Team would be able to visit at an unspecified time within the next four hours and that it is essential that I am present, for the safety of her staff. I tell her that Ellie is forlorn and passively imploded: she is a possible hazard only to herself, not imminently and only indirectly. Also this institutional safeguard takes no account of my other work: I have a busy Practice to run.

The young manager is curt and adamant: Team Policy is not negotiable. We are at an impasse: it is impossible for me to comply. I now fractiously ask if she has any ideas as to how I may get Ellie urgently cared for, at home. She brightens with a nascent possibility: if I send Ellie to St Thomas' A&E Department after 6 pm, she will be seen by the OOH Emergency Psychiatric Team there, and they will assess her, and my suggestion.

*

After 6 pm I manage to contact the Duty Psychiatrist after much searching via the Hospital Switchboard. I tell him the outline of the current crisis and some selected antecedents. He is sympathetic in manner and pragmatic in plan. I do not tell him of my freshly-exited impasse with the Crisis Team, lest this somehow invalidates my request. He cordially suggests I send Ellie to A&E, where someone from the Emergency Team will assess her. A much briefer but much more dialogic and helpful phone call, this. I express my relief and gratitude.

*

I now call Ellie: her mother answers, fatigued and expectant. I outline the plan. She responds with realistic despondency and deferral: "Ellie's now exhausted and asleep ... She's in no state to go to hospital and wait around for someone to ask her lots of questions. Can I take her tomorrow, after she's had a night's sleep?" This deferral makes sense to me, though I simultaneously sense my unfair frustration with their lack of 'compliance' to The System.

I call back the hospital Duty Psychiatrist and tell him of these developments. She will arrive the next morning at A&E. I will fax a letter with some helpful background and my reasons for recommending Home Treatment, by the Emergency Team who can assess her in A&E.

No, he says. Do not send a letter as this will be received within ordinary working hours, deemed a procedurally incorrect GP referral, returned to me with the instruction to re-contact the Crisis Team and start again. However, if I get the patient and mother to attend A&E, and make no mention of all our prior communications, it would be treated as a fresh self-referral and not sent back to me. As co-conspirator, he is inventive and supportive: he knows The System. Such stealth and deceit is essential to procure what I know is necessary for Ellie. And to return home that night. It has taken me 2½ hours.

The time later taken by Staff in A&E, and later by the Home Treatment Team, merely to assess and decide, would be much longer.

### 3. Simpler Times: The Institutional Response 1970s-80s

From the early 1970s I have had several decades working in, and then alongside, psychiatric services (the latter as a Principal GP). The response I now describe is drawn from many similar incidents in this earlier period, in which I was either active, or witness to. It is typical of the better practice of the time. The scenario is thus a fictitious graft of those old experiences onto my more recent problem with Ellie.

\*

After seeing Ellie at home, I immediately phone Dr G, the Consultant Psychiatrist at Highmount Mental Hospital. Dr G is aged about 50, and has been a consultant there for ten years. He has got to know many of the GPs on his patch and is interested in, and respectful of, the very different psychological qualities, styles and abilities that the different practitioners bring to the encounters with complex emotional distress. We have had warm and efficient problem-exchanges several times over five years. I sense he has a good sense of my human and professional strengths, deficits and (I secretly hope) vulnerabilities.

When I call Highmount I am initially put through to Linda, his secretary. She has a bright, alert and friendly manner and is clearly interested in her work. We immediately recognise the other's voice: we have a short bantering diversion, the kind of safe familiarity that keeps morale and relationships buoyant in turbulent waters. I tell Linda about my patient Ellie, in outline, and what I am hoping Dr G will arrange. She tells me that Dr G is busy on the Wards, and that he will call me in an hour.

Dr G calls me as arranged. It is calming and reassuring to hear his voice. Linda has briefly briefed him, and he invites me to tell him what else I think is most salient. His few questions are intelligently chosen, from long and wide experience. He understands a complex situation with graceful and subtle speed. My conversation with him has lasted only five minutes, but it is full and consummate.

He will get Ellie visited in the next couple of hours, he says. He's not sure who will go, either himself or his trusty, long-affiliated CPN, Patrick. Either Patrick or Dr G will call me the next morning and let me know what they have decided and implemented.

Dr G makes his expected second call to me. He had visited and spoken to Ellie and her mother for about half an hour: it was harrowing, affecting contact, and the time taken matched what he needed to know, as well as the sufferers' near-exhausted emotional resources. They had all agreed to try caring for her at home, unless she deteriorated. Patrick would visit daily, and would also liaise with Social Services. Dr G would revisit later in the week. The usual medications were specified and prescribed. Another short but full colleagueial dialogue: concise, companionable, accommodating, flexible and satisfying.

## 4. Comparisons, contrasts and comments

These different scenarios will be familiar to all older Practitioners who have retained memory and interest. Likewise, I believe, my frustrations and critique. The following brief comments are fairly random. Some problems I identify may have become insoluble: I hope I am wrong.

The old system of Consultant General Psychiatrist-managed small teams covering In-Patients, Out-Patients, Domiciliary Visiting and (even) Long-Stay wards was much more intelligently responsive, interpersonally continuous and economically-efficient. (I would accept that only better Consultant-teams from that era support my argument.)

Senior Psychiatrists in that earlier period were, when appointed, usually both more widely experienced and older than is now the case: Consultant Psychiatrists typically started their tenure aged about 40 years, having worked for many years as Physicians or General Practitioners, before turning to Psychiatry.

The equivalent today is a Practitioner almost ten years younger, with often very little medical experience. Furthermore, the psychiatric experience they have had is likely to expose them more to academic or managerial meetings, and far less to the complexities of longer-term understanding and response to individual anguish. The contemporary Consultant is thus likely to be algorithmically well-trained, but interpersonally (and Clinically) sparsely experienced and educated. This statement does not reflect the innate calibre of the practitioners, rather the consequences of the systems that train and employ them. The economics and design of training and services are now subsumed excessively to the Medical Model and a derivative Commissioning Economy. These tend to confer specious order and authority to situations poorly understood or engaged with. It is easy to understand the allure of thinking and language that seems to provide such speedy definition and clarity. In my view it usually requires considerable clinical experience to develop a subtle understanding of the limitations of the Medical Model, in order to be able to selectively and competently discard it; to make way for the more creatively empathic and imaginative aspects of growth and healing.

'Assessments' and 'Treatments' are often administered by inexperienced Multi-Disciplinary Team Practitioners, who are themselves programmed, strictured and structured by algorithms, guidelines or diktats from NICE, relevant Trusts, etc. These commissarial imperatives are themselves navigated almost entirely via the Medical Model and the Commissioning Economy.

I have an endless stream of examples of inexperienced MDT workers conducting lengthy, formulaic assessments, leaving an indigestible, long trail of bureaucracy and documentation. Amidst such dogged (sometimes zealous) compliance to The System, the patient feels exhausted, overpowered and unheard. This pattern is conveyed to me regularly. Paradoxically, the inflexible overuse of the Medical Model seems more likely with younger Clinical Psychologists, OTs, Social Workers, RMNs, etc, perhaps because they are prone to use the model anxiously and defensively. Spectres of Medical incompetence or negligence are so much easier to tame or side-step after lengthy and substantial Clinical experience. In my view these kind of Practitioners should revert to auxiliary, complementary or supportive roles in relationship to the Principal Psychiatric Practitioner ('PPP" = Consultant or Deputy) who would then be freer to 'cut to the chase'. In the previous era, when the PPP delegated to other Practitioners with skill and sensitivity, then administration and bureaucracy was light and dextrous and staff morale was much higher. People mostly did what they were good at, and felt safer and more valued.

Unanswerable questions? Impossible options? In order to reclaim and regrow some of the departing skills and wisdom (I would designate them as 'Holistic', 'Psychodynamic' or 'Humanistic'), we need to undo many recent 'advances' (which I suggest are not). Among the many conundrae, some involve training and staffing: how can we selectively undo rapid specialist training and encourage might-be psychiatrists to be immersed as (say) Physicians or GPs for several years first? Could consultant status be strengthened but delayed for several years? How could applicants happily accept this as part of an unengineered and gentle acquisition of wisdom, for the benefit of themselves, their therapeutic eco-systems, their patients? Can this possibly fit alongside the near ubiquitous streamlining and acceleration of NHS Professional career pathways? Likewise, could we dismantle current MDTs and get the non-PPP psychiatric-care workers to reclaim, and re-energise, with pride and cooperation, traditional but more limited roles, once valued but now atrophied from disuse?

No easy answers to such questions, even if desired. No Reset button.

The work of all in Public Welfare has become increasingly in thrall to doctrines and mindsets from Health and Safety, corporate, competitive industry and policing. The resulting Bureaucratyrannohypoxia has coalesced to a Culture that ensnares and suffocates us all. The fragile but rich influences of healing, humanism and holism are now almost extinguished. Likewise the better kind of confederate socialism that used to contain the NHS. How can we resuscitate and rehabilitate these?

Such questions are crucial far beyond our local responsibilities or individual career spans. I hope this open letter will provide some spark and fuel for our further thought and discussion. I look forward to both.

Ω

Letter to Director of Mental Health Services, South London & Maudsley NHS Trust, 2010

Dear Andrew Lansley, MP
(Secretary of State for Health 2011)

## Commodification, commissioning and commercialisation: the growing threats to personal healthcare

I have been an inner city Principal GP since the 1970s and have witnessed and implemented the successive changes. All have been well intentioned, and all have had adverse unintended consequences. Changes towards commodification, commissioning and commercialisation of healthcare are particularly destructive where 'soft skills' and personal investment are crucial.

We are at the edge of another tranche of accelerated changes. In the near future I fear for the integrity of my work and the personal care of my patients. Beyond that, almost certainly, I shall become a patient: I have a dread of care by agencies and teams with no personal experience or knowledge of me, and little skills or interest to invest in these.

I enclose an analytical summary of my last few years' observation and thoughts about these very difficult and important healthcare issues. *Five Executive Follies* pursues lines of enquiry that may be unfamiliar for you, but may be rewarding. It has been written very carefully and requires similar attention to best assimilate and understand. Despite your enormous volume of written communication and other work, I hope you will find time for this.

I write to stimulate thought and creative discussion. I welcome any further contact from either you, or one of your deputies.

Thank you for your attention and interest.

Ω

# Five Executive Follies

## How commodification imperils compassion in personal healthcare

Summary: Commodification, competition and commercialisation are often introduced as agents of efficiency into State welfare services. In healthcare all of these may, unwittingly, lead to a loss of 'soft skills'; personal understanding and compassion. The human and economic cost is considerable. How this happens is not obvious. This article explains.

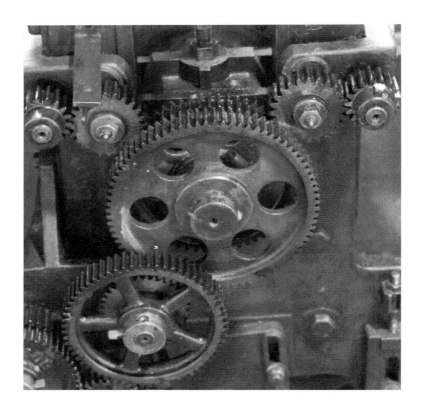

## Prologue

The threat to healthcare from inadequate resources or management has become a little-challenged truism: easy to understand and demonstrate. Healthcare is now submissive to our Management Culture: a world which then authoritatively delegates all human problems to specialists and their executive actions. All this can seem simple, sensible and correct.

The reality is more complex. Paradoxically, there is an additional and opposing, though less obvious, threat to our healthcare: an *excess* of such management, specialist activities and resources – but misplaced. This more subtle and countercultural reality is – it is proposed here – responsible for much of our current system's incapacity to imaginatively address individual variation. Such obliviousness to human diversity and complexity has serious consequences. The more stark examples of failures of physical care make headlines that are hard to understand or even believe. In contrast, failures of personal understanding, and thus therapeutic and compassionate engagement, are usually born invisibly, painfully and privately. Such are the perils of abdicating our capacity to conceive or care more holistically.

Compassion becomes an inevitable casualty whenever personal attunement or engagement are compromised. The word 'compassion' derives its meaning from a Latin root 'to suffer together', thus offering a 'transpersonal' psychology; one drawing from exchanges of resonance and imagination. This is often very different from distancing, 'objective' psychologies used unilaterally by healthcare professionals to pathologise, categorise and commodify in attempts to tightly manage healthcare. Yet there are many studies showing how an empathic bond conveying compassion is a powerful source of comfort and healing for the sufferer, and work-satisfaction (and healing) for the healer.

The skilled evocation of compassion often has powerful effects, but is a subtle activity. This was well recognised and explored by previous generations of practitioners. It now ails amidst hardy slogans of 'Increased Patient Choice' and 'Ensuring quality of care is always central'. How could this cme about? The causal paradoxes and anomalies have been poorly recognised and understood. What follows dissects and explores.

*

# Five Executive Follies: How commodification imperils compassion in personal healthcare

*The fatal metaphor of progress, which means leaving things behind us, has utterly obscured the real idea of growth, which means leaving things inside us.*
GK Chesterton, *Fancies versus Fads*, 1923

We are living longer, more complex lives. Our technological possibilities multiply. Inevitably healthcare expectations, then demands, burgeon. To manage all this, an Industrial Revolution has been unleashed in the NHS. This revolution is itself guided by a core phalanx of doctrines. These are independent of other political considerations or affiliations, and implicitly embraced by all. Such assumptions have developed from cultural changes rooted in our advanced industrialised ways of life. These predicate often unconscious values and mind-sets. Consequently, our rubric for healthcare has become increasingly of *applied sciences*, leaving *humanities* peripheral and disregarded. The tasks then become reduced to engineering tissues or behaviours, rather than extension to nurturing human understanding and contact.

The doctrines that flow from such assumed applied science and industrialisation may thus offer real help in discretion, but an added tranche of folly in excess. Like many truisms, they turn specious, then hazardous. The Law of Unintended Consequences becomes evident: industrialising healthcare, much to our perplexity, is responsible for very substantial 'collateral damage'. Despite allocating ever-increasing resources, in certain areas, our therapeutic and compassionate engagement is poorer. The progressive loss of quality and continuity of personal contact – essential elements of compassion – are crucial factors. This brief survey samples how these difficulties constellate.

Below are itemised these interlocking cardinal notions. Consequences of their over-use are portrayed. In the final section, authentic vignettes illustrate how these Five Executive Follies converge; what happens to our care.

Failure to accurately conceive the essential nature and limitations of the medical model is a primal difficulty. Unbridled objectification may soon turn to alienation. The underlying misconceptions unwittingly arise from 'category errors' that are very powerful, yet rarely distinguished or discussed. Such discernment requires unfamiliar thought about our working axioms. For this reason our first folly receives the lengthiest deliberation. The later appendix offers a tabulated summary and illustrative graphs.

**1. Medical diagnoses and treatment models are the most effective for dealing with human ailments. These methods are clear, authoritative and evidence-based. They should be precedent wherever possible.**

This is mostly and uncontentiously true when dealing with 'structural' diseases of the body, particularly where the condition is localised and acute. Common examples: hip fracture, pneumonia, appendicitis. With any of these we are grateful and satisfied with competent and courteous biomechanical attention. With other kinds of health problems this effectiveness becomes much less clear. The 'medical model' then loses its unrivalled command and precision; for example, when dealing with complaints that are not structural, but experiential, 'functional' and stress-related. What are these? They include an ocean of ill-defined but physically distressing complaints which present to GPs and various healers; they become loosely packaged with labels such as migraines, dyspepsia, dysmenorrhoea, tension headaches, IBS, PMS and ME. Then there is the vast range of human anguish – the psychiatrically classified Mental Disorders: disturbances of behaviour, appetite, mood or impulse (BAMI).

There is a useful general equation that can guide our designation and understanding:

structural change = disease; functional disorder = dis-ease.

Although the words look very similar, our optimal methods for approaching and apprehending them often need to be very different. For example: structural disease can be tightly clustered into *generic* diagnoses where individual variation and meaning are relatively unimportant. 'One size fits all.' In contrast, functional dis-ease is more likely to be *idiomorphic*: the generic pattern now less decisive, but the individual meaning and variation crucial. 'Only the wearer knows where the shoe pinches.' As we will see, erroneous conflation of the two leads to many other follies in practice, from individual consultations to national healthcare planning. Such conflation is easily done, and then often very hard to undo. Because of its importance, this subtle but powerful distinction is worth paying time and attention to understand

The dazzling success of biomedical science in tackling many structural diseases may blind our perception of its competent boundaries. Dazzled, we fail to see that overuse of medical diagnosis and treatment in areas of dis-ease becomes counter-productive. This kind of misplacement is complexly inefficient: it frequently leads to eclipse or displacement of more personal and fruitful types of dialogue and understanding – the keys to healing, growth and resolution. Without these, compassion perishes.

There are problems, too, about the integrity, the 'realness', of our research and knowledge when we confuse or conflate these two territories, of disease and dis-ease. Current currencies of quantification and 'evidence-basis' are now a shibboleth to any 'service provision'. Despite this assigned pre-eminence, such esteemed quantitative research becomes less valid when applied away from the shoreline of solid-state pathology: disease. Problems arise when investigating dis-ease because this is primarily a form of communicated experience, not a stable or simple physical state. Yet, no inner experience can be measured directly. We can only access and measure external, associated behaviours or verbal reports. This is hard for those healthcare workers in thrall to objective scientific method: they hope and believe that their measurements or observations reliably indicate private experience. But such formulated indices are, alas, never equations. Research of internal experience here becomes inescapably 'contaminated' by a myriad of personal, relational or institutional factors. For example, attempts to measure 'mood' or 'well-being' are fraught with subjective and interpersonal intrusions and distortions and can never match the clarity or precision of, say, blood electrolytes. To compound the problem, the contaminating factors (eg of conscious or unconscious suggestion, influence or wish) are themselves unmeasurable. In this welter of uncertainties, away from bodily structural disease, science can only operate with severely annotated compromises: 'pscience'. Organisationally and economically, this introduces myriad tangles to the meaning and integrity of statistics. Projects such as 'Commissioning' and 'Payment by Results' then entice specious clarity, with all its inevitable difficulties and corruptions.

All cultures are defined by a prevailing rhetoric. In our industrialised healthcare the categorised and the quantified are now hegemonic. Flawed pscience is now precedent to an unquantified vernacular, however apposite. Such statiticised pscience thus proceeds with a kind of abstracted, regal authority in areas of delicate interpersonal uncertainty. This is a growing problem, most clearly in psychiatry and primary care: here the insidious change has become cultural, and has, by definition, led to a diminution of professional awareness, analysis and debate. The interpersonal skills deriving from these perish, too.

Such areas of healthcare need to reclaim those receding and very different kinds of imaginative intelligence. For example, pscience is likely to assess a distressed person by administering a quantifiable mood questionnaire. A more holistic psychology asks: 'What is it like to be this other person; to have lived their life? What is the meaning and significance, for them, of this distress? What is the meaning and significance, for them, of me, now? What needs do I need to address that they might not (yet) be able to articulate? Answers are hardly to be found in academically studied or managerially designated psychologies. Only a personally imaginative and engaged sentience can lead us to bespoke compassion.

Isn't all this just overcomplicated and academic? No.

Why, then, is it important? Because our conventionally assumed or conferred language and knowledge largely configure our pattern of understanding and engagement with others. How we think, speak and document will determine what we do. If our language eschews personal resonance and understanding, our actions will follow suit. Any System, in excess, will offer specious clarity and certainty. We must be vigilant; an overreaching scientism will become a pyrrhic progress. Overusing the language, understanding and interventions of disease in the territory of dis-ease is such a seductive but debilitating error. Like a mislocated expedition, it leads to a massive misapplication of effort and resources. Not only does this lose us efficiency and economy. The loss of personal understanding is even more serious: unnecessary attribution of illness mentality and behaviour can be profoundly disempowering. Myopic and inapt labelling generates its own disabilities. The loss of personal language, autonomy, agency and responsibility – these are all causes and casualties of an over-reaching medical model. In our preoccupation to measure we often deskill and desensitise ourselves in the unmeasurable. A mind full of generic dicta, data and algorithms cannot heed the individual voice.

Such losses can largely account for the recurrently exposed, shocking and grotesque examples of basic failures of care in hospitals – institutions which are heavily invested with high-technology and managed care-pathways.

We are faced with a serious and perennial conundrum: in our muscular but blind resolve to treat, we may easily destroy the gentler sentience to heal and humanely care. Compassion may be powerful in effect, but it is fragile in viability: it needs a mindful and respectful space and ambience to survive.

## 2. Healthcare is important and complicated. All practitioners should be tightly monitored and controlled. Increasing healthcare management is bound to be to the patient's benefit.

Yes, but only sometimes. The caveats for this are broadly similar to the section above. For example, the rules and regulations addressing safety in a Cardiac Surgery Unit should be strictly enforced. Exceptions would be very exceptional, if ever. In contrast, such tight governance is much less helpful when attempting to relieve functional complaints. For example, a perfectionistic lonely person with tension headaches, or another incapacitated by rage and grief at the discovery of a major infidelity, or another enervated by mysterious polysymptoms since his wife became pregnant. In these functional disorders, the therapeutic effect of the practitioner depends upon imaginative skills of personal contact and suggestion. Institutional or formulaic management are likely to run counter to these: rigid management eviscerates compassionate imagination.

There are parallels here to family-life and how we bring up children. The balance we choose between rules $v$ freedom and structure $v$ spontaneity, etc, will vary with the child, its age, the situation, and so forth. Families where structure and discipline are rigid and excessive will yield children who may appear orderly and well behaved, but are stunted in their capacities for creativity, initiative, expression, joy and intimacy. Necessary conflict, too, will be turned inwards or displaced, with all the destructive effects within and without.

Organisations that are over-managed show equivalent afflictions. Such harassed groups suffer from defensive proceduralism, low-morale, high sickness rates, scapegoating, and a fascinatingly subtle range of subversion, both conscious and unconscious. Paradoxically, such depletions are retroflected casualties; the result of management compulsively 'driving' efficiency. Over-controlling parents rarely get what they intend. Compassion, too, requires our intelligent flexibility.

### 3. Mass-production and standardization must be a good thing, if it makes things more available.

We don't question this with washing-machines or ball-bearings. Entering the arena of healthcare, we can still extend this confidence to, say, pharmaceuticals, surgical materials and certain procedural treatments, eg cataract extraction. This remains true so long as individual variation, subjective complexity and personal understanding are relatively uninfluential. In contrast, chronic and functional complaints confront us with the importance of individuals' variation of experience and meaning. These all-too-human factors elude quantitative, formulaic and procedural approaches. We must here develop more flexible, 'crafted' and individually addressed responses. Centrally-programmed factory workers are not equipped for this.What are these elusive variables, and how are they important?

Much of this we know from everyday experience. For example, most of us, when distressed by personal or relationship problems, find difficulty in describing, expressing or explaining these. We are likely to have all kinds of fears about sharing or disclosure. How a listener or helper might respond becomes decisive as to whether and how we do this. In this process we are exquisitely sensitive to the subtlest interpersonal signals and changes. Example: how we feel with apparently tiny variations of voice, timing or body language with a verbal greeting or a handshake. For all their power, such nuances of interpersonal influence are almost impossible to measure or manage directly. Paradoxically, though, over-management may stifle, even extinguish, an emotionally-literate environment, which creatively respects the fragile complexity and uniqueness of each interchange. Compassion needs space and oxygen to flourish. Analogies with parenting are, again, clear and prophetic.

### 4. Competition, commissioning and commercial pressures will raise standards of care.

In industry, encouragement of these '3Cs' makes much sense: in providing technical services and physical commodities, and the manufacture and sale of objects. With complex welfare activities it, again, leads to a similar pattern of the unintended. The '3Cs' solution often becomes more problematic than the problem it is attempting to address. For example, if we attempt to commodify, and then trade, in 'packages of care', how do we pre-scribe the changing, often inexplicit, complexity of people's needs? And then any need for flexibility and sensitivity of response? How do we then standardise a package and a price? If we mandate such specification, what is the human cost of doing so?

To illustrate such problems:

Mr C is 62 years and needs a total hip replacement due to premature osteoarthritis. He is otherwise very fit, healthy, happy and actively involved in his work and large family.

Mrs D is 83 years and also needs this operation. She is a childless widow: she had a stillbirth 60 years ago and never again conceived. Her beloved husband died of cancer a year ago. She now lives alone; lonely, with stoic and brave melancholy. She was an only child and was sexually abused:

she is wary of any kind of physical care or examination. Her complex diabetes and emphysema add to her vulnerability, but she tends to deny this due to her aversion to any kind of dependency.

Clearly, Mrs D's anaesthesia, surgery, physical recovery and psychological resilience are all more likely to be problematic than Mr C's. All these processes will require intelligent and imaginative care. How can such delicate compassion be predictively and commercially contained, controlled or costed? How do we have 'diagnoses' for such kaleidoscopic but decisive human complexity? How will each separate Specialty or Trust precisely delineate and invoice its responsibilities?

What happens with a system of competitive commissioning? Practitioners become controlled by their thraldom to Trusts, and the Trusts are in thrall to optimising their profits and 'performance data'. Thus are they likely to fulfil to the letter (only) their contractual obligations. Officious practice flourishes; managers, even lawyers, direct and tailor individual practice to suit institutional and commercially negotiated 'contracts', and thus policies. These replace more humanistic or holistic practice: encounters guided by broader and longer-term views, and informed by a growing understanding of each particular individual.

Under such a system, over time, we lose vocational practitioners: those motivated primarily by the pursuit of humane enquiry and healing relationships. These become replaced by 'Teams' of management-directed, piece-work biomechanics. Chosen vocations become managed careers. Thinking and activity turn institutional, not interpersonal. Resources become increasingly commandeered for defensive and offensive organisational fights and feints: meetings about meetings – negotiation, litigation, imposing but slyly tendentious statistics, PR, 'spin'... Services that for several decades existed in a state of trusting and cooperative confederation, now become mistrustful competitors: Trusts (!).

The patient is now a commercial proposition: if he generates revenue (for the Trust), then find reasons to provide a service; if he does not generate revenue, then find reasons swiftly to discharge him somewhere (anywhere) else. 'It's not our responsibility.'

Amidst this Darwinian struggle for survival, can our compassion really be commissioned or commodified?

## 5. Specialisation is always a good thing. It provides greater expertise when and where it is needed

Yet again this is most impressively true with well-defined structural disease, but often counter-productive when dealing with more complex and less stable situations. Positive examples of the use of specialisation are clear and obvious. If we have a knee problem that requires surgery, then we want, not just an orthopaedic surgeon, but one who specialises in knees. The idea is that we can divide the body up into smaller and smaller parts and systems, and thus concentrate knowledge, effort and expertise with greater precision and efficiency. This is viable so long as we are dealing with disease that is stable and confined to a body-part or system. We can term this fragmenting specialisation 'Anatoatomisation'.

This kind of specialisation can become far from helpful when applied away from the stable, localised disease scenario. To illustrate:

Mr S is age 70 years. Two years ago he developed an aggressive form of Parkinson's Dementia, shortly after his retirement. He had been an extremely educated, fit, diligent and disciplined man, holding a senior post in international diplomacy. His multidimensional decline has been relentless and tragic. He has become an insentient and incontinent shell of his former self, recognising no one and requiring constant care. Amidst this, his beleaguered, self-sacrificing wife discovers a breast-lump, a cancer. She then has chemoradiotherapy, which itself makes her ill, in the hope of a cure. As Mrs S struggles to recover, Mr S's decline is unabated. He has unmanageable 'episodes': he freezes, falls, develops chest infections, deepening deliria. Each of these needs his admission to hospital, and each time it is to a different Ward and a different 'Team', who do not recognise him. Each team then routinely refers him on to further specialist teams: to Gerontology (for his age!), to Neurology (for Parkinson's), to Elderly Psychiatry (for Dementia), to Urology (for recurrent urine infections), to Respiratory Medicine (for chest infections). None of these teams seems to acknowledge the larger picture, and what is needed in terms of wise, humane contact; continuity, containment support and comfort. Mrs S is an intelligent woman, but now fatigued, despondent and confused by the constantly changing medical personnel, designations and venues.

'Why does he need yet another brain scan?', she wearily asks a bustling and brisk Neurology Registrar.

'Just to make sure we're not missing anything', comes his clipped reply, his tone of defensive authority primed by Trust Protocol.

Thirty years ago this unneeded and very expensive brain scan would not have been available. Nor would the panoply of specialist teams. Mr and Mrs S would have had something else: continuity of care by a known general physician on a particular ward. This broadly-based clinician and dedicated nursing staff would have provided the personal investment, familiarity, acknowledgement and understanding that were needed to nurse and palliate all of these 'episodes'. They would have seamlessly apprehended the human needs, not just of the ravaged Mr S, but also his exhausted wife. They would probably not have used the word 'compassion', but it would have been woven into their experiences, acts and utterances. Such traditional skills are easily displaced by the often specious imperative to 'specialisation'. The whole is more than the sum of its parts: compassion is a tender and fragile fruit of holism.

Ms T is a 38-year-old single woman with a son of four years. Her persona of engaging warmth and polite cooperation belies her deeply troubled and troubling history. A product and victim of, and hostage to, a painfully unhappy parental marriage, she has spent most of her life trying impotently to break free, to establish an autonomous and wholesome self. But she has not the self-esteem, the internal model, or sense of entitlement to do any of these things. She is like a blinded, enraged, captive creature convulsively throwing itself against the bars of its cage, trying to find the outside. The symptoms signalling this impacted struggle have been wide-ranging. They have been shepherded and clustered by a parade of specialists over many years: mood disturbance and instability, gastritis, eating disorders, intermittent alcoholism, impulsivity, irritable bowel syndrome, obsessive compulsive disorder, migraines, menstrual dysfunction, eczema…

Each specialist attempted to subsume, quell, or at least contain, her disturbance with their own language and circumscribed focus of the medical model. Sometimes, paradoxically, such specialisation led to her being the object of exclusion instead: once she was lost between the GP Counsellor, the Psychiatric and the Alcohol Services, who each said that one of the others should be responsible. Despite seeking helpful engagement, she was extruded by all three: 'she does not meet our intake criteria'; 'It's not our responsibility…'

Dr W, her General Practitioner, has learned over many years that such marathon, polymorphous disturbance is usually signalling some failure of personal evolution, some frustration of gratified belonging. It lies behind and beyond any specialisms, their language or measurements. He remembers an old mentor saying of his endeavours to help such people: 'You need patience with patients, and patients with patience'. But Dr

W knows now that it requires also evocative but structured encouragement, to safely uncover and decipher what lies beneath. He arranges an hour's appointment with Ms T, to try to take them both from a world of fragmented and serial specialisms, to a holistic perspective deriving from, and imbued with, personal meaning.

The polyclinic Practice Manager is alerted, and now uneasy: 'We have pressure on clinic rooms, doctor, and this kind of work takes up a lot of time, and earns no additional "points" for the Practice ... in any case, all the other doctors have said this kind of work is not your responsibility ...'

*

Is there a more crystalline coda for these Five Follies?

*

And the question arising? In a healthcare system increasingly determined by the quantifiable, the commercial and the industrial, how do we restore, and then assure, the primacy of holistic, human care – the quality and continuity of our personal contact with others? In our busy and difficult jobs, every day and in every consultation, how do we create afresh, then nurture, an ever-evanescent culture of compassion?

*

*'Is it progress if a cannibal eats with a knife and fork?'*

Stanislaw Lec, *Unkempt Thoughts,* 1962

*

APPENDIX

|  | Disease | Dis-ease |
|---|---|---|
| 1. Knowledge | Impersonal Objective, generic, clustered, data | Personal Subjective/intersubjective, Idiomorphic, bespoke |
| 2. Ideology/ paradigm | Dualism, Determinism, Biomechanics | Monism, choice, consciousness |
| 3. Resources/ transmission | External (eg drugs, instruments, radiation, manipulation, lasers) By Conduction 'Treatment' | Internal (eg immunity, growth, repair) By Induction 'Healing' |
| 4.Power/ responsibility | Dr >>> Pt | Pt [+/-Dr] |
| 5. Language | Objective, Doctors', technical, designatory Generic | (Inter)personal. Shared dialogue = co-creation Idiolectic |
| 6.Communication mode | Didactic Mostly logical/structured | Dialogue/Dialectic Often openly imaginative/evocative |
| 7. Psychology | Designatory 'Objective' Quantitatively researched | Evocative (Inter)subjective Qualitatively researched |
| 8. Role/ metaphor of Doctor/healer | Engineer, expert, teacher, manager | Gardener, guide, midwife, |

| | | compassionate fellow-traveller |
|---|---|---|
| 9. Art or Science? | Science | Art |
| 10. Accessibility to industrialisation: mass-management, , training, standardisation, mass production, commodification, measurement | High | Low |
| 11. Importance of personal contact, meaning and understanding | Low | High |

**Figure 1**: Disease v. Dis-ease; Art and Science, Treatment and Healing: comparative paradigms of effective response to human ailments

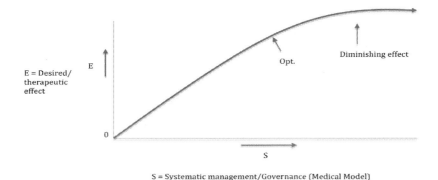

**Figure 2**: Systematic management and structural disease
Decaying exponential. Desired response proportional to systematic governance, until optimal point (Opt). Then diminishing returns. (Illustrated principle: structural disease responds relatively well to scientific strictures and structures.)

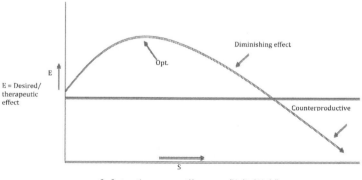

S = Systematic management/Governance (Medical Model)

**Figure 3:** Systematic/generic management and functional dis-ease
Shallower Bell Curve with reversal. Desired response to systematic governance is less. Yields earlier to ineffectiveness, then becomes counterproductive. (Illustrated principle: functional dis-ease less positively responsive to impersonally prescribed approaches. Excess application has adverse effects.)

Ω

Submitted to the Secretary of State for Health. It was subsequently published in the *Journal of Holistic Healthcare,* Vol 8. Issue 3. Dec 2011.

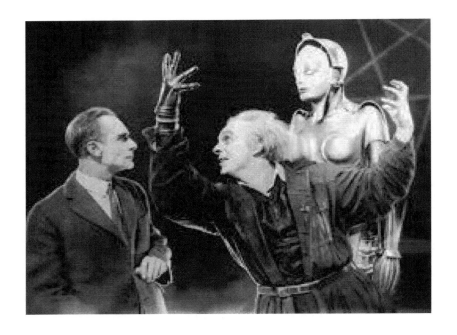

Fritz Lang *Metropolis 1927*

# Further NHS Reforms: inevitable and unintended Consequences

As the debate becomes more fraught, I want to add my voice to the fray. I have been a frontline Medical Practitioner for more than forty years, and have seen recurrent waves of reform and their very mixed results. The least disputable advances are in the realms of technology and technical competence: drugs and procedures have become more accurate and effective, practitioners mostly apposite in their delivery. Likewise, a few decades ago we all knew of doctors widely reputed as rude, curt, alcoholic, incompetent and shabby – sometimes simultaneously. In those times, with moderate luck, they would retire, without formal challenge, on a full NHS Pension. That kind of collusive incompetence is now most unlikely. These changes represent real progress.

But the institutional reconfigurations and the management devices applied to achieve these have inadvertently destroyed much of the best, in order to extirpate the worst. I experienced this 'best' in my first twenty-five years, working in NHS General Practice and Psychiatry. I was mentored by Practitioners who were vocational in their ethos and holistic in their view of their specialty. Although my administrative duties and salary were referable to one tiny sector of the NHS, my professional efforts and communications roamed with easy and pragmatic conviviality amongst colleagues from other disciplines and institutions. Despite some 'bad' practitioners, I felt mostly a welcoming and fraternal support: a kind of 'therapeutic family'. I was not then much interested in branded politics, but I wondered if this was one of the few good and viable examples of a kind of 'Confederate Socialism': a world of colleagueial exchanges that was benignly intentioned, inclusively respectful and often mutually educational and supportive. 'Medicine is a humanity guided by science': not a phrase I heard explicitly from my early mentors, but they would have readily agreed.

For the last two decades this network of interpersonal communication, support and understanding has been increasingly eroded and dismantled by various ideas to increase 'efficiency'. The galvanising panoply has included: The Internal Market; Commissioning; NHS Trusts; the widening of schematic medicalisation of complex human distress; mandating goals and targets, performance-related pay and league tables; proliferation of ever more and sharply defined specialties, then acceleration of specialist training ... and now GP Commissioning. The danger with each and all of these is that Medical Practice is propelled away from any basis as a humanely networked welfare activity, and towards an entrepreneurial kind of 'civic engineering' whose currency is commodification. Thus, increasingly, we attempt to 'manage' people and their distress without the commensurate growth of personal contact, meaning and understanding.

Notions and methods from commerce and manufacturing industries may make some useful contributions to Healthcare, but they are seriously limited. Beyond these limits they can do real damage. NHS doctors' pay and working hours are now more generous than twenty years ago; in contrast, their morale, work-satisfaction and sense of creative and compassionate engagement (with colleagues, as well as patients) are not. In a recent large meeting of senior colleagues, we were being briefed and instructed, yet again, by another executive imperative, about a complex and subtle area of care. I protested, saying I felt like an eight-year-old working in a car factory. The identification was explosive and rapturous – especially, I thought, from older colleagues schooled in the earlier culture. The comic relief was evident and welcome. The underlying reservoir of alienation, resentment, mistrust, fear and anomie remains largely unarticulated, and little understood.

Doctors are probably the most privileged among the victims of our misindustrialisation of healthcare: certainly they are the best paid. Among other welfare and NHS Healthcare workers the pay is less, but the psycho-spiritual affliction much the same. The shocking stories of elderly, frail, dry-mouthed patients lying with abject helplessness in soiled sheets, while within yards of them nurses sit rapt in electronic engagement with abstracted NHS Foundation Trust data collation tasks, are harsh symptoms of a malign Zeitgeist: the consequences of depersonalising the personal. This is what happens when we overinvest in the biomechanical, when we industrialise the procedural, but fail to see or value or understand the complexity of human needs and attachments.

The biomechanical is necessary but not sufficient in healthcare. Competition, commercialisation and commodification – the 3Cs – may contribute peripherally and in minor ways. But we must heal as well as treat; compassionately engage as well as manage. For these we need practitioners and networks fuelled and nourished by the energy and art of the interpersonal: by humanism and holism. For all its flaws (many otherwise remediable), the old NHS of 'Confederate Socialism' encouraged this in me and for me, and those around me, for twenty-five years.

I am asked: what would I now do to rehumanise our healthcare? To start, I suggest a phased, radical retreat, then reclamation. Practical examples: to abolish any kind of Internal Market, Commissioning, and thus the likes of NHS Foundation Trusts; to restore Hospital Nursing Schools, the centrality of General Physicians, and personal patient lists to General Practitioners. But the cultural tides propelling our problematic recent changes are wide and strong: the easiest course is confluence, to be swept along. Creative counterculture will always be harder.

Amidst these conundrae, as my own career nears its end, I mourn the loss of Love's Labour. I fear, too, for my future: when I become old and helpless, what kind of personal care and understanding will I receive?

$$\Omega$$

Letter to the *British Medical Journal* 2012

# 'Evidence' is both more and less than it seems

## The rise of scientism and the demise of the personal in healthcare

Dear Mr Hunt MP
(Secretary of State for Health 2012)

I am writing to you as a long-serving single-handed GP: now an almost-extinct species, but one occupying an exceptional vantage point for length and familiarity. My views, therefore, often have a different emphasis from many of the consulted professional bodies.

I heard a recent interview with you (Radio 4, 19/10/12) in which you talked of 'being led by scientific evidence'. The phrase can sound unarguably sensible and pragmatic: in healthcare it has become increasingly used as a kind of justifying slogan or even shibboleth: measure or perish. But the words 'evidence' and 'led' may be trickier than we realise: a brief analysis may clarify.

Evidence is a highly complex endeavour; its complexity grows with scrutiny. Some general principles can help us navigate: evidence occupies a spectrum of contentiousness – it is much clearer with the inanimate than the human. And with the human it is much clearer with the objectively physical than the experiential. To help tether all this we have quantifiable evidence, and this is often regarded as a 'gold-standard' of clarity and certainty. Yet in complex human healthcare it is often difficult (sometimes impossible) to quantify what we are really interested in without introducing speciousness of many kinds. Nevertheless quantifiable evidence now commands such high cultural-currency value that much 'counterfeit-currency' is produced and sought; this 'bad currency' then enters our exchanges to displace an intelligent openness to other kinds of (unquantifiable) evidence.

What does this lead to?

In my view the most serious adverse changes are those of the loss of personal attachments and their understandings. Because these are mostly impossible to measure, standardise or regulate, they cannot be readily turned into the staples of current NHS managed operations: statistical data, standardised procedures or tradeable commodities. Efforts to do so are now frequent and have often grotesquely absurd consequences: difficult and detailed questionnaires given to the rawly distressed from life-shock or bereavement; poorly understood children from painfully struggling families being didactically diagnosed with 'neurodevelopmental disorders' – these are common follies from our growing medical scientism.

In earlier times – before the ubiquity of computers and our consequent submission to the quantified and the mass-managed – it was far easier for health carers to develop attachments and personal understandings. These were often of great therapeutic value. Good practice then recognised that our capacity to heal, contain or comfort depend on professionally tempered attachments and affections: the better we know people, the better we can care for them. Current trends obstruct such possibilities: rapid rotations of staff and venues, multiple 'hit and run' specialists, generic and anonymised teams rather than named and familiar persons ... With complex and chronic ailments, in particular, these 'management systems' cannot readily offer compassionate and imaginative containment.

The culture of healthcare has rapidly and radically changed. We have incrementally displaced the ethos of a family with that of a factory: personal connections and understandings are increasingly rare; standardised procedures and utterances common. Far fewer people know the name of their GP; in their large Polyclinics GPs cannot personally remember their patients and do not even know the names of their own receptionists. In the large district hospitals Consultants do their ward-rounds with junior medical staff they have never met before, often, seeing patients for a first and only time. Patients – often alone, exposed and afraid – feel unable to express their vulnerability and needs to rule-bound and management-programmed nurses. Such anomie has burgeoned in parallel with the regal rise, then hegemony, of (quantifiable) evidence. This is not coincidental. Yet we also know that our best relationships are largely fuelled by certain kinds of faith, aspiration and ideal – and that none of these could be quantitatively 'evidenced'. We live with gratitude and wonder for such indeterminate anomalies: our faith lies at the heart of our humanity.

This brings me back to your use of the word 'led': for we should rarely be led by scientific evidence, rather we should be guided. This means we guard and retain our autonomy so that we may be informed by much else, too. For we need our broadest understandings; we need to be able to discern, and yet assimilate, very different kinds of comprehension and knowledge. In healthcare, as in much of life, wisdom is often the conciliation and choreography of options that are themselves inescapably flawed or limited.

My own slogan is 'Healthcare is a humanity guided by science'. The implication here reminds us to be, always, careful and mindful of such delicate balances and conundrae. This is not easy, yet to avoid such complexity leads to what we have now: a healthcare rich in provided resources, but cumulatively impoverished of internally generated human connection and understanding.

My voice is experienced, though old: I hope you find some freshness in the views. It would interest me greatly to continue a dialogue. If you, or one of your deputies, want to visit my inner London GP practice you can see In Vivo what has motivated and informed this letter.

Ω

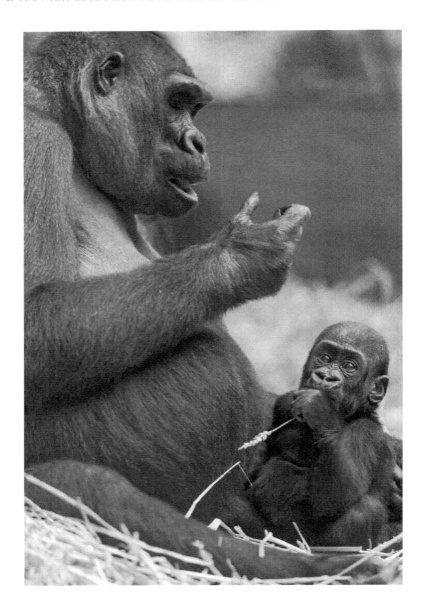

# Continuity of Care -
# Of course, but whose?

## A Sleight of Slogans
## — letter to Family Doctor Association

Continuity of Care is a phrase increasingly used to indicate a cornerstone of good practice. But the phrase is often used with very different assumptions and intent: personal and institutional continuity are often discordant. Personal care and family-doctoring are both an art and an ethos: we must beware of ultimately expensive and mass-produced imitations.

Names and titles quickly convey a designation, sometimes evaluation. Similarly, slogans attempt to transmit a message – often moral or transformative – with sharp economy, sometimes wit. Sloganeers aim to rapidly catch our interest and affiliation.

And so it was. Some years ago I was 'caught' by the title of The Small Practices Association (SPA): I joined. I was – and resolutely remain – a well-defined, small practice. Single-handed in London's centre, I sensed the rising cultural tides running against me. I steeled myself: I would have to be articulate and resilient to guard and nourish the kind of personal understandings and relationships that have been at the heart of my working lifetime's vocation. Long experience has fuelled my conviction that a small practice is best suited to the delivery of person-centred healthcare. The SPA's title vaunted (and provided) valuable support to stand against the tide.

In more recent years the SPA rebranded itself as the Family Doctor Association, the current FDA. I liked this title, too. For my work is much enriched when I can see and understand an individual's struggles and afflictions within broader frames of life-cycles and relationships: a family-perspective is essential to this. There are here some interesting and daunting parallels. In earlier years I experienced my work as being part of the broader endeavours of a kind of colleagueial healthcare 'family' – in this some individuals were close and well-known, others invisible and unknown – an extended 'family', nevertheless. Sadly, for expedient organisational then cultural reasons, doctors now usually have much less personal knowledge of patients and families, and are less likely in their work to feel affiliated into a national healthcare 'family' Both kinds of family-contact in our work are impoverished.

I mourn the loss of these subtle personal nexae. I see and fear the consequences. But there is restitution – the FDA's slogan, Continuity of Care, enlivens and encourages me: it draws from timeless principles of healing. These principles help us revise and revitalise a healthcare that is increasingly anonymised, alienated, algorithmetised – a culture that has steadily lost any individual view of people in its exponential development of the schematic and managerial. For any real reconciliation here, we need to exert a kind of healing. Central to healing processes are two triads. One develops within the individual (the intrapersonal): immunity, growth and repair. This first triad is induced by a second, which develops between individuals (the interpersonal): attachment, containment and affection.

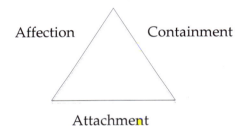

Affection    Containment

Attachment

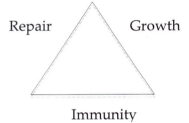

Repair    Growth

Immunity

**Figure 1:**
*Interpersonal healing inductions*
The 'family' *ethos* of
well-fared welfare
Difficult to measure
Personal

**Figure 2:**
*Intrapersonal healing inductions*
The 'family' *effects* of
well-fared welfare
Difficult to measure
Personal

Clearly, for any of these to occur, the presence of good therapeutic rapport is likely to be crucial. How can these things evolve without continuity of care? This seems a rhetorical question.

The professional responses, though, are less straightforward; we need to look carefully.

'Continuity of Care' can be constructed very differently by, say, patients, administrators and different sorts of doctors. Personal continuity is the familiar face, voice and ambience: the uniquely evolved complex of contacts, events and personal understandings. This kind of continuity is what we yearn for when a condition renders us vulnerable because of its chronicity and complexity. If we live long enough we all suffer this vulnerability, and will seek succour in personal familiarity and continuity. This succour often has a kind of organic growth, for the nourishing and warming benefits to patients of personal continuity are often equally important to practitioners. For the more humanly interested doctor, it is the relationships that keep heart and mind alive, fresh, engaged and integrated. And here is a powerful and wonderful mystery: caring for those that matter to us adds to our own lives and energies.

But there is a very different ethos of continuity of care that is increasingly vaunted by planners, managers and, now, a new generation of practitioners. This emphasises institutional and administrative impersonal continuity: here it is the designated 'Team' that delivers; any desire for personal attachment is discouraged. Personal understanding becomes an obsolescent and irrelevant impediment: data is the official currency. The intention is that anonymised healthcare professionals and patients can all be speedily referred to managed Services Care Pathways and Team Protocols. These administrative devices attempt to template a kind of in loco parentis for personally responsible and responsive care. This will, of course, take us far away from care anchored in the personally familiar. Where, then, does all this lead? Here are two examples:

Suki has deep-rooted dysthymic mental health problems that cannot be simply 'treated', even less 'cured'. Her early childhood was rent and wounded by unstable, inconsistent and incompetent parenting. What seems to work for her – very slowly – is the reverse of all these in her healthcare: kindness, consistency, patience, imaginative and respectful interest. As her GP I try to provide this by offering my personal continuity of care: her appreciation of this is subtly evident and demurely expressed.

Nevertheless, she gets mentally ill, and this is when attachments fragment and unravel. In one turbulent year she encountered the following psychiatric teams: Hospital Liaison Psychiatry, Community Mental Health, Assertive Outreach, Emergency Psychiatry, Crisis Resolution, Home Treatment, In-Patient Psychiatry, Early Discharge and Recovery. Each of these boundaried teams transferred electronic abstracted 'data' to the next team, to prime their very long and formulaic assessment. The electronic continuity might seem seamless and neatly well-functioning to a manager or detached clinician. Suki's experience is shockingly and instructively different. At the times when she most needs familiar and trusted faces, and attachments rooted in personal knowledge, she instead encounters a procession of strangers who interrogate her, often never to be seen again. She describes these often stilted disquisitions as if they are conducted for an unseen third person, but not really for her. She rarely remembers their names or designations.

I tell some senior managers and clinicians what I have heard and seen. They diplomatically imply that my view is lacking in clarity and sophistication. They tell me that Suki is the recipient of a well-honed system of 'Integrated Care': she is being managed through her 'Patient Journey'; the procession of strangers are, in fact, choreographed specialists, each tending a complex niche in this engineered journey. I think: whose language and needs are being heeded? And who decides?

I have had a part-time hospital post for many years. Much of my work has been to help patients with complex interweavings of substantial physical disease and emotional distress. I have heard patients' accounts of their medical encounters for decades. Until recent times, patients would almost always know who their GP was: often the rapport was deep, trusted and clearly valued. This is now very rare: most frequently patients know the names of their health centre, but not any particular doctor. 'I used to see Dr J, but now when I go it always seems to be someone different … the last time it was a young woman: she seemed nice enough but spent most of the time looking on the screen. No, I don't know her name …' This is typical of our increasing healthcare data-centred anonymity.

This serious loss of personal attachment has been accelerated by the abolition of Personal Patient Lists. This administrative fiat discouraged the development of particular personal bonds and replaces them with Systemic Management; when I now go to my GP I am not to think of myself as cared for by my doctor, Dr X: my care is now managed by the Hillside Primary Care Medical Centre.

There are essential differences between these contrapuntal kinds of continuity of care: the personal and the administrative. Generally planners and managers will favour and better understand administrative and systemic continuity as this can be (theoretically) delivered with detachment and objectivity. Clearly, these kinds of continuity must always be available – for no individual practitioner can provide invariable, eternal, perfect and instant personal care, or not for long! We must all be allowed absences, holidays, and the errors and vicissitudes of life. Yes, personal continuity can rarely be complete and there must always be institutional back-up plans and resources.

So, we must have both kinds of continuity of care: personal and impersonal. The problem then is how do we define, find and assure the best mix or compromise in each situation? Certain principles can guide us. Where a patient and practitioner wish for personal continuity of care for a non-acute condition – and this possibility is feasible and competent – then this should take precedence. Yet this personal continuity should be contained within, and in some ways accountable to, a systemic continuity: this is the safety-net, lest the personal continuity breaks or fails.

None of this is easy. In our risk-averse times we have become haunted by spectres of breakage and failure. And personal continuity of care – like love – is vulnerable to loss and damage. Yet to attempt to avoid these risks – by driving out personal attachments and replacing them with 'safer' generic management – may lead to different, but greater, breakages and failures. Broken spirits and hearts are common and often ineluctably important in our health and welfare. Such complex humanity eludes management and measurement: at these times we need a harbour of experienced compassion and imagination. Skilled and personal continuity of care may be the best kind of harbour we can offer.

*It is better to have loved and lost,*
*than never to have loved at all.*

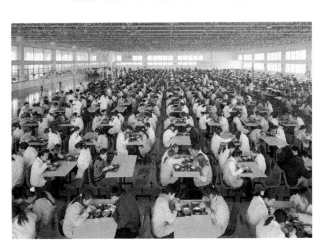

Ω

Publ. in *Family Doctor* 2012

# Balancing Healthcare
## Technical v. Personal,
## Local v. Systemic

Closures at Lewisham Hospital

I heard your important but brief debate on BBC Radio 4 on 26 January. As expected, your arguments were cogent, though polarised. What was not explicated was the inescapable conundrae we now have in contemporary healthcare: that there are, increasingly, juxtaposed principles we must balance – these are technical vs personal, objective vs (inter)subjective and science vs art. The conundrae arise most clearly when we cannot easily combine these, when they remain antithetical: then we need the wisdom of our best compromises. As you have demonstrated, finding the right balance is no easy task.

I am a long-serving, small-practice City GP with an attentive view of people and their relationships. I think we have a growing problem – paradoxically – from the indisputable success of the scientific/technical/objective in certain areas: because of these successes they have largely hegemonised our mindsets, budgets and plans in all areas of healthcare. This has then led to an inadvertent neglect of the personal/art/ (inter)subjective in healthcare: people! We have lost our balance and this is now manifest in our healthcare centres being often technology-rich but humanity-poor: shock headlines pillory the worst examples, but it is clear to me that this sinister new pattern has much to teach us.

Yes, of course it is important that we receive the best technical care, but we must attempt to do so in a humanly-scaled and responsive milieu, where people feel seen, heard, understood, connected and cared-for. These interactions are complex living processes which can only survive with the interpersonal equivalents of space, oxygen, nutrients and habitat. For these we need a 'family' environment, if we are to perform our 'factory' tasks with rooted and growing humanity.

Yes, larger regionalised Specialist Units may logistically provide better technical care, but how do we combine high volumes of technically exacting and urgently required work (that is needed for the procedures of treatment) with a personal sense of connection and understanding (that is required for the care of healing)? For when we industrialise healthcare to treat more efficiently, the care often drains away. If we are not mindful of this, it becomes inevitable.

If we take the examples of Stroke, or Coronary Care, it may make good sense to centralise and specialise skills and expensive resources, and this is probably reflected in good results. But results will be better still if personal connections and communications are regarded as an equal priority. This is even more so with chronic conditions. The required balance of centralised efficiency vs locality identifications needs careful thought: it may be very different for different people.

This is now a formidable task as the personally connected aspects of the NHS have suffered from inadvertent but parlous selective inattention. I now work in a health service where, increasingly, patients cannot name their GP or hospital consultant, doctors have little personal knowledge or understanding of their patients, colleagues do not know one another, Hospital Consultants do ward rounds with junior staff and nurses they do not know, seeing patients for a first and only time ... There are many more examples. What kind of therapeutic contacts, affections or care can develop in such a system? What happens to staff morale? Our shock-headlines provide a darker part of the answer.

The causes of such industrialised healthcare casualties are numerous, complex and sometimes obscure. The fact that very large organisations with rapid human throughput may have difficulty in positively bonding with and understanding complexly distressed individuals may be easy to discern and explain. Other decisions and events which alienate, depersonalise, dislocate and demoralise may be more obscure, but just as real. Examples? The dispersal of hospital nursing schools to Universities; the European Working Hours Directive; the amalgamation of smaller, identity-rich Medical Schools; the abolition of GP personal lists; the economic discouragement of small GP practices; the demise of the General Physician – all such have contributed to our ever more tightly managed, but anomic, healthcare.

How we reinfuse and re-enthuse our often misindustrialised healthcare with human heart and professional art, is an endless and difficult challenge, for the problems now have deep cultural roots. If we can discern our excessive uses of industrialisation, informatics, systems management, competition, commodification and commercialisation, we may be able to act with more intelligent restraint. Those smaller, more fragile and imperilled, caring aspects of healthcare may then revive and, possibly, flourish.

Small and large, generic and bespoke, art and science, universal and vernacular, all address different aspects of our complex health needs. We need matching, complex, though pragmatic, responses. There are rarely (if ever) solutions, only our wisest compromises.

I have a distilled slogan for all of this: 'Healthcare is a humanity guided by science'.

Ω

Letter to Joan Ruddock, MP and Lord Ara Darzi (ex Minister of Health) 2013

# 'Fixing the NHS is straightforward'
## Really?

Gerry Robinson in his article (Daily Telegraph, 18.2.13) tells us that 'fixing the NHS is straightforward'. He writes with optimistic alacrity of pragmatic, logistical, data-fuelled managerial devices to sharpen purview and performance. He cites management in McDonalds and Phones4U as good role models for healthcare. He conveys this as if it is bold and new.

I have been a frontline NHS doctor for more than forty years and my view is very different. For in the last two decades we have had ever-increasing infusions of such Management Modelling and Corporate redesigns, based on what works in Commerce and manufacturing industries. The resulting industrialisation of healthcare – and its guidance by the 3Cs: commissioning, competition and commodification – has led to grievous loss of humane interest, attachments and vocation in healthcare. The Mid Staffs debacle is one severe and grotesque consequent example.

My own view has become countercultural. It is that healthcare is a humanity guided by science. That humanity is an art and an ethos; these cannot simply be managed or manufactured. They are complex manifestations of education and culture more than any training and obedience. At the heart of this humanity lie the questions of why and how we should care for one another. The best answers come from milieux that can respectfully grow personal attachments, affections and understandings. The less industrial, older NHS fostered such important subtleties much more readily.

Healthcare is bedevilled by such chimera and complexity. It is dangerous folly to think we can easily short-circuit these by

651

some kind of brilliant, quasi-commercial or military-type plans or charismatic leadership. 'Straightforward'? No. 'Fixes'? There are none: we can offer only our wisest and most compassionate and dextrous compromises. Mid Staffs is not so much about simple managerial incompetence; it is more about the overgrowth of managerialism and the inadvertent asphyxiation of natural humanity.

The older NHS that mentored me may have been less scientifically efficient and managed, but it was richer in humanity and caring imagination.

Ω

Published in BMJ, 2013

# The Rise of Business Culture in the NHS:
## our consequent loss of compassionate healthcare ethos

I write in agreement with Professor Elkeles' thoughts about the dehumanised disarray in our NHS.

I, too, am a veteran NHS doctor. Thoughtful practitioners of my generation are almost always in agreement: the twenty years' development of the 'internal (healthcare) market' has not enlivened, incentivised or optimised procedural treatments, even less compassionate care. With few exceptions it has led, rather, to widespread staff anomie and demoralisation. As both cause and effect to these we have more depersonalised and formulaic care, managed increasingly in ways that are remote, defensive and officious. The business-modelled NHS costs much more, too: a complexly competitive commissioning system of autarkic Trusts etc leads to an explosion of administrative artefacts and artifices. Healthcare is a humanity: science makes great contributions. But a business? We are discovering just how specious and dangerous this misconception can be. How and why we should care for one another far exceeds any business we can manage.

Ω

Letter to the Times 2013

653

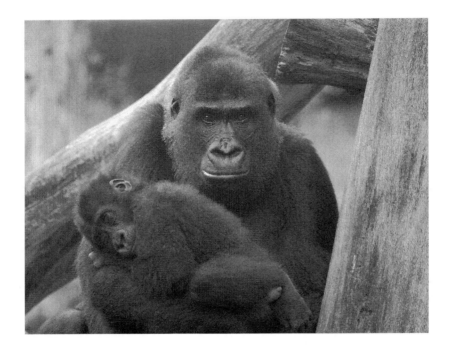

# Physis

## Healing, Growth and
## the Hub of
## Personal Continuity of Care

A thirty-nine (39) year delayed
follow-up correspondence with Sally

## 1. Explanatory introduction

Occasionally benign coincidence far exceeds mere serendipity, as if the cosmos has somehow read and responded to our intent. Receiving the letter was one of those occasions: its primally evocative and illustrative power far exceeds its apparent brevity and plain speaking. This needs some explanation.

**First the stage.**

For several years I have been increasingly resolute in pursuing qualitative research into the nature and significance of personal continuity of healthcare. I have been led to this by witnessing and enduring the consequences of its progressive loss, especially in the latter third of my professional lifetime. From this has come some understanding. For example, much of this involution derives from the fact that relationships are more difficult to code, manufacture, manage, quantify and research than, say, drugs or physical procedures. This is a conundrum. Rather than acknowledging its difficulty we have instead worsened it by creating something of an academic (then economic and administrative) oligarchy from the 'safer' confines of more easily codifiable and quantifiable research and knowledge – the shibboleths of 'Evidence Basis', a kind of nouveau riche 'Ruling Class'. This newer and narrower culture then often wreaks blind damage because subtle, and thus less measurable, aspects of care then become liable to indifferent neglect or, worse, rationalised hostility and exclusion. In this arena of collateral damage the loss of personal continuity of care is one of the most important and egregious examples. When I was a young practitioner I was encouraged to develop and nurture this earlier longer-term and personal approach. I did not then perceive the probability of its extinction.

## Now, the events.

I am perusing a letter, one of many: there are always more. My eyes scan for the sender, semi-consciously, to decide on priority and degree of attention. The name galvanises my distant memory. I then search for other details, to confirm my guess: it is correct.

I have not heard from Sally for thirty-nine years. My visual memory quickly yields her face, its expressions, thence to her mien and spirit; I remember a very sensitive, melancholic and intelligent young woman struggling with her own shadows, intensity and complexity. I cannot remember anything more precise about her symptom-constellation, or her life or family history. I suppose she would be called 'Chronic severe depressive dysthymia': a more adventurous psychiatrist might also risk 'underlying conflicts and struggles with identity formation'.

As I write this I have not refreshed, checked or garnered more details: the account is thus fresh but unrefined. My recollection is that my encounters with Sally spanned about three years and were located in three consecutive Greater London hospitals. I was then a young trainee psychiatrist, very interested in unproceduralised influences of healing. I was certainly receptive to psychotherapeutic ideas but had not (yet) any training. I was only marginally older than Sally and not that differently endowed with resources and problems. I knew this but was able – with care – to sequestrate 'it' but not myself: our roles were then clearly different – our selves and existential predicaments were not. Her letter, after four decades, indicates a further convergence of our common humanity.

Sally's letter is a pithy personal testament of great power and – I believe – importance to all healthcare professionals. Her clear and candid account is suffused with many themes, all of which merit long thought and discussion. I certainly will not attempt to designate these all for the reader, but instead here briefly highlight themes from the cultures of care that include yet transcend we two individuals.

For me, most remarkable is the evidence of how, in those previous decades, we were able to create imaginative, sensitive, flexible services. The best of these could, and did, then deliver a much more substantial person-centred continuity of care. For several years I worked with such services: they are now very rare. I remember my supervisory consultants being accommodating and encouraging to provide the flexibility of arrangements, space and time for this therapeutic relationship (and others) to run its course and bear its fruit. This was possible because there were, then, far fewer diktats, rules and bureaucratic obelisks stymying autonomous, responsible judgements of wisdom and experience. In those days coded and hegemonic psychiatric diagnosis was far less important than personal connection and understanding; care often proceeded down unmade tracks rather than prescribed tarmacked, generic Care Pathways; care was often a delicate dance improvised between individuals rather than an institutional march decreed by academic or administrative committees.

Sally today would be most unlikely to find such continuity of personal containment and accompaniment in any NHS Psychiatric (not Psychotherapy, remember) Services. What she then received may now seem extraordinary, but it was not uncommon then. I am saddened not just for patients, but also for the working welfare of current doctors: few, if any, will have the licence or latitude for such broad, deep or long contact with individuals, or garner the humanly profound and lasting satisfactions.

Some will say that we cannot now economically afford such bespoke services. I do not agree: such care is much cheaper than the kind of anomic, multi-disciplined, multi-teamed approaches that flounder with great expense and poor personal connection in the current NHS. I see this regularly and spend much of my professional time trying to repair the damage. If we do not make good human sense to one another, economic and human costs are much higher.

Sally's letter was a kind of dramatic oxymoron – a shock from the anciently familiar: amidst my current healthcare concerns it rapidly crystallised into a welcome and edifying sense. For the outside reader its private significance for us both is easily imagined. This will produce many individual resonances. Many may identify Agape: non-erotic, unpossessive, unidealised love that is probably essential to Physis. The institutional and cultural themes invite opportunities for reflection that should not be missed: hence this invitation to greater readership. After contact and discussion with Sally she agrees. This is thus a documentary presentation, and to anchor authenticity real names are used.

I have attached my reply to her largely for human interest.

The correspondence is unedited, apart from the omission of addresses. Claybury refers to Claybury Hospital, then a large psychiatric hospital in suburban East London. It closed about twenty years ago.

## 2. Letter 1

3 June 2013

Dear David Zigmond

Back in the 1970s I was a patient of yours. At first an outpatient at North Middlesex Hospital and then I became an inpatient in Claybury.

I met John at Claybury and although at the time many people advised against us getting together, we went on to have a happy 30 years. Like everyone we had our ups and downs, had three great kids, Rachel, Paul and Natalie, and now three lovely grandchildren too.

He died 3 days after that anniversary in 2006. I continued my long career in nursing which has changed so much from those early years and in the last decade I focused on palliative care which was more in tune with my own values and beliefs on patient centred care. I retired last year as all the NHS changes finally wore me down!

I'm writing not to just tell you all this information but to let you know what a difference you have made to my life. You really cared, you made me feel like I was important, not just another NHS patient. You listened and believed in me. I don't often talk about that time to many people, but when I do I say how you made me feel safe and I believed that you wouldn't leave me – and you didn't. I left and never told you what a big impact you had on my life and that I knew I would never sink into those dark depths of depression again, I felt healed. That experience influenced every area of my life and work and the person I became.

Radical changes have taken place in mental care over the years but it wasn't just about the system, I was so fortunate to have had you as my Doctor. I don't know how difficult it was in those days to keep me as a patient when you moved hospitals, but you did and it made all the difference. I've never forgotten, it's just taken me a long time and before any more time passes, I just want to say a heartfelt 'Thank you, you saved my life'.

Best wishes

*Sally Baynes*

Sally Baynes (Davies)

## 3. Letter 2

15 June 2013

Dear Sally

Thank you so much for your candid and unsentimentally heartfelt letter.

I very quickly recalled your face and your spirit though, interestingly, I cannot remember your 'clinical' details, your 'history'. It is instructive, what we retain of one another.

I find your letter remarkable for the span of time you recall and the unaffected clarity and veracity of your account. I am deeply gratified and moved that the 'cuttings' I offered you so long ago were cherished, planted and nurtured by you and have steadily borne fruit, over a lifetime. In parallel it has been my conviction, over my working lifetime, that this kind of activity should often lie at the heart of what we do for one another. In these realms most damage and most healing is human.

It sounds to me as if your 'recovery' has gone far beyond the medically mapped realms of 'symptom relief' and 'good clinical outcome'. You indicate that most wondrous and humbling transformation: you have turned your painful burden into a compassionate and healing gift, for yourself and others. It seems that this has cascaded through your marriage to two generations of family, and beyond that to your many recipients of palliative care nursing. All of this is heartening for me, too: our healing and nourishment of one another is often unobvious.

But there are shadows, too, where I also wish to join you. You refer to your 'patient-centred values and beliefs ... being worn down', leading to your retirement (from the NHS). Likewise, your reference to 'radical changes in mental healthcare' making your own previous healing experiences most unlikely now. I resonate with this: such concerns are at the centre of my vocational life.

We are here different in our adjustment: you have expediently retired to your more accessible gratifications of family and grandchildren; I remain contentiously engaged with heroic obstinacy, possibly because I do not yet have grandchildren (though the social and biological machinery looks promising).

It seems that as we get older we find solace and peace in a few simple and timeless maxims: 'Counting our Blessings ... Seeing what is there, not what is not ...'. Simple to say, yet often so difficult to live by. It sounds as if you have managed a great deal.

Your letter has particular and intense value for you and I. But I think it has messages that are universally important, especially for healthcare workers. What you talk of lies before, behind and beyond all trainings, texts, systems, manuals, data and codes which now weary and alienate so many.

With suitable safeguards, could we publish these letters?

Whatever your reply I have found it deeply satisfying to have heard from you in this way: such communications give great difficulties even deeper meaning.

With warmest wishes
David Zigmond

Ω

(Private correspondence with an ex-patient, 2013 – with her consent for publication)

# NHS Savings?

## Abolish the Internal Market

The Internal Market is a failing experiment aiming to submit complex Welfare to monetarism and commerced industrialisation. Our earlier federal system addressed human and economic needs with much greater directness and honesty.

Recently, Sir David Nicholson, NHS Chief Executive, raised alarmed questions about how the NHS can possibly be paid for in the near future.

Throughout a working lifetime as a GP I have carefully watched many changes. I now have a pragmatic but retro-radical suggestion: we should abolish the entire Internal Market and thus such subordinate institutions and devices as the purchaser-provider split, autarkic and competing Trusts, payment by results and Commissioning. All of this may be well intended but is a failing experiment to apply commerce and Monetarism to complex welfare.

The human and economic costs of this defederalised system are very high. As fragmentation and boundaries increase, so do procedural, bureaucratic and financial complexity and delay. Competition, or its threat, decreases professional synergy and replaces it with expensively expedient tactics and presentations: glossy brochures, specious statistics, mistrustful feints, 'gaming' the systems and being guided more by technical legality than humanistic ethos. I have hundreds of examples documenting these,[1] but rarely (if ever) discern clear benefits of defederalisation.

Here are two commonplace and recent examples. First: my locality GPs have cumulatively invested hundreds of hours tendering competitive plans for an Out of Hours Centre: this was a politically prescribed project of no real value: it evaporated without sense or trace. Second: at a mental-health centre I attended a dreary, droning, dead-eyed meeting where eight fractiously obedient practitioners discussed for half an hour a patient who none of them had ever met; in particular whether, or not, the referral was procedurally correct. Until recent times this would have been dealt with by a friendly five-minute phone call by an experienced practitioner with good sense and courtesy. Time and energy were then saved; helpful relationships fostered.

Such losses and follies may seem comically grotesque to an outsider: as an insider I know the enormity of the consequences: the costs to people as well as budgets – such is the maturing culture of corporatized and marketised Welfare.

The old, federal, 'Socialist' NHS did not have these problems. Yes, it had others but I think they were more honest and more soluble.

Ω

Published as a letter to the *Guardian*, 16 July 2013

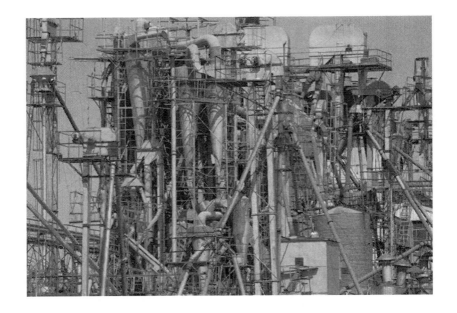

# How Care Pathways obliterate Care

## More industrial follies from the NHS

Overschematisation in complex welfare will usually yield results quite different from those intended.

Recently many seemed shocked by the malign metamorphosis of the Liverpool Care Pathway. For here we have an attempt to mass-produce and standardise compassionate palliative care for the terminally ill then contorting to a designed absence of care that combines shocking insensitivity, psychopathic expedience (hastening death to vacate usable bed-space) and chilling indifference to the suffering of the dying and their relatives. I am not shocked but wearily despondent: I work in a health service where 'progress' is increasingly defined by the displacement of the best, discriminating personal healthcare by didactic, 'expert-committee' generated systems which attempt to command quality by prescribing some kind of uniform plan. Industrialisation of dying sounds stark; it is. Most such schemes are doomed to very serious losses of personal connection and imaginative compassionate understanding. In any matters of human complexity institutional schemes and human understandings are often countervailed, unless we take great care.

The story of the Liverpool Care Pathway is like a Brothers Grimm fairy story even more unfit for children. It is an example of what can happen if we do not take that care. For the care of the dying is a poignant and delicate dance: each encounter requires unique responses of contact, utterances, understandings and technicalities. This is fine and fragile work that calls on any practitioner's capacities of empathic imagination quite as much as technical knowledge. It is the discriminating weaving of these that makes up the art of Medicine. With the characteristic follies and losses of our times we have largely crushed or displaced both the habitats and activities of such art in our healthcare in an attempt to get factory-like efficiency, compliance and uniformity.

Healing and palliation are complex interactions that arise from human kinship, not object-like management. Mind-sets and management modes from industry or commerce have very limited contributions to make to complex welfare. It is when their influence exceeds this that we have the toxic moral vacuum phenomena of Mid-Staffs or the Liverpool Care Pathway.

Ideas that seem easy in areas of great human complexity usually have a large and horrible price. As the philosopher Alfred North Whitehead said: 'seek simplicity, then always mistrust it'.

Ω

Published in the *Daily Telegraph*, 23 July 2013

# The High Price
# of Commodified Healthcare

Commerce, industrial manufacture and monetarism are seriously flawed bases for Welfare provision. This brief letter presents another snapshot of what is happening.

.

On one evening in the last week there were two separately channelled TV programmes addressing yet more apparent incompetence in NHS Healthcare. Each of the two programmes focused at opposite ends of a spectrum: the 111 Service for acute and short-term directive contact and then psychiatric services for the complexly distressed, for longer-term care. From this wide span of missed and miscommunications what common themes emerge?

The programmes' portrayals were consistent with my many decades' experience as an NHS doctor. What we are witnessing is the loss of a healthcare culture of personally invested connections and understandings. This has happened through attempts to emulate industrial manufacture and commercial trade. Before twenty years ago there was much good practice that was free of the current errors. For example, I was part of a GP out-of-hours rota which – together with our telephonists – provided a much more skilled, competent and personable service with little administrative clutter or expense. Likewise, when I worked as a psychiatrist I was able to offer personal continuity of care over many years with the commensurate containing, and healing effects: this was humanly rich yet financially economical. These lost patterns of healthcare extended beyond sensitive and sensible care for patients, they were – indirectly though substantially – sources of human nourishment and enlivenment for healthcarers too: the doctors I know may now be paid more, but they have less personal work satisfaction.

In complex human Welfare if employees do not really like their work they are unlikely to ever do it well, whatever the strictures and structures. A commercially or industrially modelled system becomes – perversely – humanly disconnected, then harmful and economically wasteful. The evidence for the failure of this approach is now ineluctable: it is a doomed project. We now need to largely dismantle these well intended but corrupting devices: autarkic and competing Trusts; commercial subcontracting; payment by results; hegemonic Goals and Targets, algorithms, Care Pathways and statistics-before-sense. We need to understand and reclaim the underlying motivational and vocational psychology of our work: why and how should we care for one another?

Our complex human bonds may then be better honoured.

Ω

Published in the *Guardian*, 7 August 2013

# Psychiatry?

## Everyone is right – but not for long

Psychiatry and physical medicine are often contiguous, sometimes continuous. This is subtle and precarious, for careless conflation can be harmful: we need vigilant discernment to prevent this.

.Will Self has done us all a service by provoking an interesting and telling correspondence ('Psychiatry, drugs and mental healthcare's future', (Guardian letters 8.8.13). What is demonstrated is that Psychiatry is like its erstwhile Rorschach (inkblot) projective tests: it can plausibly represent – even 'justify' – almost any of our fears, hopes, explanatory notions, preoccupations or prejudices. We can easily people it, too, with heroes and villains.

Yet if we heed certain distinctions we can avoid much confusion. For the territory and predicaments of psychiatry are often different from prevailing physical medicine. Psychiatry engages a protean realm of dis-ease, whereas much of medicine is more stably anchored to a solid world of disease. Dis-ease – our more undifferentiated human ailments – contains much that cannot be satisfactorily objectified or measured, as well as offering us endless puzzles of coexistent contradictions: these are due to the fact that our dis-ease is often a pre-verbal signalling system to ourselves and others that all is not well, that we are disequilibrated.

Both kinds of veterans – the Psychiatrist (Professor David Goldberg) and patient (Trish Oliver) – write with convincing sense of the massive blessings of psychiatric medication applied when dis-ease is so great that it is not just contiguous to, but seems continuous with, disease: this is 'major mental illness' and its designation is often problematic because this must rely mostly on human experience and judgement. Unlike physical medicine, attempts at objective testing of dis-ease often turn out to be more flawed than useful.

Most of us seeking help with substantial psychological distress do not have such major mental illness and require not didactically structured treatments but dialogically evocative forms of containment and healing. The former (treatments) may be accessible to standardisation, measurement and mass-production, the latter (healings) generally cannot.

Why is all this important? Because it leads to a predicament for current NHS Healthcare whose increasingly industrial, measurement-fuelled ethos will tend to favour the prescriptive treatment interventions appropriate to cure disease, rather than the imaginatively attuned healing encounters that may help us transcend dis-ease. This accounts for an increasing, sometimes tragic, discrepancy: as our technical treatments get better, our personal care gets lost. This is reflected in many of our recent grotesque headlines of institutional neglect and abuse. The over-prescription of psychoactive drugs is a commoner example, less dramatic but still important. Such skewed professional activity is often telling us that we are losing our best balance between the science of manipulation and the art of understanding. Yes, prescriptive and designatory psychiatry can provide great benefits, but its limits always need artful and humane discernment.

Good healthcare is a humanity guided by science. That humanity is an art and an ethos. Any wisdom we can bring to bear will be in the blending and balancing of these: the constitution of such wisdom must always extend beyond our formulae.

$$\Omega$$

Letter to the *Guardian* 2013

# NHS Healthchecks

## more automation and less intelligence

The front-page story *NHS checks on over-40s condemned as 'useless'* (20 August) and subsequent letter (*Healthcheck checks*) can lead us to additional valuable insights into virtuously squandered resources and depleted staff morale in the NHS.

In the last two decades of my work as a GP my original role as a skilled, holistic, personal and family physician has been steadily displaced by imperatives to perform government-dictated generic and measurable procedures: a tick-box world for healthdroids. Goals and targets are now firmly welded to contractual payments to ensure conformity. Such obedience costs not just money and skilled time, but also the doctor's intelligent and imaginative discretion and – eventually – the experience and ability to make humane and sophisticated judgements.

The current overtreatment of 'high' blood pressure is a common example of such perverse consequences. GPs are now paid according to how many high blood pressures they can lower: *ergo* they are driven to treat a measurement, not the patient. This has created serious secondary problems, particularly among the frail-elderly whose prescriptively over-lowered (for them) blood pressure then often leads to dizziness, falls, collapse and serious injuries – always distressing, sometimes fatal.

What is getting lost in such mass-produced and formulaic testings and treatments are the erstwhile aspects of care that are intelligently discerning, personal and bespoke. This is not just injurious to patients and budgets – practitioners, too, become diminished, deskilled and demoralised. This happens because our sense of meaningful contact and satisfaction grows from the autonomous exercise of such skills: they comprise the now ailing heart and art of medical practice. Importantly, these are closely akin to compassion. The process of these losses may be insidious, but the consequences are more stark. We are already finding that the more we reduce vocational healthcarers to act as centrally-programmed healthdroids, the more horror healthcare headlines we have coming to us.

Ω

Letter to the *Times* 2013

# Re-establishing Personal Bonds and Understandings in NHS Care

Dear Jeremy Hunt
(Secretary of State for Health)

I am a veteran inner London single-handed GP with a working lifetime's interest in humanistic aspects of healthcare, its bonds and milieux.

I listened to your Conference speech last week and was heartened by some of your messages. Previous Health Secretaries have management-spoke almost entirely of strategies, goals and targets, new regulations and control and monitoring systems. But you, refreshingly, have expanded the language and thus the perspective. You talk of the culture of values, the nature of the personal bonds and attitudes, and how these constitute the personal care that so often lies behind and beyond generic treatments.

In the early 1970s I had several thoughtful and compassionate mentors who modelled and encouraged imaginative and person-centred care. As a young practitioner I was led to see how overly bio-mechanistic healthcare encounters impoverished both human understanding and therapeutic opportunities. My interest and concerns about this led to my long train of qualitative research and writing.

What I did not foresee in my early career was how much worse the human disconnections would become: I had not predicted the impact, for example, of computers, informatics or systems management. The benefits these bring are early, evident and alluring; the human price is more subtle and delayed.

In your speech you anchored your human-scale concern to practical proposals. One of these is of particular interest to me: your wish to restore and revitalise personal investment and continuity of care by reinstating GP Personal Lists for the elderly. I think this is salutary and pragmatic: a good foundation-stone. But I would like to see this re-found foundation widened to all age groups who have chronic, complex or protean difficulties – for it is this large healthcare territory that must have personal bonds and understandings to make therapeutic effects likely.

The current NHS has become better at technology-based treatments where cure is likely, but worse at humanity-based care where cure is unlikely or impossible. The former may parallel the optimism of youth; the latter is the fate of age. Care and cure often require different kinds of heart and mind-sets: this often requires a flexible, delicate weave – and this becomes impossible with systems that are over-systematised and over-prescriptive. I have explored and written about these problems for several decades. If you are interested I have attached a small sample of articles, with some brief notes of guidance at the end of this letter.

In your speech you described how much you had learned from your brief work engagements on the frontline of the NHS. Here is an invitation for a similar and deepening experience: come to my small inner-city General Practice and see my attempts at long-term, personal continuity of healthcare and the adversaries I have in institutions, politics and culture.

Meanwhile, thank you again for your humane and humanising contributions and plans: I hope you hold office long enough for them to grow securing roots.

Ω

Letter to Secretary of State for Health 2013

# Loneliness in the Ailing Elderly: social and healthcare responses

Dear Jeremy Hunt
(Secretary of State for Health)

I heard of your comments recently. I am grateful that you are, again, broadening the language and thought from the systemic and managerial to include the humanistic and ethical.

I am a small-practice GP with decades of experience working long term with the kinds of problems you refer to: I would like to share some of my understandings.

I am sure you have far too much to read, but I am attaching two writings that are almost certainly different from your usual fare: they are personal narratives, written in a spirit of scientific enquiry, by a veteran frontline NHS doctor. The first, The Psychoecology of Gladys Parlett was written in 1988 and more prophetic than I intended. The second, Five Executive Follies, was written much more recently, for your predecessor, Andrew Lansley: it demonstrates and explains what has happened in the last two decades, since Gladys Parlett.

Of course, I shall be interested in any thoughtful response.

Ω

Letter to Secretary of State for Health 2013

# Dr Frankenstein's Reprise

## Industrialisation of personal healthcare: adverse effects of sequestered psychiatric in-patient services

Dear Dr Dratcu
(Consultant, In-patient Psychiatrist)

I am writing to you as a long-serving GP with a long but now increasingly consternated interest and experience in Mental Health. For many years I have accumulated both dismay from, and interest in, the riddle of our increasing personal disconnection in healthcare.

This letter is very long: this reflects not just the length of my observation and reflection, but also the protean complexity and multivalence of our tasks. Crucially, I believe it is our expedient oblivion and then short-circuiting of these essential subtleties that has led to many of our current errors. So this long missive is a small act of correction.

Yet though this letter may be unusually demanding, I hope it will be equally rewarding through attention. It is one of several I have written about areas of endangered or eroded personal care. For several years I have worked in a system where mental health services have become more humanly disconnected despite, apparently, good administrative coherence. Patients' experiences of psychiatric admissions provide clear examples of this.[1] The first part of this letter portrays the problems I encounter. Later I provide some little-discussed explanations and finally my ideas about the now very difficult restoration.

It is important that I first clarify that this letter is not a personal or professional criticism of you or any of your staff, though it is a critique of the system we are operating and the culture it leads to. All the difficulties I describe may include, but extend far beyond, any individual practitioner. Though addressed to you, I am intending communication to be stimulated more widely.

*

First, let me tell you something of the background to this letter, and outline a more general view of our mutual problems: for many stymies we have in psychiatry, including your territory of acute admissions, are a constituent of this larger, ailing, puzzled jigsaw.

I am one of your local GPs. I am working in an NHS that is increasingly troubled by its own designs: by generating a more and more industrial-type system of rigidly boundaried fragments, defined by administratively categorised specialisations. The costs of the resulting human disconnection are high, but its subtlety also leads to expedient ignorance: over-systematised and depersonalised care has developed its own life and momentum: sleep-walking like a Frankenstein's Monster among the perplexed and vulnerable.

My concern about such healthcare misindustrialisation extends to all more pastoral areas of healthcare – those where the charismatic blessings of rapidly successful technology-based cure is unlikely: this constitutes much of mental health services and General Practice. I have been recently engaging with colleagues in these areas to stimulate creative debate. Amidst these wider concerns and efforts, the activities of sequestered In-Patient psychiatry continue to provide me regularly with graphic examples of the consequences of our healthcare follies. I have written previously to other mental health executives detailing some of my own and patients' experiences: I urge you to read them.[1]

Second, let me introduce myself. I am a veteran inner-city GP servicing a small practice in Bermondsey, your catchment area. In the first half of my career I did much qualitative research into healthcare human connections; what is therapeutic and what not, then why and how[2]. In more recent years this interest has become bound to my consternation that modern systems of diagnosis-centred management, in their attempt to confer precision and efficiency, are often overused and then become countertherapeutic.[3] This is obviously the reverse of what is intended, and further attempts to rectify the problems with similar methods will compound and compact the human disconnection. This is the corrosive paradox and conundrum we have generated throughout pastoral healthcare. This letter is part of my mission to widen and broaden thought and discussion.

*

Now I would like to return to our problems with acute psychiatric admissions.

I am currently caring for four patients who, in the last year, describe urgent in-patient psychiatric care at the Maudsley Hospital. Their individual stories converge with similar experiences of care: the emergent themes – of being cared for with impoverished personal understanding at times of intense vulnerability – are growing with our current accelerated systemisation.[4] Increasingly we have a system ill-equipped to offer havens of comfort, containment and personal understanding to enable natural processes of healing and recovery. Instead the overwhelmed, the dis-integrated, the disequilibrated – the acutely mentally ill – are hurried between relays of assessment and risk management teams: staff who usually have no prior or subsequent relationship with the patient.[5] All of this may make much sense to management. It does not for patients: for their inchoate agitations or utterances of distress – and then the personal understandings of meaning necessary to heal such breakdown – require a rapport involving personal continuity, patience and imagination: these are unlikely to survive on a conveyor-belt of short-term objectification. No kind of institutional or academic cleverness can substitute for personally evolved healing relationships.[6]

My argument here is separate from, though may be amplified by, those of scarcity of resources. There is, currently, a media conveyed interest in the lack of acute psychiatric beds.[7] This may also be a serious problem, but different to what I am addressing: my four patients were all 'lucky' to be promptly admitted to a local unit (The Maudsley Hospital). My questions here are not about funding or procurement, but the nature of such care. My view here is that in mental health it is often the failure or disruption of human bonds that sicken, and it is through certain kinds of careful human bonds and understandings that we heal.[8] Technical language and procedures may sometimes help such humanities, but rarely should they displace them.

\*

I used to work both in, and with, psychiatric services that offered mental healthcare based on far greater personal continuity and thus understanding. Because of this, the previous services were more economically viable, too: a psychiatrist and his team who have developed a trusting, nuanced and personally understanding rapport with a patient are likely to have far greater therapeutic leverage and success than a rapid carousel of centrally-directed strangers, however well trained. But this is what we have now: the attempt to model such pastoral care on airports, surgical techniques or car factories leads to the abject disconnected 'care' described by my four patients.[9]

\*

We cannot recreate the past, yet with intelligent analysis it has much to teach us. My early career experiences in now-vanished, better Mental Hospitals taught me much about the subtle values of longer-term personal bonds and understandings; of flexible and intelligent capacities for containment and asylum; and – conversely – the folly of sharp, excessive packaging – our expedient resort to rigid diagnoses and institutional care pathways. Such early lessons in thoughtful eclecticism guided and enriched my working lifetime, had decades of enthusiastic agreement among my peers and are supported by much historic documentation.[10] Sadly and importantly such lessons are increasingly lost or disregarded – this is one definition of cultural change.[11]

*

So, how can we transpose or transplant these lessons to our current situation? Here are some notions, caveats and suggestions to help us reconfigure mental health services in a way that restores my working maxim: Healthcare is a humanity guided by science. That humanity is an art and an ethos.

In Principle, we need to understand:

- How and why have we brought about these difficulties? I think much can be explained by a little discussed, but seminally important, shift of axioms in teaching and academia throughout mental healthcare. We have abandoned the previous equilibrium between phenomenology (a description and clustering of how things are, or appear) and semiotics (what things might mean).
- Phenomenology is more compatible with objective and scientific discourse and understanding. Semiotics is necessary for imaginative human understanding. So, phenomenology is more concerned with treatment: healing must draw largely from semiotics. A balance and easy exchange between the two is necessary for holism. Compassionate care is mostly impossible without holism.
- Partly due to the rise of computers, and then the seductive (often treacherous) opportunities to industrialise mental

healthcare, there has been an increasingly demanding rhetoric to displace semiotics (an unmeasurable art) by phenomology (a measurable proto-science, though often speciously so).

- Without intelligent discrimination this can easily lead to the follies of scientism: to services whose zealous attempts to make a science of manipulation is often at the expense of the art of individual understanding.

- We need to return to a personal continuity of care – sometimes over long periods. This can provide much better individual understanding and thence to humanly nuanced diagnosis and therapeutic influences. (The exceptions to this are always instructive and interesting.)

- Personal continuity of care is more an understanding and arrangement between consenting adults than a procedure decided by a Central Directorate.

- Nevertheless personal continuity – even when desired, optimal and unproblematic – must always be 'safety-netted' by background administrative and institutional continuity.

- Generally, when working well, personal continuity of care should be a pre-eminent and anchoring principle.

## In Practice this means:

- Bringing back Consultant General Psychiatrists who would be responsible for running a team (these used to be called 'Firms' and typically consisted of the Consultant, one or two grades of trainees, a Psychiatric Social Worker, Community Psychiatric Nurse, Clinical Psychologist, Occupational Therapist and then his in-patient Ward Staff).[12]

- This Consultant Psychiatrist would be responsible for a geographical area and therefore would get to know families, streets, local myths and rumour, GPs, Social Workers, Health Visitors and District Nurses.[13]

- By having their own core-staff and in-patient Ward, the Psychiatrist, and the more long-serving members of the team, are then able to provide a much more personally-knowledged and engaged service.

- This locality-based, consultant-led team would provide the bulk of widely ranging psychiatric help for most patients who need it. The team would be responsible for the whole span of most patients' likely care: out-patient clinics, home visits (assessment, monitoring and therapeutic), day-patient and in-patient care.[14]

- For very refractory or unusual cases there would be tertiary centres to refer to.[15]

- This consultant and their team would then have the advantage of personal knowledge and understanding to make dextrous and effective decisions. For example, a psychiatrist with long experience of a patient is much more able to quickly and accurately evaluate a difficult and unstable situation and, say, admit the patient, or have the CPN visit regularly or get them an urgent Day Centre place, supervised by an OT. (This was much of my experience in the setting of large Mental Hospitals in early 1970s. Care was – comparatively – much more efficient, person-centred and seamlessly initiated and integrated. Holism was not explicitly talked about, but easily enacted. Staff conflict, tension and sickness was much less and morale much higher: people liked their work.)

- It is, therefore, not just patients who will benefit. Work satisfaction is much greater when personal investment is more valued and attachments last long enough to bear fruit that can be witnessed and savoured. Staff who derive warmth and satisfaction from their difficult tasks will work much better. This has benefits for both management and the economy.

- The dismantling of administrative barriers to more holistic and personal healthcare is needed throughout the NHS where pastoral care is elemental. For example, there are strong arguments for reinstating GP personal lists and hospital General Physicians.[16]

- The kind of Consultant Psychiatrist that I envision re-establishing resembles also the better old kind of General Practitioner in terms of their breadth of skill, accumulation of personal knowledge and long-term vernacular commitment. They would thus be more experienced, and thus older, on appointment. Their professional influences would derive as much from vocational education as hegemonic training.[17] This raises further issues about medical recruitment, training v education, and the design and finance of career structures: all need further complex analysis.[18]

*

I do hope you will read this letter with something of the thought and spirit that has gone into it. I certainly do not expect a long written reply, but I would like to begin some informal discussions. I am also inviting this from our Mental Healthcare Commissioners and Medical Director.

Ω

## Notes and References:

[1] In this long letter I have not included a description or analysis of individual accounts that have provided me with grist and motivation. Similar stories can be found in earlier writings, which I have numerically referenced and are easily accessible via my Home Page. This applies also to related and cited healthcare themes.

Previous letters to senior colleagues might interest you. They are:

- *Eric: Another victim of Hypertrophic Obstructive Management Coagulopathy:* A letter to the Medical Director, South London and Maudsley NHS Trust (2012)

- *Bureaucratyrannohypoxia:* An open letter to Mental Health Services Director (2010)

The particular patients who talked with me of their depersonalised and unattuned in-patient experiences are willing to talk to you and other responsible healthcare workers.

[2] My interest in this has spanned a long career. See, for example:

- *Three Types of Encounter in the Healing Arts: Dialogue, Dialectic and Didacticism* (1987)

- *The Front Door of Psychotherapy: Aspects from General Medical Practice* (1989)

- *Why Would Anyone Use an Unproven Therapy? Treasures in the Mist* (2010)

[3] See, for example:

- *Idiomorphism: the Lost Continent. How diagnosis displaces personal understanding* (2011)

- *Institutional atrocities: The malign vacuum from industrialised healthcare* (2013)

[4] *Continuity of Care: Of course, but whose? A Sleight of Slogans: Letter to Family Doctor Association* (2012)

[5] *If you want good personal healthcare, see a Vet. Caveats for holistic healthcare Part II* (2012)

[6] *Sense and Sensibility: The danger of Specialisms to holistic, psychological care* (2011)

[7] Dr Martin Baggaley recently talked to the media about the loss of psychiatric in-patient beds. He was there talking of *quantity*: my

concerns here are *qualitative* and different, though they may be parallel.

[8] *Mother, Magic or Medicine? The Psychology of the Placebo* (1984)

Thirty years ago this article expressed a kind of imaginative, yet disciplined, *intersubjective* analysis often pursued by thoughtful practitioners. This kind of thought has become nearly extinct in the last twenty years. In my view this is largely due to our indiscriminate use of electronic informatics. This has generated an unwise and uncompromising rhetoric of *objectification*, whose language is data. Unmindfully unleashed, such data have a similar relationship to human imagination and relationships as swarms of locusts have to human habitats and crops – see *Words and Numbers: Servants or Masters? Caveats for holistic healthcare Part 1* (2012).

[9] I documented this change in culture, and its human casualties in Psychiatry: *Love's Labour's Lost. The pursuit of The Plan and the eclipse of the personal* (2010)

[10] I have many documents to itemise and date these changes. Two of them I have contextualised in:

- *Language is not just data: it is a custodian of our humanity* (2013)
- *Physis: healing, growth and the hub of personal continuity of care A thirty-nine (39) year delayed follow-up correspondence with Sally* (2013)

[11] *Institutional atrocities: The malign vacuum from industrialised healthcare* (2013)

[12] My earliest experiences in Psychiatry – in an old Victorian Mental Hospital in the early 1970s – provided an excellent (comparatively) personal service of this kind. Its positive influence has been indelible for me. See *Psychiatry: Love's Labour's Lost. The pursuit of The Plan and the eclipse of the personal* (2010)

[13] The conception of the old general psychiatric team could be redesigned. Obviously they would not operate from a large Mental Hospital. Smaller, more numerous In-Patient units would be close to Day Centres, Out-Patients etc, ideally within easy walking distance. Geographical proximity and easy personal contact with colleagues lead to much better colleagueial understanding and relationships – see *Eric: Another victim of Hypertrophic Obstructive Management Coagulopathy* (2012).

[14] These reincarnated General Psychiatrists would function much like the better GPs of this earlier period: they guide and care for many different kinds of patients over long periods, will often delegate to known colleagues but retain an overarching interest, personal knowledge and responsibility.

This kind of sense of caring containment was mostly more therapeutic for patients: work satisfaction for the professionals was commensurate with this.

[15] This worked well in the 1970s. Only a small fraction of more puzzling and refractory cases would be sent to a tertiary centre (eg for Severe and Uncontained Psychosis, Eating Disorder or for long-term Psychotherapy). This is paralleled elsewhere in the NHS: see note 16.

[16] See my examples at the end of *Five Executive Follies: How commodification imperils compassion in personal healthcare* (2011)

There is a parallel argument to reinstate the erstwhile kind of General Physician who would provide the vast bulk of hospital-based secondary medical care. They (as before) would only refer on a small fraction of more complex work. Currently, older people are often under multiple medical specialists, each for a fairly common condition. Very often patients cannot name the speciality, even less the specialist: there are all kinds of losses here – of personal bonds and understandings that are essential to comfort and healing; to speedy, accurate professional judgements that come from personal familiarity; of efficiency that comes from uncomplex administration; of efficiency that comes from good work satisfactions from satisfying personal bonds.

General Practice, since the abolition of Personal Lists and the accretion and demise of small Practices, has very similar problems.

[17] Consultants many years ago were usually less formally trained but more informally educated. They were older and thus had longer and wider experience. This may have been less neatly compact for managers but produced many unsystematic blessings.

See *No Country for Old Men: The Rise of Managerialism and the New Cultural Vacuum* (2009)

[18] There is a welter of problems in all this. What are the alternatives to the current severe academic meritocracy to gateway Medical Schools? How can we best encourage education (learning by enquiry) without losing the hard essentials of training (assurance by instruction)? If (as I would argue) Psychiatric Consultants should have longer and wider prior experience of healthcare and life, how would we encourage this without loss, to them, of money or motivation?

$$\Omega$$

Letter to the Medical Director, In-patient Psychiatry, Maudsley Hospital, South London, 2014

**Post-scripted appendix: Early reply from Dr Dratcu**

6 November 2013

Dear Dr Zigmond

It was a pleasure talking to you on the telephone. I am honoured that you have decided to share your thoughts with me. I am also very pleased to see that you have such wide and longstanding interest in, and understanding of, the ever changing framework within which mental health services operate, and the implications of this to our patients.

You have written a very detailed document and I apologise for not addressing it point by point. May I nonetheless start by saying that many of the concerns you have raised are exactly the same that I and a significant numbers of my colleagues frequently entertain about developments in mental healthcare provision within the NHS. We are all aware of the fragmentation of mental health services in recent years and its pitfalls. We are also aware of the challenges that many management-driven approaches may engender in our interaction with our patients. In an age where IT and databases increasingly encompass everything we do, there is indeed a risk that all this may culminate in what you describe as "increasing personal disconnection and industrialisation of healthcare".

These are clearly broad issues that go far beyond mental healthcare alone, and for which we are unlikely to have easy answers. With your permission, and as we discussed on the telephone, the best course of action for me at the moment is to divulge your message to my colleagues.

Kind regards

Luiz Dratcu

Dr Luiz Dratcu, MD PhD FRCPsych
Consultant Psychiatrist, Maudsley Hospital

# Qualifications
# may be less than useful

D. Stewart's letter ('Qualifications aren't everything', Independent, 2 November 2013) conveys much robust sense and sensibility. Our world of Welfare services is increasingly strangled and obstructed by excessive and rigid technical requirements. As a veteran GP in the NHS I have seen how damaging this has been. NHS healthcarers are now more highly trained and qualified than ever, but this is often at the expense of humane and vocational spirit. Our technical treatments are undoubtedly better, but our personal and pastoral care is often worse. The now-frequent headlines of healthcare-horrors are tips of icebergs: under the surface we will find much more.

Yes, technical procedures need specific training and qualifications. But the complex needs we have in our care and guidance of one another requires much more, and that more is often very different. Compassionate interest and imagination are subtle and natural fruits. They may be induced, encouraged and modelled, but then cannot be directly or didactically instructed or assessed.

More worrying, an attempt to technicalise personal care and understanding will often destroy them. More of something 'good' is sometimes worse.

Ω

Letter to the *Independent* 2013

# We need an Appointment with Dr Finlay

A recent article by Stephen Moss ('Pills, bills and bellyaches: a peek behind the scenes at a GP surgery', *The Guardian*, 3/11/13) is a vivid Hogarthian portrait of a frontline of our current NHS.

As a long-serving inner-city GP there is much I can endorse, amplify or dispute. One strand is of interest and illuminates much else. Health Secretary Jeremy Hunt is reported as pressuring *simultaneously* for a return to a traditional 'family doctor' ethos (which I strongly support) and an instant, Skyping, emailing, extended hours service (which I find inimical). It seems clear to me that one service cannot do both, and that an emphasis on the latter will destroy the former. Personally sensitive and imaginative care requires certain kinds of understanding, and these can come only from attentive human contacts and bonds.

The article then notions the various types of GP arrangements: consortia, businesses, partnerships and polyclinics. These are considered as options for future service delivery. What is not returned to is the *small* practice with its strong vocational ethos and long vernacular roots. The better examples of these could, and did, provide much better human contact, understanding and containment than the current large-scale alternatives. Small practices may not have advantages of economies of scale but they can save much – in both human and economic terms – by restoring subtle and important human connections and understandings.

When my small, single-handed practice closes it will be dissolved into something much larger and less personally sentient and responsive. In my old age it is most unlikely that I will receive the kind of care I have been able to offer for so long.

I will want it.          Ω

Published on *BMJ blog*, 2013

# Dementia is not only (or even) a Disease: it is a Signal of our Community Cohesion

In recent weeks there has been much written about dementia, including articles by your correspondent Max Pemberton (*Dementia sufferers must have specialist care*, 2/12/13) and the Health Secretary (*Why I truly believe this generation can be the one to overcome dementia*, 29/11/13). While I certainly agree with their analysis and concern about the size and seriousness of the problem, my understanding of the nature of the problem is importantly different.

Both write of dementia as if it can be tackled head on – 'to beat dementia' – as we have done substantially with HIV and some cancers. But there are crucial (if unwelcome) differences: much dementia is a natural correlate of advanced age and not necessarily a pathological variation. Partly due to medical technology and partly due to social mobility we are living longer, but then have prolonged and slow declines in relative social isolation. This is now the usual and embedding matrix of dementia.

Medical technology currently has little to directly offer to most such cases of dementia. What helps much more is responsive, sensitive and imaginative guidance and containment. This is pastoral healthcare and welfare: twenty years ago the better GPs, district nurses and social workers were able to do this much better than now. Personal continuity of care – one of the best contributions to such welfare – has been made almost extinct by the successive devices of managerial systematisation and industrialisation of healthcare.

No, we do not need a massive new tranche of dementia clinics, consultants and brain-scanners: we need to retrieve the kind of social workers, GPs and general hospital physicians who can build personal relationships with patients, their families and communities – often over many years. No, we cannot 'beat dementia', and substantially may never do so. But we can, and should, offer professionally wise and compassionate counsel and containment to people we can get to know, understand and care about. This is good, personal, pastoral medical care of a traditional kind. Its retrieval sounds less inspiring and glamorous than 'beating dementia', but it is more realistic and thus achievable.

Ω

Letter published in the *Daily Telegraph*, December 2013

# Thank Goodness we now have business-sense to safeguard our Welfare

Commercially injected Welfare Services are managing a magical amalgam: combining venal corporate capitalism with leaden, officious, State bureaucracy. Here is one tiny example: we can expect much more.

*

We are living in worryingly ingenious times. Example: I have just paid fifty pounds to a large profit-making Corporation, subcontracted by the local council, for them to issue me with a Certificate, in order for them to collect my non-clinical refuse. They know that my clinical waste is disposed of by another (non-commercial) agency. Because I am a GP I am posed certain questions to certify my good citizenship and thus guarantee public safety: I must answer that I will not put such things as used dressings, sharp surgical instruments, excised body parts, unwanted organs, bodily fluids or dead babies in the general waste. They will not collect my waste without their (my) Certificate, which I can only purchase from them. They do not check the accuracy of my answers.

This is a brilliant conflation of venal, opportunistic, corporate capitalism and laden, vacuous, officious bureaucracy: it exemplifies much that is most specious, profligate and foolish in our commercially injected welfare services. Whatever happened to medical office effluent before such corporate vanguards were there to protect us, and the Certificates issued to 'prove' it?

Ω

Published in the *Independent*, 27 January 2014

# Failure of Personal Continuity of Care in Mental Health Services.

## The high cost to patient and practitioner welfare and the health economy

Dear Mr Lamb
(Minister for Care, Dep. of Health)

I am a long-serving GP with much additional experience working alongside and within mental health services.

Recently, I heard you talking on the Today programme (6.5.14). You were responding to concerns about our services' difficulty in providing good quality response and containment for the acutely mentally distressed.

It is a common view that our major problems are primarily due to inadequate resources, training or management. This may be partly true. But I think there is a more important though more subtle problem: the progressive loss of personal continuity of care throughout the NHS. I have watched this with growing alarm for many years: my long view motivates this long letter.

Our loss of more personal types of understanding and care is not easy to understand. It is a kind of 'collateral damage': its evolution is insidious, complex and paradoxical. For example, it can seem incontestably beneficial to always increase the schematic and 'objective' in our healthcare: but pastoral healthcare (ie our human responses to all those problems that do not have quick and definitive fixes) is chimeric, and these measures can then easily displace or destroy its many kinds of meaningful but fragile bonds: our relationships. This often happens without much awareness: we later awake and are shocked by their absence. Our current mental health services – both acute and chronic – are replete with such paradoxes: of how density of schematic management is often inversely proportional to therapeutic meaning for the patient. Every working day I do what I can to rectify many exigencies from this. I have forged for myself and my patients a precarious respite to do this: I have battled to retain a stable small practice. So, for many years I have still, with some difficulty, provided a kind of countervailant personal perspective and continuity: this kind of vantage is now very rare.

*

Throughout pastoral healthcare our best therapeutic engagements come from personal understandings. And these must come from growing bonds, each of which – like each individual – has both commonality and uniqueness. By not heeding this we are creating many more problems. For such personal bonds fare poorly in services that are complexly remote, highly managed, sharply boundaried and fragmented. The human casualties from this make for some shocking stories: I have witnessed and documented many. Yet these industrial kinds of services design do have a better place: for example, they are much more compatible with clearly anatomised physical disease – though even there we are finding serious problems emerging; even the most biomechanical needs some carefully bespoke care.

*

Pastoral and biomechanical healthcare are countervailant, yet complementary and synergistic. They are apparently opposite, yet we must combine them in innumerable ways. The art of evoking this synergy is a good definition of holism. But such holistic practice is now ailing and imperilled, for recent schematised healthcare reforms have often deracinated our personal bases of pastoral care. Inevitably, we then lose our more holistic views and understandings. In General Practice and Psychiatry – my areas of work – the losses are most clear and grievous.

*

How can we repersonalise our now humanly enucleated pastoral care? In the wide spectrum of the NHS the remedial principles converge, but the applications vary. Yet whatever the variation, we need to retain this seminal anchoring principle: personal continuity of care. For it is primarily from the development of personal attachment, affection and understanding that healing and palliation can take root. What we are now witnessing is serial examples of how all of this disintegrates in large, fragmented organisations that tend to standardised procedures. So, what specifically can we do to restore NHS Psychiatric Services? Here, in outline, are my summarised suggestions and bridging explanations:

- We need to bring back Consultant general psychiatrist-led 'Firms' (this is an old term for consultant-led teams).
- These teams would be locality-based and would take the vast majority of the wide variety of more severe mental and behavioural distress.
- The Consultant, with necessary deputies, would take overall responsibility for the complete cycle of mental healthcare from first contact to (provisional) discharge. (The bracketed word is necessarily important, if unwelcome.)
- The Consultant's Firm would have three major 'limbs': for Out-Patient consultations, for Home Visiting and for In-Patient Care. These three limbs would have some cross-flow and overlapping of staff (eg a patient is likely to be seen by the same practitioner(s) in a clinic, a ward, a Day-Centre, or at home).
- Most importantly, patients could move dextrously between different aspects or phases of care (Out-Patient, Day-Care, In-Patient and Home-based) with the kind of speedy and intelligent sensitivity that can come from personal continuity.

- Such personal continuity confers personal and economic benefits. Lengthy, cumbersome-yet-blind, bureaucratic assessments, procedures and documents become unnecessary. This cuts administrative burdens, costs, errors and frustrations drastically. Patients, generally, feel more contained, understood and comforted by people with whom they have an enduring bond. Staff have the slow, deep 'parental' satisfactions of seeing things through – the therapeutic effects of personal continuity are not confined to the patient!
- Obviously the Consultant Psychiatrist needs help with all this. The typical Firm would also contain trainee and deputy psychiatrists, psychologists, nurses, occupational therapists and social workers. As in well-functioning families there is, generally, easy and apt overlap and interchangeability of roles, though some important areas of sequestration.
- Most therapeutic encounters would thus be delivered and monitored within the Firm. When other skills are required (eg for more intensive psychotherapy, Day-Centres, or more unusual or refractory cases) the Consultant would (with the help of their other professional staff) make tertiary referrals to more specialised units.
- The Consultant's Firm would therefore be looking after patients in Clinics, In-Patient Units, Day Centres and at home. Ideally all of these are easily commutable from one another.
- Much psychiatric work is with people whose complaints fluctuate over many years. A relapse can be much more humanely and effectively responded to and contained by staff who already have developed bonds of personal knowledge and understanding.
- Likewise In-Patient discharges are likely to be far less problematic if a patient continues to receive guidance and support by the same team that tended them in times of greater distress.

- Of course, personal continuity of care is never complete or perfectible. It is a value and a guiding principle. In the untidy and buffeted real world all kinds of compromises are inevitable or advisable.
- The General Psychiatrists' work would thus resort to a wider base of more 'parental' personal responsibility. Their professional development and appointment would depend, as in previous eras, more on length and breadth of experience and education. This is in contrast to what we have now: a pressure to successive, modular, technical-type trainings to accelerate earliest promotion. (This itself raises many questions about the selection and process of medical trainings v education.)

*

What do I base these ideas on, and why do I think they will work?

From the early 1970s I worked in Psychiatry for many years. In that time we were able to provide much better personal continuity and quality of care than is generally available now. This more personally continuous care was not only more meaningful and satisfying for staff and patients, it was also more efficient: our decisions had greater speed, sensitivity and appositeness. This was less expensive.

Almost all my cohorts from that period take this view. They are, however, at retirement age and most are too beleaguered or weary to argue: their resonance with these views now exceeds their public articulation.

If you are interested in reading about particular scenarios and patient-situations, together with my expanded analysis of the problems and our responses, then I would like you to read my letters and submissions to senior managers and clinicians of our Mental Health Services. They are available via my Home Page.

In addition I have collected hundreds of relevant NHS documents over many years. Each one provides salutary and graphic evidence for these ideas.

I want to end this letter with another paradox and an ensuing invitation. The paradox: I prefer pithy, live dialogue to prolix, abstract documents. The invitation: my Practice is ten minutes of easy Underground travel from (or to) Westminster. If you, or one of your deputies, wish to discuss these matters, it would please me greatly.

Ω

Letter to the Minister of State for Care, Dep. of Health 2014

# Renationalisation of the Rail Services?
## Why not, instead, start with the NHS?

Recently the media has told us that the Labour Party is considering a long-journeyed return: back to the nationalisation of rail services. Some claim this will offer better long-term value, efficiency and safety.

Many would welcome this, but there is a puzzling anomaly: why do we not, instead, start with the NHS? For, surely, the contentious market principles of competitive commissioning are better suited to human transport than human healthcare. This is an important distinction, and our failure to recognise the difference between the mechanical and the human has led to a new tranche of serious NHS problems.

For twenty-five years we have had successive governments push through legislation to extend the control, reach and leverage of the NHS Internal Market. Yet almost all senior practitioners with long prior experience agree about the human and economic cost consequent to our depersonalised fragmentation of the NHS. This has been engineered by such commercialising devices as competitive commissioning and autarkic NHS Trusts. Cumulatively they have been highly destructive to both the quality of continuity of care, and the morale and trust of staff. The Royal Colleges have consistently taken this view. From my own long-serving GP practice I have hundreds of documented cases to illustrate these organisational follies.

Personal knowledge and continuity of care may matter little in the carriage of passengers. It matters a great deal in the care of the complex human interweavings of the ailing body, mind and spirit. The NHS Internal Market is like Communism: a failed ideological experiment. Such ideologies may start with some aspirational ideas of merit, but these must always be diluted and titrated. For they are only partial and conditional truths, and our failure to heed the difference between guidance and dominance has led to our failed massive social experiments.

Yes, a reconstituted national British Rail could possibly offer us greater economy, choice and comfort. What an intelligently refederalised NHS would offer us would be much more. Here is another anomaly: why now do we hear no substantial challenge to the existence of the Internal Market from our usually glad-to-be-contentious opposition politicians?

Ω

Published by *Open Democracy* 2014

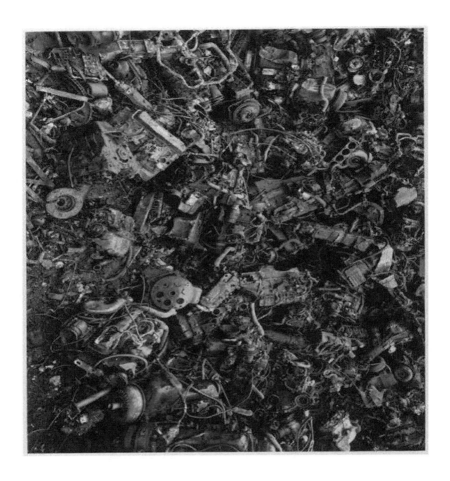

### The End: Reality and Bathos.
Redundant motor engines dump. USA

# The Author

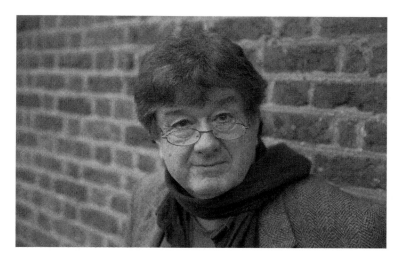

**David Zigmond** initially trained in Medicine in the 1960s. For several decades he has worked in the NHS as a small-practice GP, and as a large hospital psychiatrist and psychotherapist. Alongside these he has maintained a practice as a private psychotherapist. From these long tenures he has explored the nature and importance of relationships, imagination and personal meaning throughout healthcare. These have fuelled and guided his view and practice of holistic medicine. His long-spanned teaching and writing have been committed to develop and secure these values.

He helped launch the British Holistic Medical Association in the 1980s and has remained active in developing this approach. This anthology contains many of his contributions.

## Other Books on Health
## by New Gnosis Publications

**Wilberg, Peter** *The Illness is the Cure - 2nd extended edition: an introduction to Life Medicine and Life Doctoring - a new existential approach to illness,* 2014

**Wilberg, Peter** *from Psychosomatics to Soma-Semiotics: Felt Sense and the Sensed Body in Medicine and Psychotherapy,* 2010

**Wilberg, Peter** *Being and Listening: Counselling, Psychoanalysis and the Ontology of Listening,*2013

**Wilberg, Peter** *Heidegger, Medicine and 'Scientific Method': The Unheeded Message of the Zollikon Seminars,* 2012

**Wilberg, Peter** *Meditation and Mental Health: an introduction to Awareness Based Cognitive Therapy,* 2010

**Wilberg, Peter** *The Therapist As Listener: Martin Heidegger And The Missing Dimension Of Counselling And Psychotherapy Training,* 2008

**Zigmond, David** *The Psychoecology of Gladys Parlett – Hidden personal meaning in healthcare*(If you want good personal healthcare – See a Vet, Volume 1) 2015

**Zigmond, David** *From Family to Factory – Lost personal meaning in healthcare* (If you want good personal healthcare – See a Vet, Volume 2) 2015

**Zigmond, David** *Bureaucratyrannohypoxia - The struggle for personal meaning in healthcare* (If you want good personal healthcare – See a Vet, Volume 3) 2015

Printed in Great Britain
by Amazon